Raven Press Series In Physiology

Basic Medical Endocrinology
Second Edition

Raven Press Series in Physiology
William F. Ganong, M.D., Series Editor

Raven Press Series In Physiology

Basic Medical Endocrinology

Second Edition

H. Maurice Goodman, Ph.D.
Professor and Chairman
Department of Physiology
University of Massachusetts
Medical School
Worcester, Massachusetts

Raven Press   New York

Raven Press, Ltd., 1185 Avenue of the Americas, New York, New York 10036

Made in the United States of America

Library of Congress Cataloging-in-Publication Data

Goodman, H. Maurice
    Basic medical endocrinology / H. Maurice Goodman.—2nd ed.
      p. cm.—(Raven Press series in physiology)
    Includes bibliographical references and index.
    ISBN 0-7817-0106-6 (hardcover).—ISBN 0-7817-0105-8 (pbk.)
    1. Endocrinology. 2. Endocrine glands—Physiology. I. Title. II. Series
    [DNLM: 1. Endocrine glands—physiology. 2. Hormones—physiology.
WK 102 G653b 1994]
QP187.G589 1994
616.4—dc20
                                            94-4602
                                            CIP

9 8 7 6 5 4 3 2 1

To my wife Sandra and our children who bring joy to living

To my mentors, Ernst Knobil, Ted Astwood, Fred Hisaw, and Gjerding Olsen whose words and accomplishments continue to inspire
and To my students, past, present, and future who give meaning to this effort.

Contents

PART II. INTEGRATION OF HORMONE FUNCTIONS

Fatty Acid Cycle • Overall Regulation of Blood
Glucose Concentration • Integrated Actions of
Metabolic Hormones *Adipose Tissue/Muscle/Liver/
Pancreatic islets* • Regulation of Metabolism during
Feeding and Fasting *Postprandial period/
Postabsorptive period/Fasting* • Hormonal Interactions
During Exercise *Short-term maximal effort/Sustained
aerobic exercise* • Suggested Reading

PART III. REPRODUCTION, GROWTH, AND DEVELOPMENT

Preface to the First Edition

This volume is the product of more than 25 years of teaching endocrine physiology to first-year medical students. Its focus is human endocrinology with an emphasis on cellular and molecular mechanisms. In presenting this material, I have tried to capture some of the excitement of a dynamic, expanding discipline that is now in its golden age. It is hoped that this text provides sufficient understanding of normal endocrine physiology to prepare the student to study not only endocrine diseases but the cellular and molecular derangements that disrupt normal function and must therefore be reversed or circumvented by rational therapy. It is further hoped that this text provides the necessary background to facilitate continuing self-education in endocrinology.

Endocrinology encompasses a vast amount of information relating to at least some aspect of virtually every body functions. Unfortunately, much of the information is descriptive and cannot be derived from first principles. Thorough, encyclopedic coverage is neither appropriate for a volume such as this one, nor possible at the current explosive rate of expansion. On the other hand, limiting the text to the bare minimum of unadorned facts might facilitate memorization of what appear to be the essentials this year but would preclude acquisition of real understanding and offer little preparation for assimilating the essentials as they may appear a decade hence. I therefore sought the middle ground and present basic facts within enough of a physiological framework to foster understanding of both the current status of the field and those areas where new developments are likely to occur while hopefully avoiding the pitfall of burying key points in details and qualifications.

The text is organized into three sections. The first section provides basic information about organization of the endocrine system and the role of individual endocrine glands. Subsequent sections deal with complex hormonal interactions that govern maintenance of the internal environment (Part II) and growth and reproduction (Part III). Neuroendocrinology is integrated into discussions of specific glands or regulatory systems throughout the text rather than being treated as a separate subject. Although modern endocrinology has its roots in gastrointestinal (GI) physiology, the gut hormones are usually covered in texts of GI physiology rather than endocrinology; therefore there is no chapter on intestinal hormones. In the interests of space and the reader's endurance, a good deal of fascinating material was omitted because it seemed either irrelevant to human biology or insufficiently understood at this time. For example, the pineal gland has intrigued generations of scientists and philosophers since Descartes, but it still has no clearly established role in human physiology and is therefore ignored in this text.

Human endocrinology has its foundation in clinical practice and research, both of which rely heavily on laboratory findings. Where possible, points are illustrated in the text with original data from the rich endocrine literature to give the reader a feeling for the kind of information on which theoretical and diagnostic conclusions are based. Original literature is not cited in the text, in part because such citations are distracting in an introductory text, and in part because proper citation might well double the length of this volume. For the reader who wishes to gain entrée to the endocrine literature or desires more comprehensive coverage of specific topics, review articles are listed at the end of each chapter.

H. Maurice Goodman
1988

Preface

In the five years that have passed since the first edition of this text the information explosion in endocrinology has continued unabated, and may have even accelerated. Application of the powerful tools of molecular biology has made it possible to ask questions about hormone production and action that were only dreamed about a decade earlier. The receptor molecules that initiate responses to virtually all of the hormones have been characterized and significant progress has been made in unraveling the events that lead to the final cellular expression of hormonal stimulation. As more details of intracellular signaling emerge, the complexities of parallel and intersecting pathways of transduction have become more evident. We are beginning to understand how cells regulate the expression of genes and how hormones intervene in regulatory processes to adjust the expression of individual genes. Great strides have been made in understanding how individual cells talk to each other through locally released factors to coordinate growth, differentiation, secretion, and other responses within a tissue. In these regards endocrinology and immunology share common themes and have contributed to each other's advancement.

In revising the text for this second edition of *Basic Medical Endocrinology* I have tried to incorporate many of the exciting advances in our understanding of cellular and molecular processes into the discourse on integrated whole body function. I have tried to be selective, however, and include only those bits of information that deepen understanding of well-established principles or processes, or that relate to emerging themes. Every chapter has been updated, but not surprisingly, progress has been uneven, and some have been revised more extensively than others. After reviewing the past five years of literature in as broad an area as encompassed by endocrinology one cannot help but be humbled by the seemingly limitless capacity of the human mind to develop new knowledge, to assimilate new information into an already vast knowledge base, and to apply that knowledge to advancement of human welfare.

H. Maurice Goodman
1993

1

Introduction

As animals evolved from single cells to multicellular organisms, individual cells took on specialized functions and became mutually dependent on each other to satisfy their own needs and the needs of the whole organism. Survival thus hinged on integration and coordination of their individual specialized functions. Increased specialization of cellular functions was accompanied by decreased tolerance for variations in the cellular environment. Control systems evolved that allowed more and more precise regulation of the cellular environment, which in turn, permitted the development of even more highly specialized cells, such as those of higher brain centers, whose continued function requires that the internal environment be maintained constant within narrow limits—no matter what conditions prevail in the external environment. Survival of the individual requires a capacity to adjust and adapt to hostile conditions in the external environment, and survival of the species requires the coordination of reproductive function with those factors in the internal and external environment that are most conducive to survival of the offspring. Crucial to meeting these needs for survival as a multicellular organism is the capacity of specialized cells to coordinate their activities through some sort of communication.

Cells communicate with each other by means of chemical signals. For communication with the relatively few adjacent cells, these signals may be substances that form part of the cell surface, or they may be molecules that pass from the cytosol of one cell to that of another through gap junctions. To communicate with the vast number of more distant cells, chemical signals are released into the extracellular environment and are recognized by other cells that react to them in a characteristic manner. These signals may be simple molecules, such as modified amino acids, or they may be more complex peptides, proteins, or steroids. When cells are near each other, signals may travel from one cell to another by simple diffusion through the extracellular fluid. Such communication is said to occur by *paracrine*, or local, secretion. Sometimes cells respond to their own secretions, and this is called *autocrine* secretion. For cells that are too far apart for the slow process of diffusion to permit meaningful communication, the chemical signal may enter the circulation and be transported by the blood to all parts of the body. The release of chemical signals into the blood stream is referred to as *endocrine* (or internal) secretion, and the signal secreted is

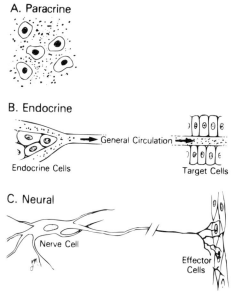

A. Paracrine

B. Endocrine

General Circulation

Endocrine Cells   Target Cells

C. Neural

Nerve Cell

Effector
Cells

FIG. 1. Chemical communication between cells. **A:** Paracrine method. The secretory product, shown as *black dots,* reaches the nearby target cell by diffusion through the extracellular fluid. **B:** Endocrine method. The secretory product reaches distant cells by transport through the circulation. **C:** A neural secretory product released from terminals of long cell processes reaches target cells distant from the nerve cell body by diffusion across the synaptic cleft.

called a *hormone.* We may define a hormone as *a chemical substance that is released into the blood in small amounts and that, after delivery by the circulation, elicits a typical physiological response in other cells* (Fig. 1).

Because the hormone becomes diluted in the huge volume of blood and extracellular fluid, achieving meaningful concentrations (10^{-10} to 10^{-7} M) usually requires coordinated secretion by a mass of cells, an *endocrine gland.* Endocrine glands have the common feature of releasing their secretory products directly into the blood stream. This feature distinguishes them from *exocrine glands,* which deliver their products through ducts to the outside of the body or to the lumen of the gastrointestinal tract. Classical endocrine glands include the pituitary, thyroid, adrenals, parathyroids, gonads, and islets of Langerhans. It has become apparent, however, that this list is too short. Virtually every organ, including the brain, kidney, and heart, has an endocrine function in addition to its more commonly recognized role.

Another mechanism has also evolved to breach the distance between cells and allow rapid communication. Some cells developed the ability to release their signals locally from the tips of long processes that extend great distances and nearly touch cells that receive the signals. This mechanism, of course, is the manner by which nerve cells communicate with each other or with effector cells. By releasing their signals (neurotransmitters) so close to the receptor cells, nerve cells achieve both exquisite specificity and economy in the quantity of transmitter needed to provide a meaningful concentration within a highly localized space. Although use of the action potential to trigger secretion is not unique to nerve cells, the electrical wave that travels along the axons enables these cells to transmit information rapidly over great distances between the perikarya and the nerve terminals. Despite these specialized features of nerve cells, it is important to note that the same cellular mechanisms are used for signal production and release as well as for reception and response during neural, endocrine, and paracrine communication. The distinctions between these modes of communication are limited only to the means of signal delivery to the target cells, and even these distinctions are blurred in some cases. Sometimes neurotransmitters diffuse considerable distances and act in a paracrine fashion or even enter the blood and act as hormones, in which case they are called *neurohormones*. Moreover, the same chemical signals may be secreted by both endocrine and nerve cells. Nature is parsimonious in this regard. Many peptides that have classically been regarded as hormones or neurohormones may also serve as paracrine regulators in a variety of tissues. Although adequate to cause localized responses, the minute quantities of these substances produced extraglandularly are usually too small to enter the blood and interfere with endocrine relationships.

In this text, we limit our discussion principally to that aspect of cellular communication that is carried out by the classical endocrine glands and their hormones and that constitutes the science of endocrinology. Part I deals with basic information about various endocrine glands and their hormones. In Part II, we consider the interaction of hormones and the integration of endocrine function in homeostatic regulation. Throughout, our emphasis is on normal function, and reference to disease is limited to those aspects that are logical extensions of normal physiology or that facilitate our understanding of normal physiology. Endocrine disease is not simply a matter of too much or too little hormone; rather, disease occurs when there is an inappropriate amount of hormone for the prevailing physiological situation or when there is an inappropriate response by the target tissues to a perfectly appropriate amount of hormone. Some aspects of endocrine disease are too poorly understood to be put in the context of normal physiology and are best left for a more detailed text of pathology or medicine.

Endocrinology is a subject that, unfortunately, involves a sometimes bewildering array of facts, not all of which can be derived from basic principles. To help organize and digest this necessarily large volume of material, the student might find the following outline of goals and objectives helpful.

A. The student should be familiar with the following:
   1. Essential features of feedback regulation
   2. Essentials of competitive binding assays
B. For each hormone, the student should know the following:
   1. Its cell of origin
   2. Its chemical nature, including
      a. Distinctive features of its chemical composition
      b. Biosynthesis
      c. Whether it circulates free or is bound to plasma proteins
      d. How it is degraded and removed from the body
   3. Its principal physiological actions
      a. At the whole body level

b. At the tissue level
c. At the cellular level
d. At the molecular level
e. The consequences of inadequate or excess secretion
4. What signals or perturbations in the internal or external environment evoke or suppress its secretion
   a. How those signals are transmitted
   b. How that secretion is controlled
   c. What factors modulate the secretory response
   d. How rapidly the hormone acts
   e. How long it acts
   f. What factors modulate its action

BIOSYNTHESIS OF HORMONES

The classical hormones fall into three categories: (1) derivatives of the amino acid tyrosine; (2) steroids, which are derivatives of cholesterol; and (3) peptides and proteins, which comprise the most abundant and diverse class of hormones. Table 1 lists some examples of each category. A large number of other small molecules, including derivatives of amino acids and fatty acids, function as neurotransmitters or paracrine signals but fall outside the scope of the classical hormones. The relevant

TABLE 1. *Chemical nature of the classic hormones*

Tyrosine derivatives	Steroids	Peptides (<20 amino acids)	Proteins (>20 amino acids)
Epinephrine	Testosterone	Oxytocin	Insulin
Norepinephrine	Estradiol	Vasopressin	Glucagon
Dopamine	Progesterone	Angiotensin	Adrenocorticotropic hormone
Triiodothyronine	Cortisol	Melanocyte-stimulating hormone	Thyroid-stimulating hormone
Thyroxine	Aldosterone	Somatostatin	Thyrotropin-releasing hormone
	Vitamin D		Follicle-stimulating hormone
			Luteinizing hormone
			Gonadotropin-releasing hormone
			Growth hormone
			Prolactin
			Corticotropin-releasing hormone
			Growth hormone-releasing hormone
			Parathyroid hormone
			Calcitonin
			Chorionic gonadotropin
			Choriosomatomammotropin

details of hormone synthesis and storage, particularly for the amino acid and steroid hormones, are presented in the discussion of each gland, but the steps in protein biosynthesis, storage, and secretion common to all protein and peptide hormones are sufficiently general for this largest class of hormones to warrant some discussion here.

All protein and peptide hormones are synthesized on ribosomes as larger molecules (prohormones and preprohormones) than the final secretory product. As they come off the ribosomes, the proteins destined for secretion have a hydrophobic sequence of amino acids at their amino terminal end (Fig. 2). This so-called signal sequence allows them to enter the cisternae of the endoplasmic reticulum and be translocated to the Golgi apparatus, where they are processed and packaged for export. Postsynthetic processing includes cleavage of the long polypeptide chain to remove the signal peptide. For some hormones, cleavage at appropriate other loci removes those amino acid sequences that may have functioned to orient folding of the molecule so that disulfide bridges form in the right places. Clipping the protein may yield more than one biologically important molecule from a single precursor, as seen with the corticotropin family of hormones (Chapter 2). For some secretory peptides, the final clipping occurs in the secretory granules with the result that one or more other molecules are released into the circulation along with the hormone. Other processing of peptide hormones may include glycosylation (addition of carbohydrate chains to asparagine residues) or coupling of subunits.

Defects in processing of normal precursor molecules cause some rare, exotic inherited diseases. It is more common to find precursor molecules in the circulation, sometimes in large amounts. This situation may be indicative of hyperactivity of endocrine cells or even aberrant production of hormone by nonendocrine tumor cells. Often such hormone precursors have biological activity, and their effects may be the first manifestation of neoplasia.

Postsynthetic processing to the final biologically active form is not limited to peptide hormones. Other hormones may be formed from their precursors after secretion. Postsecretory transformations to more active forms may occur in the liver, kidney, fat, or blood, as well as in the target tissues themselves. For example, thyroxine, the major secretory product of the thyroid gland, is converted extrathyroidally to triiodothyronine, which is thought to be the biologically active form of the hormone. Testosterone, the male hormone, is converted to dihydrotestosterone within some target tissues and may even be converted to the female hormone, estrogen, in other tissues. These peripheral transformations, beside confounding the student of endocrinology, are additional sites that are vulnerable to derangement and, hence, must be considered as possible causes of endocrine disease.

STORAGE AND SECRETION

Hormones are stored, sometimes in large quantities, in their glands of origin, a factor that facilitated their original isolation and characterization. Protein hormones

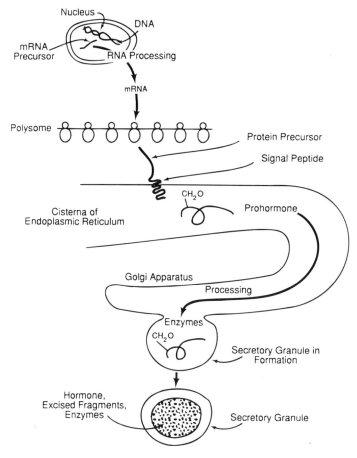

FIG. 2. Synthesis and processing of the peptide and protein hormones. The DNA that encodes a hormone is transcribed to RNA, which is processed, and released from the nucleus as messenger RNA (mRNA). In the cytosol, mRNA binds to ribosomes and is translated to form a large precursor of the secretory product. After entering the cisterna of the endoplasmic reticulum, the signal peptide sequence of the newly synthesized protein is removed, carbohydrate (CH_2O) may be added, and the prohormone is transferred to the Golgi apparatus for packaging into secretory granules, which may also contain enzymes responsible for the final processing of the hormone, and any excised fragments of the prohormone.

are stored in membrane-bound vesicles or granules and are secreted by *exocytosis.* In this process, storage granules are translocated to the cell surface and their surrounding membranes fuse with the plasma membrane. The area of fusion then breaks down opening the storage vesicle to the extracellular fluid (Fig. 3). The movement of the storage granule to the cell surface and membrane fusion usually require an influx of calcium, both from internal organelles and the extracellular fluid. Changes in protein conformation secondary to protein phosphorylation or dephosphorylation

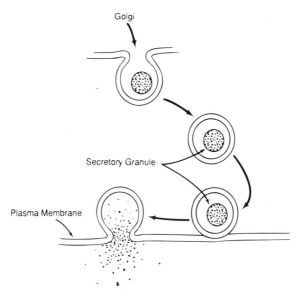

Golgi

Secretory Granule

Plasma Membrane

FIG. 3. Exocytosis. In response to signals for secretion, secretory granules are translocated to the cell surface. Membrane surrounding the granule fuses with the plasma membrane opening the granule to the extracellular fluid.

may also play a role in some cells. It is obvious that the synthesis of hormones must be coupled in some way with their secretion, so that cells can replenish their supply of hormones. A common cellular event might simultaneously signal both release and synthesis, or some cells may be able to monitor how much hormone is stored and begin synthesis when hormone stores fall below some critical level.

The tyrosine derivatives, epinephrine and norepinephrine, are stored in membrane-bound vesicles within the adrenal medulla, and the mechanism governing their secretion is analogous to that described for the protein and peptide hormones. The manner of storage and secretion of the thyroid hormones is unique and is discussed in Chapter 3. There is little storage of steroid hormones—too little, in fact, to allow a study of whether these hormones are also secreted by exocytosis. Because they are lipid soluble, steroid hormones may simply diffuse across the plasma membrane down their concentration gradient.

HORMONES IN THE BLOOD

Most hormones circulate in the blood in free solution at low nanomolar (10^{-9} M) or even picomolar (10^{-12} M) concentrations. Steroid hormones and thyroid hormones, whose solubility in water is limited, circulate bound specifically to large carrier proteins. Some protein and peptide hormones may also circulate bound to specific proteins. Bound hormones are in equilibrium with a small fraction, sometimes less than 1%, in free solution in plasma. Generally, only unbound hormones get out of the capillaries to produce their biological effects or be degraded. Protein binding protects against loss of hormone by the kidney, slows the rate of hormone degradation by decreasing cellular uptake, and buffers changes in free hormone concentrations. Recent evidence suggests that, in some instances, binding proteins may affect hormonal responses by facilitating or impeding delivery of hormones to particular cells. Because biological responses are related to the concentration of hormone that reaches target cells, rather than the total amount in blood, increases in abundance of binding proteins that occur during pregnancy, for example, or decreases seen with some forms of liver or kidney disease may produce changes in the total amounts of hormones in the blood even though free, physiologically important concentrations may be normal.

Most hormones are destroyed rapidly after secretion and have a half-life in blood of less than 30 minutes. The half-life of a hormone in blood is defined as that period of time needed for its concentration to be reduced by one half, and this depends on its rate of degradation and on the rapidity with which it can escape from the circulation and equilibrate with the fluids in extravascular compartments. Some hormones, e.g., epinephrine, have half-lives on the order of seconds, while thyroid hormones have half-lives on the order of days. The half-life of a hormone in the blood must be distinguished from the duration of its hormonal effect. Some hormones produce effects virtually instantaneously, and the effects may disappear as rapidly as the hormone is cleared from the blood. Other hormones produce effects only after a lag time that may last minutes or even hours, and the time the maximum effect is seen may bear little relation to the time of maximum hormone concentration in the blood. Additionally, the time for decay of a hormone effect is also highly variable; it may be only a few seconds, or it may require several days. Some responses persist well after hormonal concentrations have returned to basal levels. Understanding the time course of a hormone's survival in the blood as well as the onset and duration of its action is obviously important for understanding normal physiology, endocrine disease, and the limitations of hormone therapy.

HORMONE DEGRADATION

Implicit in any regulatory system involving hormones or any other signal is the necessity for the signal to disappear once the appropriate information has been conveyed. Recall that neurotransmitters are either rapidly destroyed in the synaptic cleft or taken up by nerve endings. Little if any hormone is thought to be ''used up'' when producing biological effects, and the remainder must therefore be inactivated and excreted. The degradation of hormones and their subsequent excretion are processes that are just as important as their secretion. The inactivation of hormones occurs enzymatically in the blood or intercellular spaces, in liver or kidney cells, or in the target cells themselves. Inactivation may involve complete metabolism of the hormone so that no recognizable product appears in the urine, or it may be limited to some simple one- or two-step process, such as the addition of a methyl group or glucuronic acid. In the latter cases, recognizable degradation products are found in the urine and can be measured to obtain a crude index of the rate of hormone production.

MECHANISMS OF HORMONE ACTION

Because all hormones travel in the blood from their glands of origin to their "target" tissues, all cells must be exposed to all hormones. However, under normal circumstances, tissues respond only to their appropriate hormones. Such *specificity* of hormone action appears to reside in the ability of *receptors* in the target tissue to recognize only their own signal. We may define a hormone receptor as *a unique molecular grouping in or on a cell that interacts with a hormone in a highly specific manner such that a characteristic response or group of responses is initiated.*

Characteristics of Receptors

Hormone receptors are proteins or glycoproteins that are able to (a) distinguish their hormone from other molecules that may have very similar structures, (b) bind to the hormone even when its concentration is exceedingly low (10^{-8} to 10^{-12} M), and (c) undergo a conformational change when bound to the hormone such that (d) a biochemical event occurs and initiates the cellular response. These aspects of receptor function may reside within a single molecule or in separate subunits of a receptor complex. Hormone receptors are found on the surface of target cells or in the interior, usually in the nucleus. Receptors that reside in the plasma membrane span its entire thickness with the hormone recognition component facing outward. Components on the cytosolic face communicate with other membrane or cytosolic proteins. Receptors may be uniformly distributed over the entire surface of a cell or they may be confined to some discrete region, such as the basal surface of renal tubular epithelial cells.

Only a few thousand receptor molecules are usually present in a target cell, but the number is not fixed. Cells can adjust the abundance of hormone receptors and, presumably, their responsiveness to hormones, according to changing physiological circumstances. Some receptors may only be expressed at certain stages of a cell's life cycle or when the cell is stimulated by other hormones. Many cells adjust the number of receptors expressed in accordance with the abundance of the signal that activates them. Frequent or intense stimulation may cause a cell to decrease or *down regulate* the number of receptors expressed. Conversely, cells may *up regulate* receptors in the face of rare or absent stimulation or in response to other signals. Membrane receptors are internalized either alone or bound to their hormones (receptor-mediated endocytosis) and, like other cellular proteins, are broken down and replaced many times over during the lifetime of a cell. Some cells recycle receptors between the plasma membrane and internal membranes, and they can vary the rate of transfer and, hence, the relative abundance of receptors on the cell surface. Intracellular receptors are synthesized and degraded like other cellular proteins and probably also participate in multiple signaling cycles. In addition to adjusting receptor abundance, cells may temporarily activate or inactivate receptors by adding or removing phosphate and perhaps acetyl groups.

Hormonal Actions Mediated by Intracellular Receptors

The cholesterol derivatives (steroid hormones and vitamin D) are lipid soluble and are thought to enter cells by diffusion through the lipid bilayer of the plasma membrane. Similarly, the thyroid hormones, which are α-amino acids, have large nonpolar constituents and penetrate cell membranes both by diffusion and carrier-mediated transport. These hormones bind to receptors that are located principally, and perhaps exclusively, in the cell nucleus and produce most (but probably not all) of their effects by altering gene expression. Hormone-bound receptors, in turn, bind to specific nucleotide sequences, called *hormone response elements*, in regulated genes and enhance or repress their transcription. The end result of stimulation with these hormones is a change in the genomic readout, which may be expressed in the formation of new cellular proteins or as a modification of the rate of synthesis of proteins already in production. The sequence of events shown in Fig. 4 is probably applicable to all steroid hormones.

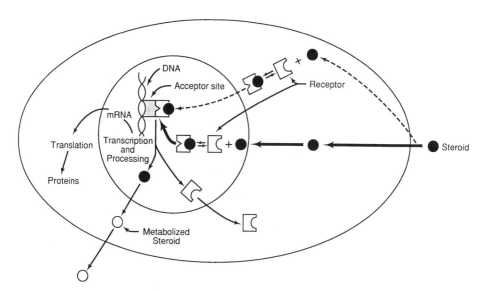

FIG. 4. General model of steroid hormone action. Steroid hormones penetrate the plasma membrane and bind to intracellular receptors found largely in the nucleus. The hormone–receptor complex then binds to specific hormone response elements in DNA to initiate transcription and formation of the proteins that express the hormonal response. The steroid hormone is cleared from the cell after metabolic degradation. From Clark, J.J., Schrader, W.T., and O'Malley, B.W. Mechanisms of steroid hormone action (1985): In: *Williams Textbook of Endocrinology*, 7th ed., edited by Wilson, J.D. and Foster, D.W., W.B. Saunders, Philadelphia, pp. 33–75.

Steroid hormone receptors are closely related proteins whose similarities in certain amino acid sequences and the arrangement of functional domains suggest they arose in evolution from a common ancestral protein. The deoxyribonucleic acid (DNA)-binding domain is a cysteine-rich region that is complexed with two molecules of zinc to form the "zinc finger" loops that grasp the DNA. This domain is flanked by peptide sequences that are required for activation of transcription. The hormone-binding domain is near the carboxy terminus. In the unstimulated state, steroid hormone receptors are noncovalently complexed with other proteins including a dimer of the 90,000 Dalton heat-shock protein (Hsp 90), which attaches adjacent to the hormone-binding domain (Fig. 5). Heat-shock proteins are abundant cellular proteins that are found in prokaryotes and all eukaryotic cells and are so named because their synthesis abruptly increases when cells are exposed to high temperatures or other stressful conditions. Hsp 90 is thought to maintain the receptor in a configuration that is capable of binding the hormone and incapable of binding to DNA. The transformation of the receptor to its active form that follows hormone binding involves a conformational change and dissociation from Hsp 90 and the

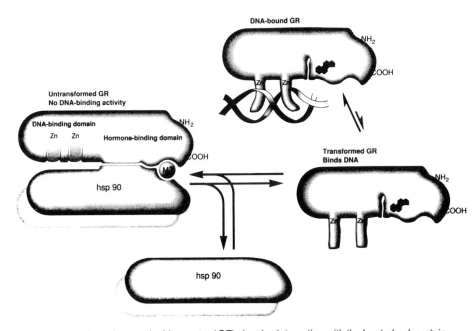

FIG. 5. Model of the glucocorticoid receptor (*GR*) showing interaction with the heat-shock protein (*Hsp 90*). Attachment of a dimer of Hsp 90 to the hormone-binding domain of the inactive GR is stabilized by molybdate (*M*). The addition of hormone causes a conformational change in the GR so that the transformed free receptor hormone complex can bind to DNA, most likely as a dimer. (Dimer not shown). Upon dissociation from DNA, the GR may be metabolically destroyed or reassociated in an energy-dependent fashion with Hsp 90 and recycled back to its inactive form. Modified from Scherrer, L. C., Dalman, F.C., Massa, E., et al. (1990): Structural and functional reconstitution of the glucocorticoid receptor-Hsp90 complex. *J. Biol. Chem.*, 265:21397.

other proteins. Activated receptors bind to hormone-response elements (HREs) throughout the genome as dimers and initiate or repress transcription of the affected genes to their ribonucleic acid (RNA) counterparts.

The receptors for thyroid hormone and vitamin D belong to the same family of proteins as the steroid receptors. Unlike the steroid hormone receptors, thyroid hormone and vitamin D receptors bind their HREs in DNA even in the absence of hormone and do not form complexes with Hsp 90 and other proteins. These receptors are able to regulate gene transcription only after binding their hormones. Thus, binding of the receptors to HREs is not sufficient in itself to initiate a response. Other changes to the receptor must also result from hormone binding, including, perhaps, changes in the phosphorylated state of the receptor or in its ability to interact with other nuclear proteins called transcription factors. Just how RNA synthesis is enhanced or repressed and the role of other nuclear-activating factors in this process are subjects of current intense investigation.

A number of steps lie between activation of transcription and changes in cellular behavior. These include processing the newly synthesized RNA, exporting it to cytosolic sites of protein synthesis, protein synthesis itself, protein processing, and translocation of the protein to appropriate loci within the cells. The final protein makeup of the cell is also determined by the rates of RNA and protein degradation. Except for possible effects on the rates of RNA degradation, it appears that these steps are not directly influenced and that the actions of the hydrophobic hormones are confined to regulation of transcription. However, because each of these steps must occur sequentially and because each is time consuming, the biological responses to stimulation by these hormones require a lag period of at least 30 minutes.

Hormone-receptor binding is reversible. As blood levels decline, the hormone dissociates from its receptors and is cleared from the cell by diffusion into the extracellular fluid, usually after metabolic conversion to an inactive form. Unloaded steroid receptors dissociate from their DNA binding sites and either recycle into new complexes with Hsp 90 and other proteins through some energy-dependent process or are replaced by new synthesis. The RNA transcripts of hormone-sensitive genes are broken down, usually within minutes to hours of their formation. Without continued hormonal stimulation of their synthesis, the RNA templates for hormone-dependent proteins disappear, and these proteins can no longer be formed. The proteins themselves are degraded with half-lives that may range from seconds to days. Thus, continued hormonal effects may be seen long after the hormone has been cleared from the cell.

Hormonal Actions Mediated by Surface Receptors

The Second Messenger Concept

Because the hydrophilic hormones (peptides, proteins, and some amino acid derivatives) interact reversibly with receptors on the outer surface of target cells, they must rely on intermediate molecules called *second messengers* to transmit hormonal commands to the cellular organelles and enzymes responsible for producing the response. Second messengers also amplify signals. A single hormone molecule interacting with a single receptor may result in the formation of tens or hundreds of second messenger molecules, each of which might activate an enzyme that, in turn, catalyzes formation of hundreds to thousands of molecules of product. For the most part, responses that are mediated by second messengers are achieved by regulating the activity rather than the amount of enzymes in target cells, usually by adding a phosphate group. The resulting conformational change increases or decreases enzymatic activity. Enzymes that catalyze the transfer of the terminal phosphate from adenosine triphosphate (ATP) to a hydroxyl group in serine or threonine residues in proteins are called *protein kinases. Protein phosphatases* remove phosphate groups from these residues. Unlike responses that require synthesis of new cellular proteins, responses that result from phosphorylation–dephosphorylation reactions occur very quickly, and therefore, second messenger-mediated responses are usually turned on and off without appreciable latency.

Although many hormones act through surface receptors, to date, only a few substances have been identified as second messengers. This is because receptors for many different extracellular signals utilize the same second messenger. When originally proposed, the hypothesis that a single second messenger might mediate the actions of many different hormones, each of which produces a unique pattern of cellular responses, was met with skepticism. The idea did not gain widespread acceptance until it was recognized that the special nature of a cellular response to any agent is determined by the particular machinery with which a cell is endowed rather than by the signal that turns on that machinery. Thus, when activated, a hepatic cell makes glucose, and a smooth muscle cell contracts or relaxes.

The Cyclic Adenosine Monophosphate System

The first of the second messengers to be recognized, and the most thoroughly studied, is cyclic adenosine $3',5'$-monophosphate (cyclic AMP, Fig. 6). The broad outlines of cyclic AMP-mediated cellular responses to hormones are shown in Fig. 7. After a hormone, such as glucagon, binds to its receptors, cyclic AMP is formed from ATP within hepatocytes by the action of the enzyme, adenylyl cyclase. Communication between the receptor, which binds to the hormone, and adenylyl cyclase is achieved by way of a protein that binds guanine nucleotides and, therefore, is called a G protein. The G proteins are comprised of three nonidentical subunits: α, β, and γ. Binding of the hormone to the receptor prompts the α subunit to replace its guanosine diphosphate (GDP) with guanosine triphosphate (GTP) and dissociate from the β,γ subunits. Free α_{GTP} has three functions: (a) it activates adenylyl cyclase; (b) it decreases the affinity of the receptor, resulting in the release of bound hormone; and (c) it hydrolyzes GTP to GDP, which allows the α subunit to reassociate with

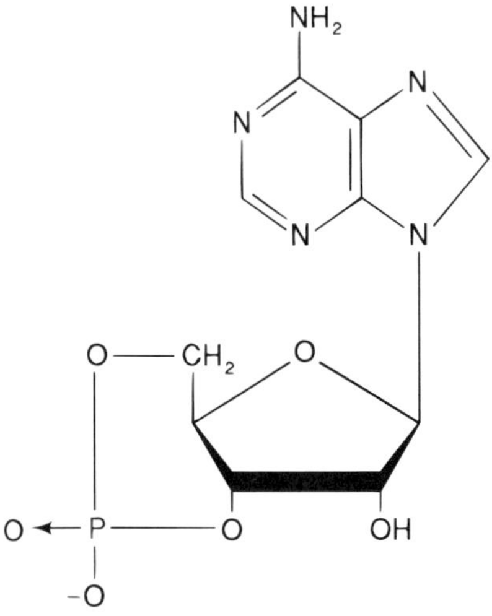

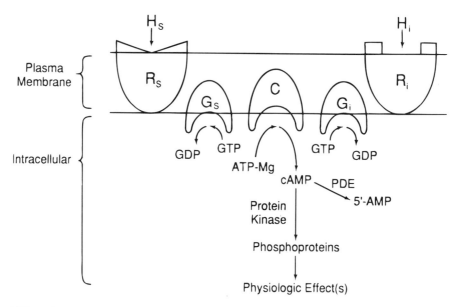

FIG. 6. Cyclic AMP.

FIG. 7. Adenylyl cyclase system. H_s, stimulating hormone; H_i, inhibiting hormone; R_s and R_i, recognition components of the receptor complex; G_s and G_i, guanosine nucleotide binding proteins; C, catalytic component of the complex that catalyzes the formation of cyclic AMP; *PDE*, cyclic nucleotide phosphodiesterase, which inactivates cyclic AMP. From Spiegel, A. M., Gierschik, P., Levine, M. A., and Downs, R. W., Jr. (1985): Clinical implications of guanine nucleotide-binding proteins as receptor-effector couplers. *N. Engl. J. Med.*, 312:26–33.

the β,γ subunits, thereby recharging the system for another encounter between the hormone and the receptor.

Some hormones, e.g., somatostatin, inhibit the formation of cyclic AMP. Their actions are produced in an analogous fashion and involve a G protein that inhibits adenylyl cyclase. Because the guanine nucleotide-binding proteins may be either stimulatory or inhibitory, they are called G_s and G_i. Whether a G protein is stimulatory or inhibitory is determined by the nature of the α subunit since G_s and G_i share the same β and γ subunits. G proteins are part of a large and phylogenetically ancient family of proteins whose functions include activation of certain ion channels in cell membranes and transduction of signals in photoreceptors.

Cyclic AMP transmits the hormonal signal by activating the enzyme protein kinase A. When cellular concentrations of cyclic AMP are low, the catalytic subunit of protein kinase A is firmly bound to its regulatory subunit, which keeps it in an inactive state. Cyclic AMP which is formed in response to a hormone–receptor interaction binds reversibly to the regulatory subunit, causing it to dissociate from the catalytic subunit, which is now free to act. Cyclic AMP that is not bound to the regulatory subunit is degraded to 5'-AMP by the enzyme cyclic AMP phosphodiesterase. With the restoration of basal concentrations of cyclic AMP, the regulatory subunits of protein kinase A lose their cyclic AMP and reassociate with the catalytic subunits, thereby inactivating them (Fig. 8). Proteins phosphorylated by protein kinase A are restored to their resting, dephosphorylated state by the action of phosphoprotein phosphatase, which is constitutively active.

In addition to regulating the activities of enzymes already present in cells, cyclic AMP can signal long-term changes that require changes in genetic expression. It does so in a manner that is reminiscent of the actions of steroid and thyroid hormones. Genes that are susceptible to regulation by cyclic AMP contain response elements comprised of particular nucleotide sequences that are recognized by transcription

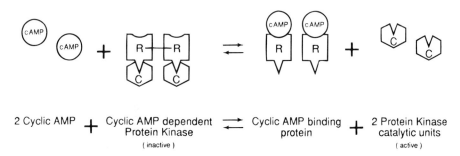

2 Cyclic AMP + Cyclic AMP dependent ⇌ Cyclic AMP binding + 2 Protein Kinase
Protein Kinase   protein   catalytic units
(inactive)   (active)

FIG. 8. Activation of protein kinase A by cyclic AMP. Inactive protein kinase consists of two catalytic units (*C*), each of which is bound to a regulatory unit (*R*). When cyclic AMP binds to the regulatory unit, the catalytic unit is released and thereby activated. A decrease in cyclic AMP allows the regulatory unit to rebind to the catalytic unit. From Roth, J. and Grunfeld, C. (1985): Mechanism of action of peptide hormones and catecholamines. In: *Williams Textbook of Endocrinology*, 7th ed., edited by Wilson, J.D. and Foster, D.W., WB Saunders, Philadelphia, pp. 76–122.

factors called cyclic AMP response element binding proteins. These transcription activation factors are substrates for protein kinase A and become active when phosphorylated.

Cyclic Guanosine Monophosphate

Though considerably less common than cyclic AMP, cyclic guanosine $3',5'$-monophosphate (cyclic GMP) plays an analogous role. Guanylyl cyclase and cyclic GMP-dependent protein kinase activities are present in many cells. Increased formation of cyclic GMP in vascular smooth muscle is associated with relaxation and may account for vasodilator responses to the atrial natriuretic hormone. Guanylyl cyclase activity is an intrinsic property of the transmembrane receptor for atrial natriuretic hormone and is activated without the intercession of a G protein.

The Calcium–Calmodulin System

Calcium has long been recognized as a regulator of cellular processes and triggers such events as muscular contraction, secretion, polymerization of microtubules, and activation of various enzymes. The concentration of free calcium in the cytoplasm of resting cells is low, usually less than 1 μM. When cells are stimulated by some hormones, their cytosolic calcium concentration rises promptly, increasing perhaps 1,000-fold. This is accomplished by the release of calcium from intracellular storage sites, mainly within the endoplasmic reticulum, and by the influx of calcium from the extracellular fluid. Although calcium can directly activate some proteins, it generally does not act alone. Virtually all cells are endowed with a protein called *calmodulin,* which reversibly binds four calcium ions. When complexed with calcium, the configuration of calmodulin is modified in a way that enables it to bind to certain enzymes, usually protein kinases, and thereby activate them. Together, calmodulin and calcium serve as a "tertiary" messenger, since yet another messenger is needed to carry information from the cell surface to the endoplasmic reticulum to trigger the release of calcium from its storage sites. Calcium is removed from the cytosol by membrane-bound calcium "pumps," which may resequester it in intracellular storage sites or transfer it to the extracellular fluid in exchange for sodium. When cytosolic calcium is restored to its low resting level, calcium is released from calmodulin, which then dissociates from the various enzymes it has activated.

The Phosphatidylinositol–Diacylglyceride–Inositol 1,4,5 Trisphosphate System

When some hormones bind to their receptors on the surface of cells, they activate the enzyme, phospholipase C through the agency of a G protein. Phospholipase C splits the membrane phospholipid, phosphatidylinositol 4,5 bisphosphate, into diacylglyceride (DAG) and inositol 1,4,5 trisphosphate (IP_3), both of which behave

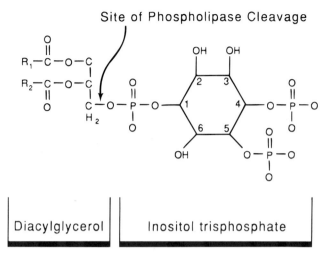

FIG. 9. Phosphatidylinositol-bisphosphate. When cleaved by phospholipase C, IP_3 and DAG are formed.

as second messengers (Figs. 9 and 10). The IP_3 mobilizes calcium from storage sites in the endoplasmic reticulum, and DAG activates protein kinase C. Protein kinase C has also been called the calcium, phospholipid-dependent protein kinase because it requires both phosphatidylserine and calcium to be fully activated. Diacylglycerol promotes the translocation of inactive protein kinase C from the cytosol to membranous components of the cell, probably the plasma membrane, where it can interact with phosphatidylserine. The increase in calcium concentration resulting from the simultaneous action of IP_3 complements DAG in activating protein kinase C.

The IP_3 is cleared from cells by stepwise dephosphorylation to inositol. The DAG is cleared by conversion to phosphatidic acid by addition of a phosphate group. Phosphatidic acid may then be converted to a triglyceride or resynthesized into a phospholipid. Tris-phosphoinositides of the plasma membrane are regenerated by combining inositol with phosphatidic acid followed by stepwise phosphorylation of the inositol.

The phosphatidylinositol precursor of IP_3 and DAG is particularly rich in a 20-carbon polyunsaturated fatty acid called arachidonic acid. This fatty acid is typically found in ester linkage with carbon 2 of the glycerol backbone of phospholipids. The liberation of arachidonic acid is the rate-determining step in the formation of the thromboxanes, the prostaglandins, and the leukotrienes (see Chapter 4). These compounds, which are produced in virtually all cells, diffuse across the plasma membrane and behave as local regulators of other cells. Thus, the same hormone–receptor interaction that produces DAG and IP_3 as second messages to communicate with cellular organelles frequently also results in the formation of arachidonate derivatives that inform neighboring cells that a response has been initiated. It is important to

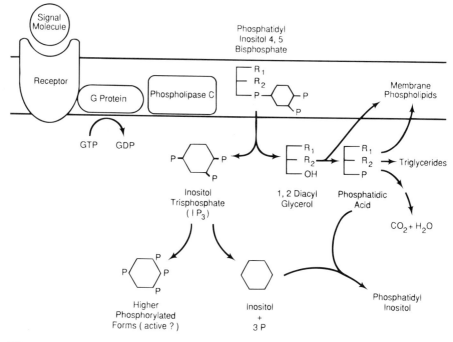

FIG. 10. Turnover of phosphatidylinositol 4,5-bisphosphate. Interaction of receptors with hormones activates phospholipase C, which cleaves the phospholipid to DAG and IP_3. The DAG can be phosphorylated to form phosphatidic acid, which can then be transformed back to phosphatidylinositol. The inositol component is then sequentially phosphorylated to restore the original phosphatidylinositol-bisphosphate. (From Nishizuka et al. *Recent Prog. Horm. Res.*, 40:301, 1984.)

recognize that phosphatidylinositol is only one of several membrane phospholipids that contain arachidonate. Arachidonic acid is also released by the actions of the enzyme phospholipase A_2 on more abundant membrane phospholipids.

Second Messages and Cellular Integration

Some cells have several classes of receptors on their surfaces and simultaneously receive excitatory, inhibitory, or a conflicting mixture of excitatory and inhibitory inputs from different hormones. Target cells integrate all inputs by summing them algebraically and then respond accordingly. For example, in the hepatocyte, both glucagon and epinephrine stimulate adenylyl cyclase, each by way of its own receptor. The effects of these signals combine to produce a more intense activation of adenylyl cyclase than would result from either one. Some cells have more than one class of receptor for a single agent, and each class is coupled to a different second messenger system. Thus, hepatic cells and pancreatic beta cells have both α and β receptors for epinephrine. After binding to epinephrine, α_1 receptors in hepatocytes communicate with cytosolic enzymes by way of DAG and IP_3, and the β receptors communicate through cyclic AMP. Both second messenger systems activate the enzyme glycogen phosphorylase, which breaks down glycogen. The two receptor-activated pathways thus converge and reinforce each other. In the pancreatic beta cell, epinephrine binds to yet another receptor, the α_2 receptor, which is coupled to adenylyl cyclase through a G_i, and to β receptors, which are coupled to adenylyl cyclase through a G_s (Fig. 7). The two receptors thus transmit conflicting information, but in this case, the inhibitory influence of the α_2 receptor is ''stronger'' and prevails.

Receptor Tyrosine Kinases

Some hormones, notably insulin and the growth factors, use a different kind of protein kinase to initiate their intracellular actions. When these hormones bind to the extracellular domain of their receptors, configurational changes transmitted through the membrane activate a protein kinase intrinsic to the cytosolic component of the receptor. The receptor kinase catalyzes phosphorylation of hydroxyl groups on tyrosine rather than the serine or threonine residues of proteins that are the sites of phosphorylation catalyzed by protein kinases A and C and the calmodulin-dependent protein kinases. Receptor tyrosine kinases may activate a cascade of protein kinases that phosphorylate serine residues. They also autophosphorylate and thereby amplify or prolong their activity.

REGULATION OF HORMONE SECRETION

For hormones to function as carriers of critical information, their secretion must be turned on and off at precisely the right times. The organism must have some way of knowing when there is a need for a hormone to be secreted and when that need has passed. The necessary components of endocrine regulatory systems include the following:

1. Detector of an actual or threatened homeostatic imbalance.
2. Coupling mechanism to activate the secretory apparatus.
3. Secretory apparatus.
4. Hormone.
5. End-organ capable of responding to the hormone.
6. Detector to recognize that the hormonal effect has occurred and that the hormonal signal can now be shut off (usually the same as component 1).
7. Mechanism for removing the hormone from target cells and blood.
8. Synthetic apparatus to replenish the hormone in the secretory cell.

As we discuss hormonal control, it is important to identify and understand the components of the regulation of each hormonal secretion because (a) derangements in any of the components are the bases of endocrine disease and (b) manipulation of any component provides an opportunity for therapeutic intervention.

Negative Feedback

The secretion of most hormones is regulated by negative feedback. Negative feedback means that some consequence of hormone secretion acts directly or indirectly on the secretory cell in a negative way to inhibit further secretion. A simple example from everyday experience is the thermostat. When the temperature in a room falls below some preset level, the thermostat signals the furnace to produce heat. When room temperature rises to the preset level, the signal from the thermostat to the furnace is shut off, and heat production ceases until the temperature again falls. This is a simple closed-loop feedback system and is analogous to the regulation of glucagon secretion. A fall in blood glucose detected by the alpha cells of the islets of Langerhans causes them to release glucagon, which stimulates the liver to release glucose and thereby increase blood glucose concentrations (Fig. 11). With restoration of blood glucose to some predetermined level or set point, further secretion of glucagon is inhibited. This simple example involves only secreting cells and responding cells. Other systems may be considerably more complex and involve one or more intermediary events, but the essence of negative feedback regulation remains the same, i.e., *hormones produce biological effects that directly or indirectly inhibit their further secretion.*

A problem that emerges with this system of control is that the thermostat maintains a constant room temperature only if the natural tendency of the temperature is to fall. If the temperature were to rise, it could not be controlled by simply turning off the furnace. This problem is at least partially resolved in hormonal systems because, at physiological set points, the basal rate of secretion usually is not zero. In the example given, when there is a rise in blood glucose concentration, glucagon secretion can be diminished and therefore diminish the impetus on the liver to release glucose. Some regulation above and below the set point can therefore be accomplished with just one feedback loop; this mechanism is seen in some endocrine

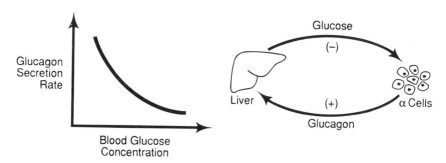

FIG. 11. Negative feedback of glucose production by glucagon. −, inhibits; +, stimulates.

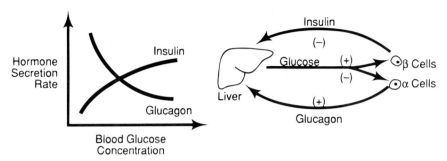

FIG. 12. Negative feedback regulation of blood glucose concentration by insulin and glucagon. −, inhibits; +, stimulates.

control systems. Regulation is more efficient, however, with a second, opposing loop, which is activated when the controlled variable deviates in the opposite direction. In the example of regulation of blood glucose, that second loop is provided by insulin. Insulin inhibits glucose production by the liver and is secreted in response to an elevated blood glucose level (Fig. 12). Protection against deviation in either direction is often achieved in biological systems by the opposing actions of antagonistic control systems.

Closed-loop negative feedback control as described can maintain conditions only at a state of constancy. Such systems are effective in guarding against upward or downward deviations from some predetermined set point, but changing environmental demands often require temporary deviations from constancy. This can be accomplished in some cases by adjusting the set point and, in other cases, by a signal that overrides the set point. For example, epinephrine secreted by the adrenal medulla in response to some emergency inhibits insulin secretion and increases glucagon secretion even though the concentration of glucose in the blood may already be high. Whether the set point is changed or overridden, deviation from constancy is achieved by the intervention of some additional signal from outside the negative feedback system. In most cases, that additional signal originates with the nervous system.

Hormones also initiate or regulate processes that are not limited to steady or constant conditions, and they also frequently involve the nervous system. Virtually all of these processes are self-limiting, and their control resembles negative feedback, but of the open-loop type. For example, oxytocin is a hormone that is secreted by hypothalamic nerve cells whose axons terminate in the posterior pituitary gland. Its secretion is necessary for the extrusion of milk from the lumen of the mammary alveolus into the secretory ducts so that the infant suckling at the nipple can receive milk. In this case, sensory nerve endings in the nipple detect the signal and convey afferent information to the central nervous system, which in turn, signals the release of oxytocin from axon terminals in the pituitary gland. Oxytocin causes contraction of the myoepithelial cells, resulting in delivery of milk to the infant. When the infant is satisfied, the suckling stimulus at the nipple ceases.

Positive Feedback

Positive feedback means that some consequence of hormonal secretion acts on the secretory cells to provide augmented drive for secretion. Rather than being self-limiting, as with negative feedback, the drive for secretion becomes progressively more intense. Positive feedback systems are unusual in biology because they terminate with some cataclysmic, explosive event. A good example of a positive feedback system involves oxytocin and its other effect, i.e., causing contraction of uterine muscle during childbirth (Fig. 13). In this case, the stimulus for oxytocin secretion is dilation of the uterine cervix. Upon receipt of this information through sensory nerves, the brain signals the release of oxytocin from nerve endings in the posterior pituitary gland. The enhanced uterine contraction in response to oxytocin results in greater dilation of the cervix, which strengthens the signal for oxytocin release and so on until the infant is expelled from the uterine cavity.

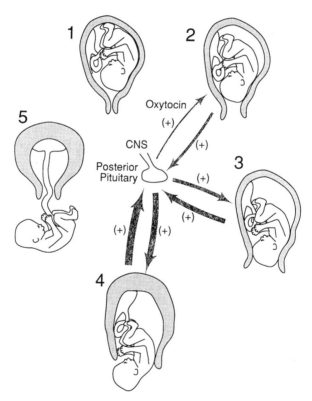

FIG. 13. Positive feedback regulation of oxytocin secretion. **1:** Uterine contractions at the onset of parturition apply mild stretch to the cervix. **2:** In response to the sensory input from the cervix, oxytocin is secreted from the posterior pituitary gland, and stimulates (+) further contraction of the uterus, which, in turn stimulates secretion of more oxytocin. **3:** This leads to further stretching of the cervix and even more oxytocin secretion (**4**) until the fetus is expelled (**5**).

MEASUREMENT OF HORMONES

Whether it is for the purpose of diagnosing a patient's disease or research to gain understanding of normal physiology, it is often necessary to measure how much hormone is present in some biological fluid. Chemical detection of hormones in blood is difficult. With the exception of the thyroid hormones, which contain large amounts of iodine, there is no unique chemistry that sets hormones apart from other bodily constituents. Furthermore, hormones circulate in blood in minute concentrations, 10^{-7} M or less, which further complicates the problem of their detection. Consequently, the earliest methods developed for measuring hormones are bioassays and depend on the ability of a hormone to produce a characteristic biological response. For example, induction of ovulation in the rabbit in response to an injection of urine from a pregnant woman is an indication of the presence of the placental hormone chorionic gonadotropin and is the basis for the rabbit test which was used for many years as an indicator of early pregnancy. Before hormones were identified chemically, they were quantified in units of the biological responses they produced. For example, a unit of insulin is defined as one-third of the amount needed to lower the blood sugar in a 2-kg rabbit to convulsive levels within 3 hours. Although bioassays are now seldom used, some hormones, including insulin, are still standardized in terms of biological units.

Competitive Binding Assays

As knowledge of hormone structure increased, it became evident that peptide hormones are not identical in all species. Small differences in amino acid sequence, which may not affect the biological activity of a hormone, were found to produce antibody reactions with prolonged administration. Hormones isolated from one species were recognized as foreign substances in recipient animals of another species. Antibodies can recognize and react with tiny amounts of the foreign material (antigens) that evoked their production, even in the presence of large amounts of other substances that may be similar or different. Techniques have been devised to permit detection of antibody–antigen reactions even when minute quantities of antigen (hormone) are involved.

Radioimmunoassay

The reaction of a hormone with an antibody results in a complex with altered properties; it may be precipitated out of solution or behave differently when subjected to electrophoresis or adsorption to charcoal or other substances. A typical radioimmunoassay takes advantage of the fact that iodine with a high specific radioactivity can be incorporated readily into tyrosine residues of peptides and proteins and thereby permits detection and quantitation of tiny amounts of a hormone.

To perform a radioimmunoassay, a sample of plasma containing an unknown amount of hormone is mixed in a test tube with a known amount of antibody and a known amount of radioactive iodinated hormone. The unlabeled hormone present in the plasma competes with the iodine-labeled hormone for binding to the antibody. The more hormone present in the plasma sample, the less iodinated hormone can bind to the antibody. Antibody-bound radioactive iodine is then separated from unbound iodinated hormone by a variety of physicochemical means, and the amount of hormone present in the plasma can be inferred by comparison with a standard curve (Fig. 14).

Although this procedure was originally devised for protein hormones, radioimmunoassays are now available for all of the known hormones. The production of specific antibodies to nonprotein hormones can be induced by first attaching these compounds to some protein, e.g., serum albumin. For hormones that lack a site capable of incorporating iodine, such as the steroids, another radioactive label can be used or a chemical tail containing tyrosine can be added.

The major limitation of radioimmunoassays is that *immunological* rather than *biological* activity is measured by these tests because the portion of the hormone molecule recognized by the antibody probably is not the same as the portion recognized by the hormone receptor. Thus, a protein hormone that may be biologically inactive may retain all of its immunological activity. For example, the biologically active portion of parathyroid hormone resides in the amino terminal one-third of the molecule, but the carboxy terminal portion formed by partial degradation of the hormone has a long half-life in blood and accounts for nearly 80% of the immunoreactive parathyroid hormone in human plasma. Until this problem was understood and appropriate adjustments were made, radioimmunoassays grossly overestimated the content of parathyroid hormone in plasma (see Chapter 8). Similarly, biologically inactive prohormones may be detected. By and large, discrepancies between biological activity and immunoactivity have not presented insurmountable difficulties and, in several cases, even have led to increased understanding.

Radioreceptor Assays

A modification of the radioimmunoassay has been devised using the specific binding of the water-soluble hormones to cell membranes rather than antibodies. This method has the theoretical advantage of measuring only biologically active hormone because receptor binding reflects binding to the biologically active site of the hormone rather than the immunoreactive site. The procedures involved, however, are sufficiently complex that radioreceptor binding is rarely used for routine hormone measurements.

Hormone Levels in Blood

It is evident now that hormone concentrations in blood plasma fluctuate from minute to minute and may vary widely in the normal individual over the course of

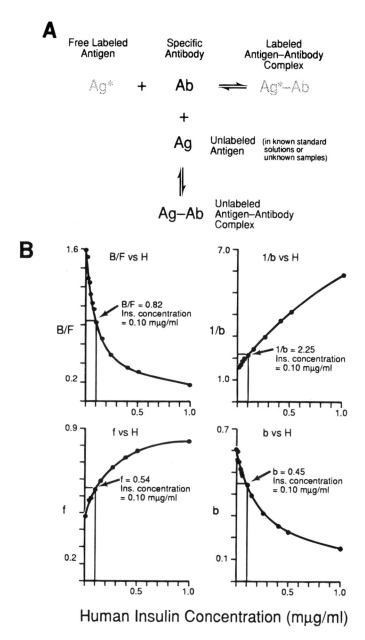

FIG. 14. A: Competing reactions that form the basis of the radioimmunoassay. **B:** Various forms of plotting standard curves based on the addition of known amounts of unlabeled insulin. *B/F*, ratio of bound to free hormone (*H*). The plot shown in the *upper left* is the usual method of plotting the standard curve. *b*, bound; *f*, free. From Berson, S.A. and Yalow, R.S. (1973): Measurement of hormones-Radioimmunoassay. In: *Methods of Investigative and Diagnostic Endocrinology*, edited by Berson, S.A. and Yalow, R.S., North Holland, Amsterdam 1973, pp. 84–135.

a day. Hormone secretion may be episodic, pulsatile, or follow a daily rhythm (Fig. 15). In most cases, it is necessary to make multiple serial measurements of hormones before a diagnosis of a hyper- or hypofunctional state can be confirmed. Endocrine disease occurs when the concentration of hormone in the blood is inappropriate for the physiological situation rather than because the absolute amounts of hormone in the blood are high or low. It is also becoming increasingly evident that the pattern

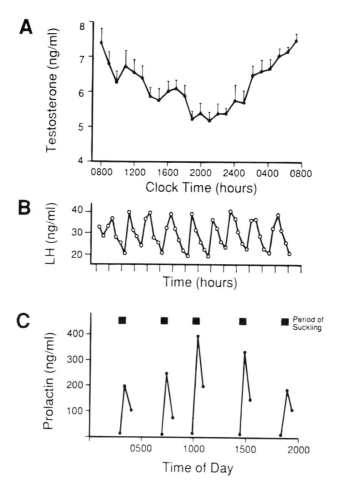

FIG. 15. Changes in hormone concentrations in the blood may follow different patterns. **A:** Daily rhythm in testosterone secretion. From Bremner, W.J., Vitiello, M.V., and Prinz, P.N. (1983): Loss of circadian rhythmicity in blood testosterone levels with aging in normal men. *J. Clin Endocrinol. Metab.*, 56:1278. **B:** Hourly rhythm of luteinizing hormone (LH) secretion. From Yamaji, T., Dierschke, D.J., Bhattacharya, A.N., et al. (1972): The negative feedback control by estradiol and progesterone of LH secretion in the ovariectomized rhesus monkey. *Endocrinology*, 90:771. **C:** Episodic secretion of prolactin. From Hwang, P., Guyda, H., and Friesen, H. (1971): Radioimmunoassay for human prolactin. *Proc. Natl. Acad. Sci. U S A*, 68:1902.

of hormone secretion, rather than the amount secreted, may be of great importance in determining hormone responses. This subject is discussed in detail in Chapter 11. It is noteworthy that, for the endocrine system as well as the nervous system, additional information can be transmitted by the frequency of signal production as well as by the signal itself.

SUGGESTED READING

Catt, K. J. (1987): Molecular mechanisms of hormone action: control of target cell function by peptide, steroid and thyroid hormones. In: *Endocrinology and Metabolism*, 2nd ed., edited by Felig, P., Baxter, J. D., Broadus, A. E., and Frohman, L. A., pp. 82–65, McGraw-Hill, New York.

Exton, J. H. (1985): Role of calcium and phosphoinositides in the actions of certain hormones and neurotransmitters. *J. Clin. Invest.*, 75:1753–1757.

Gorski, J., Welshons, W. V., Sakai, D., Hansen, J., Walent, J., Kassis, J., Shull, J., Stack, G., and Campen, C. (1986): Evolution of a model of estrogen action. *Recent Prog. Horm. Res.*, 42:297–322.

LeRoith, D., Delahunty, G., Wilson, G. L., Roberts, C. T., Jr., Shemer, J., Hart, C., Lesniak, M. A., Shiloach, J., and Roth, J. (1986): Evolutionary aspects of the endocrine and nervous systems. *Recent Prog. Horm. Res.*, 42:549–582.

Pollard, H. B., Ornberg, R., Levine, M., Kelner, K., Morita, K., Levine, R., Forsberg, E., Brocklehurst, K. W., Duong, L., Lelkes, P. I., Heldman, E., and Youdim, M. (1986): Hormone secretion by exocytosis with emphasis on information from the chromatin system. *Vitam. Horm.*, 42:109–197.

Smith, D. F., and Toft, D. O. (1993): Steroid receptors and their associated proteins. *Mol. Endocrinol.*, 7:4–11.

Spiegel, A. M., Gierschik, P., Levine, M. A., and Downs, R. W., Jr. (1985): Clinical implications of guanine nucleotide-binding proteins as receptor-effector couplers. *N. Engl. J. Med.*, 312:26–33.

Spiegel, A. M., Shenker, A., and Weinstein, L. S. (1992): Receptor-effector coupling by G proteins: implications for normal and abnormal signal transduction. *Endocr. Rev.*, 13:536–565.

Walters, M. R. (1985): Steroid hormone receptors and the nucleus. *Endocr. Rev.*, 6:512–543.

2

Pituitary Gland

OVERVIEW

The pituitary gland has usually been thought of as the "master gland" because its hormonal secretions control the growth and activity of three other endocrine glands: the thyroid, adrenals, and gonads. Because the secretory activity of the master gland is itself controlled by hormones that originate in either the brain or the target glands, it is perhaps better to think of the pituitary gland as the relay between the control centers in the central nervous system and the peripheral endocrine organs. The pituitary hormones are not limited in their activity to regulation of endocrine target glands; they also act directly on nonendocrine target tissues. Secretion of all of these hormones is under the control of signals arising in both the brain and the periphery.

MORPHOLOGY

The pituitary gland is located in a small depression in the sphenoid bone, the *sella turcica,* just beneath the hypothalamus, and is connected to the hypothalamus by a thin stalk called the *infundibulum.* It is a compound organ consisting of a neural or *posterior lobe* derived embryologically from the brainstem, and an anterior portion, the *adenohypophysis*, which derives embryologically from the primitive foregut. The cells located at the junction of the two lobes comprise the *intermediate lobe*, which is not readily identifiable as an anatomical entity in humans (Fig. 1).

Histologically, the anterior lobe consists of large polygonal cells arranged in cords and surrounded by a sinusoidal capillary system. Most of the cells contain secretory granules, although some are only sparsely granulated. Based on their characteristic staining with standard histochemical dyes and immunofluorescent stains, it is possible to identify the cells that secrete each of the pituitary hormones. It was once thought that there was a unique cell type for each of the pituitary hormones, but it is now recognized that some cells may produce more than one hormone. Although particular cell types tend to cluster in central or peripheral regions of the gland, the

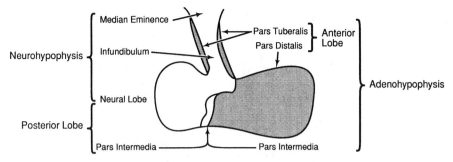

FIG. 1. Human pituitary gland in midsagittal section. Redrawn from Xuereb, G.P., Prichard, M.M.L., and Daniel, P.M. (1954): The arterial supply and venous drainage of the human hypophysis cerebri. *Q. J. Exp. Physiol.*, 39:199.

functional significance, if any, of their arrangement within the anterior lobe is not known.

The posterior lobe consists of two major portions: the infundibulum, or stalk, and the infundibular process, or neural lobe. The posterior lobe is richly endowed with nonmyelinated nerve fibers that contain electron-dense secretory granules. The cell bodies from which these fibers arise are located in the bilaterally paired *supraoptic* and *paraventricular nuclei* of the hypothalamus. These cells are characteristically large compared to other hypothalamic neurons and, hence, are called *magnocellular*. The secretory material synthesized in cell bodies in the hypothalamus is transported down the axons and stored in bulbous nerve endings within the posterior lobe. Dilated terminals of these fibers lie in close proximity to the rich capillary network whose fenestrated endothelium allows the secretory products to enter the circulation readily.

The vascular supply and innervation of the two lobes reflect their different embryological origins and provide important clues that ultimately led to an understanding of their physiological regulation. The anterior lobe is sparsely innervated and lacks any secretomotor nerves. This fact might argue against a role for the pituitary as a relay between the central nervous system and peripheral endocrine organs, except that communication between the anterior pituitary and the brain is through vascular, rather than neural, channels.

The anterior lobe is linked to the brainstem by the *hypothalamohypophyseal portal system* through which it receives most of its blood supply (Figs. 2 to 4). The superior hypophyseal arteries deliver blood to an intricate network of capillaries, the *primary plexus*, in the median eminence of the hypothalamus. Capillaries of the primary plexus converge to form long hypophyseal portal vessels, which course down the infundibular stalk to deliver their blood to capillary sinusoids interspersed among the secretory cells of the anterior lobe. The inferior hypophyseal arteries supply a similar capillary plexus in the lower portion of the infundibular stem. These capillaries drain into short portal vessels, which supply a second sinusoidal capillary network within the anterior lobe. Nearly all of the blood that reaches the anterior lobe is

Hypothalamus

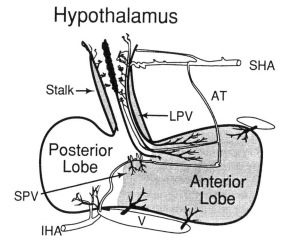

FIG. 2. Vascular supply of the human pituitary gland. Note the origin of long portal vessels (*LPV*) from the primary capillary bed and the origin of short portal vessels (*SPV*) from the capillary bed in the lower part of the stalk. Both sets of portal vessels break up into sinusoidal capillaries in the anterior lobe. *SHA* and IHA, superior and inferior hypophyseal arteries, respectively; *AT*, trabecular artery which forms an anastomotic pathway between SHA and IHA; *V*, venous sinuses. Redrawn from Daniel, P.M. and Prichard, M.M.L. (1966): Observations on the vascular anatomy of the pituitary gland and its importance in pituitary function. *Am. Heart J.*, 72:147.

carried in the long and short portal vessels. The anterior lobe receives only a small portion of its blood supply directly from the paired trabecular arteries, which branch off the superior hypophyseal arteries. In contrast, the circulation in the posterior pituitary is unremarkable. It is supplied with blood by the inferior hypophyseal arteries. Venous blood drains from both lobes through a number of short veins into the nearby cavernous sinuses.

The portal arrangement of blood flow is important because blood that supplies the secretory cells of the anterior lobe first drains the hypothalamus. Portal blood can thus pick up chemical signals released by neurons of the central nervous system and deliver them to the secretory cells of the anterior pituitary. As might be anticipated, because hypophyseal portal blood flow represents only a tiny fraction of the cardiac output, only minute amounts of neural secretions are needed to achieve biologically effective concentrations in pituitary sinusoidal blood when delivered in this way. More than 1,000 times more secretory material would be needed if it were dissolved in the entire blood volume and delivered through the arterial circulation. This arrangement also provides a measure of specificity to hypothalamic secretion because pituitary cells are the only ones exposed to concentrations that are high enough to be physiologically effective.

PHYSIOLOGY OF THE ANTERIOR PITUITARY GLAND

There are six anterior pituitary hormones whose physiological importance is clearly established. They include the hormones that govern the functions of the

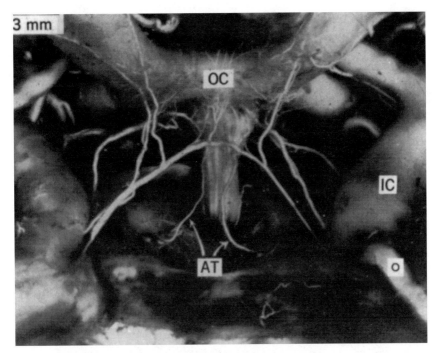

FIG. 3. Neoprene latex cast of the vasculature of the human pituitary stalk viewed from the front. *OC*, optic chiasm; *IC*, internal carotid artery; O, ophthalmic artery; *AT*, trabecular artery. From Xuereb, G.P., Prichard, M.M.L., and Daniel, P.M. (1954): The arterial supply and venous drainage of the human hypophysis cerebri. *Q. J. Exp. Physiol.*, 39:199.

thyroid and adrenal glands, the gonads, and the mammary glands, as well as bodily growth. They have been called "trophic" or "tropic" from the Greek *trophos,* to nourish, or *tropic,* to turn toward. Both terms are generally accepted. We thus have, for example, thyrotrophin, or thyrotropin, which is also more accurately called thyroid-stimulating hormone (TSH). Table 1 lists the anterior pituitary hormones and their various synonyms. The various anterior pituitary cells are named for the hormones they contain. Thus, we have thyrotropes, corticotropes, somatotropes, and lactotropes. Because a substantial number of growth hormone (GH)-producing cells also secrete prolactin (PRL), they are called somatomammotropes. Some evidence suggests that somatomammotropes are an intermediate stage in the interconversion of somatotropes and lactotropes. The two gonadotropins are found in a single cell type, called the gonadotrope.

All of the anterior pituitary hormones are polypeptides, proteins, or glycoproteins. They are synthesized on ribosomes and translocated through various cellular compartments where they undergo posttranslational processing. They are packaged in membrane-bound secretory granules and secreted by exocytosis. The pituitary gland stores relatively large amounts of these hormones, sufficient to meet physiological demands for many days. Over the course of many decades, these hormones were

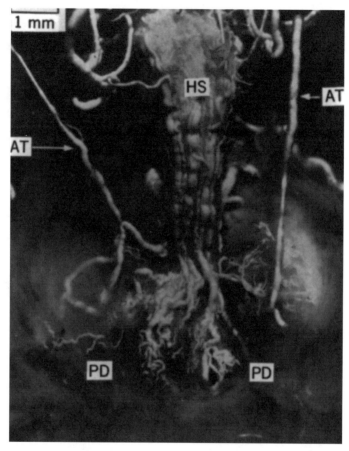

FIG. 4. Anterior aspect of the human pituitary stalk (*HS*) with the vasculature injected with neoprene latex. *AT*, paired trabecular arteries; *PD*, pars distalis. From Xuereb, G.P., Prichard, M.M.L., and Daniel, P.M. (1954): The arterial supply and venous drainage of the human hypophysis cerebri. *Q. J. Exp. Physiol.*, 39:199.

extracted, purified, and characterized. Now, even the structures of their genes are known, and we can group the anterior pituitary hormones by families.

Glycoprotein Hormones

The glycoprotein hormone family includes TSH, whose only known physiological role is to stimulate secretion of thyroid hormone, and the two gonadotropins, follicle-stimulating hormone (FSH) and luteinizing hormone (LH). Although named for their function in women, both gonadotropic hormones are crucial for the function of the testes as well as the ovaries. In women, FSH promotes growth of ovarian follicles,

TABLE 1. *Hormones of the anterior pituitary gland*

Hormone	Target	Major actions in humans
Glycoprotein family		
Thyroid-stimulating hormone (TSH), also called thyrotropin	Thyroid gland	Stimulates synthesis and secretion of thyroid hormones
Gonadotropins		
Follicle-stimulating hormone (FSH)	Ovary	Stimulates growth of follicles and estrogen secretion
	Testis	Acts on Sertoli cells to promote maturation of sperm
Luteinizing hormone (LH), also called interstitial cell-stimulating hormone (ICSH)	Ovary	Stimulates ovulation of ripe follicle and formation of corpus luteum; stimulates estrogen and progesterone synthesis by corpus luteum
	Testis	Stimulates interstitial cells of Leydig to synthesize and secrete testosterone
Growth hormone/prolactin family		
Growth hormone (GH), also called somatotropic hormone (STH)	Most tissues	Promotes growth in stature and mass; stimulates production of insulin-like growth factor (IGF-I), stimulates protein synthesis, usually inhibits glucose utilization and promotes fat utilization
Prolactin	Mammary glands	Promotes milk secretion and mammary growth
Proopiomelanocortin family (POMC)		
Adrenocorticotropic hormone (ACTH), also known as adrenocorticotropin or corticotropin	Adrenal cortex	Promotes synthesis and secretion of adrenal cortical hormones
β-Lipotropin, β-endorphin	?	Physiological role not established

and in men, it promotes formation of spermatozoa by the germinal epithelium of the testis. In women, LH induces ovulation of the ripe follicle and formation of the corpus luteum from the remaining glomerulosa cells in the collapsed, ruptured follicle. It also stimulates the synthesis and secretion of the ovarian hormones estrogen and progesterone. In men, LH stimulates secretion of the male hormone, testosterone, by the interstitial cells. Consequently, it has also been called interstitial cell-stimulating hormone, but this name has largely disappeared from the literature. The actions of these hormones are discussed in detail in Chapters 11 and 12.

The three glycoprotein hormones are synthesized and stored in the pituitary basophils, and as their name implies, each contains sugar moieties covalently linked to asparagine residues in the polypeptide chains. All three are comprised of two peptide subunits, designated α and ß, which are not covalently linked. The α subunit of all three hormones is identical in its amino acid sequence and appears to be the product of a single gene located on chromosome 6. The ß subunits of each are somewhat larger and confer physiological specificity. The ß subunits are encoded in separate genes located on different chromosomes, but there is a great deal of homology in their amino acid sequences. Both subunits contain carbohydrate moieties that are considerably less constant in their composition than are their peptide chains. The α subunits are synthesized in excess over the ß subunits, and hence, it is synthesis of ß subunits that appears to be rate limiting for production of glycoprotein hormones. Pairing of the two subunits begins in the rough endoplasmic reticulum and continues in the Golgi apparatus, where processing of the carbohydrate components of the subunits is completed. The loosely paired complex then undergoes spontaneous refolding in the secretory granules into a stable, active hormone. However, free α and the ß subunits of all three hormones may be found in blood plasma, but none of the subunits is biologically active alone.

The placental hormone, human chorionic gonadotropin (hCG), is closely related chemically and functionally to the pituitary gonadotropic hormones. It, too, is a glycoprotein and consists of an α and ß chain. The α chain is a product of the same gene as the α chain of pituitary glycoprotein hormones. The peptide sequence of the ß chain is identical to that of LH except that it is longer by 32 amino acids at its carboxyl terminus. Curiously, although there is only a single gene for each ß subunit of the pituitary glycoprotein hormones, the human genome contains seven copies of the hCG ß gene, all located on chromosome 19 in close proximity to the LH ß gene. Not surprisingly, hCG has biological actions that are similar to those of LH, as well as a unique action on the corpus luteum (Chapter 13).

Growth Hormone and Prolactin

Growth hormone (GH) is required for attainment of normal adult stature (see Chapter 10), and produces metabolic effects that may not be directly related to its growth-promoting actions. These actions include mobilization of free fatty acids from adipose tissue and inhibition of glucose metabolism in muscle and adipose tissue. The role of GH in energy balance is discussed in Chapter 9. GH is secreted throughout life and is the most abundant of the pituitary hormones. The human pituitary gland contains between 5 and 10 mg of GH, an amount that is 20 to 40 times greater than that of adrenal corticotropic hormone (ACTH), and 50 to 100 times greater than that of PRL. Because its effects are exerted throughout the body, GH has also been called the *somatotropic hormone* or *somatotropin*. Structurally, GH is closely related to another pituitary hormone, PRL, which is required for milk production in postpartum women (see Chapter 13). The functions of PRL in men or nonlactating women are not firmly established, but a growing body of evidence suggests that it may stimulate cells of the immune system. These pituitary hormones are closely related to the placental hormone human chorionic somatomammotropin (hCS), which has both growth-promoting and milk-producing activity in some experimental systems. Because of this property, hCS is also called human placental lactogen. Although the physiological function of this placental hormone has not been established with certainty, it may be to regulate maternal metabolism during pregnancy and prepare the mammary glands for lactation (see Chapter 13).

Growth hormone, PRL, and hCS appear to have evolved from a single ancestral gene that duplicated several times. The human haploid genome contains two GH and three hCS genes all located on the long arm of chromosome 17, and a single PRL gene located on chromosome 6. These genes are similar in the arrangement of their transcribed and nontranscribed portions as well as their nucleotide sequences. All are comprised of five exons separated by four introns located at homologous positions. All three hormones are large single-stranded peptides containing two internal disulfide bridges at corresponding parts of the molecule. Also, PRL has a third internal disulfide bridge. GH and hCS have about 80% of their amino acids in common, and a region 146 amino acids long is similar in human GH and PRL. Only one of the GH genes is expressed in the pituitary, but because an alternative mode of splicing of the ribonucleic acid (RNA) transcript is possible, two GH isoforms are produced. The larger form is the 22-kilodalton molecule (22K GH), which is about ten times more abundant than the smaller, 20-kilodalton molecule (20K GH) which lacks amino acids 32 to 46. The other GH gene appears to be expressed only in the placenta and is the predominant form of GH in the blood of pregnant women. It encodes a protein that apparently has the same biological actions as the pituitary hormone, although it differs from the pituitary hormone in 13 amino acids and may be glycosylated.

Considering the similarities in their structures, it is not surprising that GH shares some of the lactogenic activity of PRL and hCS. However, human GH also has about two thirds of its amino acids in common with the GH molecules of cattle and rats, but humans are completely insensitive to cattle or rat GH and respond only to the GH produced by humans or monkeys. This requirement of primates for primate GH is an example of *species specificity*, which may be limited to the actions of GH in human beings and monkeys. Other animals respond perfectly well to GH derived from the pituitary glands of unrelated species, and humans respond to the other pituitary hormones of nonprimate origin. Because of species specificity, human GH was in short supply until the advent of genetic engineering.

Adrenocorticotropin Family

Portions of the cortex of the adrenal glands are controlled physiologically by ACTH, which is also called corticotropin or adrenocorticotropin. This family of pituitary peptides includes α- and ß-melanocyte-stimulating hormones (MSH), ß- and α-lipotropin (LPH), and ß-endorphin. Of these, ACTH is the only peptide whose physiological role in humans is established. The MSHs, which disperse melanin pigment in melanocytes in the skin of lower vertebrates, have little importance in humans. The peptide ß-LPH is named for its stimulatory effect on mobilization of lipids from adipose tissue in rabbits, but the physiological importance of this action is uncertain. The 91-amino acid chain of ß-LPH contains, at its carboxyl end, the

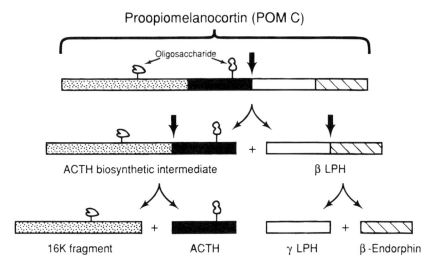

FIG. 5. Proteolytic processing of POMC in anterior pituitary cells. From Mains, R.E. and Eipper, B.A. (1979): Synthesis and secretion of corticotropins, melanotropins, and endorphins by rat intermediate pituitary cells. *J. Biol. Chem.*, 254:7885.

complete amino acid sequence of ß-endorphin (from *end*ogenous m*orphin*e), which reacts with the same receptors as morphine.

The ACTH-related peptides constitute a family because (a) they contain regions of homologous amino acid sequences and (b) they all arise from the transcription and translation of the same gene (Fig. 5). The gene product is called pro-opiomelano-cortin (POMC), which after removal of the signal peptide, consists of 239 amino acids. The molecule contains ten doublets of basic amino acids (arginine and lysine in various combinations), which are potential sites for cleavage by trypsin-like endo-peptidases. The product of the POMC gene is expressed by cells in the anterior lobe of the pituitary, the intermediate lobe, and the central nervous system, but tissue-specific differences in the way the molecule is processed after translation give rise to differences in the final secretory products. Thus the predominant products of anterior pituitary cells are ACTH, ß-LPH, and ß-endorphin, whereas the intermediate lobe in some animals gives rise principally to α- and ß-MSH. Because the intermedi-ate lobe of the pituitary gland of humans is thought to be nonfunctional, except perhaps in fetal life, it is not discussed further. It is noteworthy that final processing of POMC probably occurs in the secretory granule. Therefore ß-LPH and ß-endor-phin are secreted along with ACTH and are found in the blood plasma.

REGULATION OF ANTERIOR PITUITARY FUNCTION

Secretion of the anterior pituitary hormones is regulated by the central nervous system and hormones produced in peripheral target glands. Input from the central nervous system provides the primary drive for secretion, and peripheral input plays a secondary, though vital, role in modulating secretory rates. Secretion of all of the anterior pituitary hormones except PRL virtually ceases in the absence of stimulation from the hypothalamus, which can be produced, for example, when the pituitary gland is removed surgically from its natural location and reimplanted at a site remote from the hypothalamus. The persistent high rate of secretion of PRL under these circumstances indicates, not only that the pituitary glands can revascularize and survive in a new location, but also that PRL secretion is normally under tonic inhibitory control by the hypothalamus. In this chapter, we discuss only general aspects of the regulation of anterior pituitary function. A detailed description of the control of the secretory activity of each hormone is given in subsequent chapters in conjunction with a discussion of its role in regulating physiological processes.

Hypophysiotropic Hormones

As already mentioned, the central nervous system communicates with the anterior pituitary gland by means of neurosecretions released into the hypothalamohypophyseal portal system. These neurosecretions are called *hypophysiotropic hormones*. The fact that only small amounts of the hypophysiotropic hormones are synthesized, stored, and secreted frustrated efforts to isolate and identify them for nearly 25 years. Their abundance in the hypothalamus is less than 0.1% of that of even the scarcest pituitary hormone in the anterior lobe.

The first of the hypothalamic neurohormones to be isolated was the tripeptide thyrotropin-releasing hormone (TRH). It was isolated, identified, and synthesized almost simultaneously in the laboratories of Roger Guillemin and Andrew Schally, who were subsequently recognized for this monumental achievement with the award of a Nobel Prize. Guillemin's laboratory processed 25 kg of sheep hypothalami to obtain 1 mg of TRH. Schally's laboratory extracted 245,000 pig hypothalami to yield only 8.2 mg of this tripeptide. The structure of the gene and the messenger RNA that encode TRH have been studied, and curiously, each prohormone molecule contains six copies of TRH all encoded in exon 3. The TRH-producing neurons that control TSH secretion appear to be located within the *paraventricular nuclei* of the hypothalamus, but TRH is also found in neurons scattered throughout the central nervous system and probably mediates a variety of responses. The actions of TRH in the regulation of the TSH secretion are discussed further in Chapter 3.

The presently known hypophysiotropic peptides are listed in Table 2. The simple neurotransmitter dopamine appears to satisfy most of the criteria for a PRL-inhibiting factor whose existence was suggested by the persistent high rate of PRL secretion by pituitary glands transplanted outside the sella turcica. It is likely that there is also a PRL-releasing hormone. Secretion of FSH and LH is under the control of a single hypothalamic decapeptide, gonadotropic hormone releasing hormone (GnRH), which is sometimes called LH releasing hormone for its ability to promote release of LH. Endocrinologists originally had some difficulty accepting the idea that both

TABLE 2. *Hypophysiotropic hormones*

Hormone	Amino acids	Physiological actions on the pituitary
Corticotropin-releasing hormone (CRH)	41	Stimulates secretion of ACTH, β-LPH, and β-endorphin
Gonadotropin-releasing hormone (GnRH), originally called luteinizing hormone-releasing hormone (LHRH)	10	Stimulates secretion of FSH and LH
Growth hormone-releasing hormone (GHRH), somatocrinin	40 or 44	Stimulates GH secretion
Somatotropin release-inhibiting factor (SRIF), somatostatin	14 or 28	Inhibits secretion of GH
Prolactin-stimulating factor (?)	?	Stimulates prolactin secretion
Prolactin-inhibiting factor (PIF)	Dopamine	Inhibits prolactin secretion
Thyrotropin-releasing hormone (TRH)	3	Stimulates secretion of TSH and prolactin

ACTH, adrenocorticotrophic hormone; LPH, lipotropin; FSH, follicle-stimulating hormone; LH, luteinizing hormone; GH, growth hormone; TSH, thyroid-stimulating hormone.

gonadotropins are under the control of a single hypothalamic releasing hormone because FSH and LH appear to be secreted independently under certain circumstances. Most endocrinologists have now abandoned the idea that there must be a separate FSH-releasing hormone because other factors can account for the partial independence of LH and FSH secretion. The GnRH is secreted in discrete pulses at regular intervals from neurons located in the anterior hypothalamus. The frequency of pulses stimulating gonadotropes determines the ratio of FSH and LH secreted. In addition, target glands secrete hormones that selectively inhibit either FSH or LH secretion. These complex events are discussed in detail in Chapters 11 and 12.

Secretion of GH is controlled by both a releasing hormone (GHRH) and a release-inhibiting hormone, somatostatin, which is also called somatotropin release-inhibiting factor. The GH releasing hormone is a member of a family of gastrointestinal and neurohormones that includes vasoactive intestinal peptide and glucagon. Curiously, processing the prohormones for each of these regulators of GH secretion can give rise to two forms of the final secretory product. Somatostatin is also produced and secreted by cells in the pancreas (see Chapter 5) and the gastrointestinal tract. A considerable number of other brain peptides, including several that are closely related in structure to gastrointestinal hormones, have also been isolated from the hypothalamus, but their physiological roles have not been defined.

Although, in general, the hypophysiotropic hormones affect the secretion of one or another pituitary hormone specifically, TRH can increase the secretion of PRL at least as well as it increases the secretion of TSH. The physiological meaning of this experimental finding is not understood. Under normal physiological conditions, PRL and TSH appear to be secreted independently, and increased PRL secretion is not necessarily seen in circumstances that call for increased TSH secretion. However, in laboratory rats and possibly human beings as well, suckling at the breast increases both PRL and TSH secretion in a manner suggestive of increased TRH secretion. In the normal individual, somatostatin may inhibit the secretion of other pituitary hormones in addition to GH, but again, the physiological significance of this action is not understood. With disease states, the specificity of responses of various pituitary cells for their own hypophysiotropic hormones may break down, or some cells might even begin to secrete their hormones autonomously.

Experimental verification of the existence of hypophysiotropic hormones in the hypothalamus and hypophyseal portal blood has been obtained using sensitive immunohistological and immunoassay techniques. More recently *in situ* hybridization has been used to localize messenger RNA hypothalmic neurons. The hypothalamus receives input from many structures within the brain. Such techniques, coupled with early experiments involving electrical stimulation or introduction of discrete lesions to interrupt fiber tracts or destroy nuclei, allowed mapping of some of the centers that relay signals or govern production or release of the hypothalamic hormones. Immunocytological studies have also revealed that these peptides as well as many other neuropeptides are widely distributed in the central nervous system in structures that appear to be neurosecretory granules in nerve terminals. Some neurons contain more than one neuropeptide, along with a classical low molecular weight neurotransmitter. In addition to their actions as hypophysiotropic hormones, neuropeptides are thought to function as neurotransmitters and as pre- and postsynaptic modulators of neuronal activity. Some have been found to influence behavior or memory. The same or closely related peptides are also found in many locations outside the central nervous system, especially in the gut and its embryological derivatives. Conversely, many peptide hormones originally discovered for their actions outside of the nervous system also appear to be produced by neurons and are stored within synaptic vesicles in central and peripheral neurons.

Hypophysiotropic hormones increase both the secretion and synthesis of pituitary hormones. In doing so, hypothalamic peptides interact with specific receptors on the surfaces of pituitary cells. Although some hypothalamic hormones increase the formation of cyclic adenosine monophosphate (AMP) in pituitary target cells, the exact role of the cyclic nucleotide in promoting secretion is still a matter of debate. The inositol trisphosphate–diacylglyceride second messenger system may function as an alternative, or in addition, to cyclic AMP in signaling hormone secretion in some cells. The release of hormones almost certainly is the result of an influx of calcium, which triggers and sustains the process of exocytosis. The actions of the hypophysiotropic hormones on their target cells in the pituitary are considered further in later chapters.

Feedback Control of Anterior Pituitary Function

We have already indicated that the primary drive for secretion of all of the anterior pituitary hormones except PRL is stimulation by the hypothalamic releasing hor-

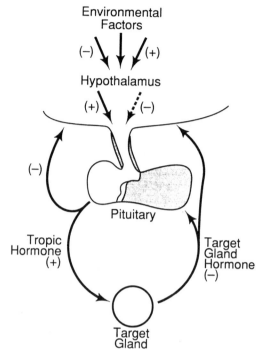

FIG. 6. Regulation of anterior pituitary hormone secretion. Environmental factors may increase or decrease pituitary activity by increasing or decreasing hypophysiotropic hormone secretion. Pituitary secretions increase the secretion of target gland hormones, which may inhibit further secretion by acting at either the hypothalamus or the pituitary. Pituitary hormones may also inhibit their own secretion by a short feedback loop. From Goodman, H.M. (1980): The Pituitary Gland. In: *Medical Physiology*, 14th ed., edited by Mountcastle, V.B., Mosby, St. Louis.

mones. In the absence of the hormones of their target glands, secretion of TSH, ACTH, and the gonadotropins gradually increases many fold. The secretion of these pituitary hormones is subject to negative feedback inhibition by the secretions of their target glands. Regulation of the secretion of the anterior pituitary hormones in the normal individual is achieved through the interplay of the stimulatory effects of releasing hormones and the inhibitory effects of the target gland hormones (Fig. 6).

Regulation of the secretion of pituitary hormones by hormones of target glands could be achieved equally well if negative feedback signals acted at the level of (a) the hypothalamus to inhibit secretion of hypophysiotropic hormones or (b) the pituitary gland to blunt the response to hypophysiotropic stimulation. Actually, some combination of the two mechanisms applies to all of the anterior pituitary hormones except PRL. The control of TSH secretion in the adult human comes closest to the second model, in which negative feedback regulation is exerted virtually exclusively in the pituitary gland. There appears to be little if any effect of thyroid hormone on the rate of TRH secretion from the hypothalamus. Rather, thyroid hormone is thought to act on thyrotropes to decrease their sensitivity to TRH by a mechanism dependent on gene transcription and translation (see Chapter 3).

In experimental animals, it appears that secretion of GnRH is variable and highly sensitive to environmental influences, e.g., day length or even the act of mating. In humans and other primates, the secretion of GnRH after puberty closely resembles that of TRH. It has been shown experimentally in rhesus monkeys and human subjects that all the complex changes in the rates of FSH and LH secretion characteristic of the normal menstrual cycle can occur when the pituitary gland is stimulated by pulses of GnRH delivered at a constant rate and amplitude. For such changes in pituitary secretion to occur, changes in secretion of target gland hormones that accompany ripening of the follicle, ovulation, and luteinization must modulate responses of gonadotropes to GnRH (Chapter 12). Other evidence suggests that target gland hormones may also act at the level of the hypothalamus to regulate GnRH secretion. It is almost certain that, even in humans, GnRH secretion is subject to environmental influences.

The rate of corticotropin releasing hormone (CRH) secretion is profoundly affected by changes in both the internal and external environment. Physiologically, CRH is secreted in increased amounts in response to nonspecific stress. Even in the absence of the adrenal glands, and hence the inhibitory effects of its hormones, ACTH secretion is known to increase in response to stress, indicating that CRH secretion must have been increased. Nevertheless, adrenal cortical hormones do exert a negative feedback effect on pituitary corticotropes where they decrease transcription of POMC and the ability of CRH to increase cyclic AMP production. Adrenal cortical hormones also act at the level of the hypothalamus and decrease CRH synthesis and secretion into the hypophyseal portal vessels (see Chapter 4).

The control of GH secretion is more complex because it is under the influence of both a releasing hormone and a release-inhibiting hormone. In addition, although GH does not have a discrete target gland that secretes a hormone, it nevertheless is under negative feedback control from peripheral tissues. As is discussed in detail in Chapter 10, GH evokes production of a peptide, called insulin-like growth factor (IGF) which mediates the growth-promoting actions of GH. This peptide exerts powerful inhibitory effects on GH secretion by decreasing the sensitivity of somatotropes to GHRH. It also acts at the level of the hypothalamus to increase the release of somatostatin and to inhibit the release of GHRH.

The modulating effects of target gland hormones on the pituitary gland are not limited to inhibiting secretion of their own provocative hormones. Target gland hormones may modulate pituitary function by increasing the sensitivity of other pituitary cells to their releasing factors or by increasing the synthesis of other pituitary hormones. Hormones of the thyroid and adrenal glands are required for normal responses of the somatotropes to GHRH. Similarly, estrogen secreted by the ovary in response to FSH and LH increases PRL synthesis and secretion.

In addition to feedback inhibition exerted by target gland hormones, some authors have obtained evidence that pituitary hormones may inhibit their own secretion. In this so-called *short-loop feedback system,* pituitary cells respond to increased concentrations of their own hormones by decreasing further secretion. The physiological importance of short-loop feedback systems has not been established, nor has that of the postulated *ultrashort-loop feedback* in which high concentrations of hypophysiotropic hormones may inhibit their own release.

PHYSIOLOGY OF THE POSTERIOR PITUITARY GLAND

The posterior pituitary gland secretes two hormones. Both are nonapeptides whose structures are closely related and differ by only two amino acid residues. These hormones almost certainly evolved from a single ancestral molecule. The genes that encode them occupy adjacent loci on chromosome 20, but they are in opposite transcriptional orientation. They are *oxytocin*, which means ''rapid birth'' in reference to its action to increase uterine contractility during parturition, and *vasopressin*, in reference to its ability to contract vascular smooth muscle and thus raise blood pressure. Because the human hormone has an arginine in position 8 instead of the lysine found in the corresponding hormone originally isolated from pigs, it is called arginine vasopressin (AVP). Each of the posterior pituitary hormones has other actions in addition to those for which it was named. Oxytocin also causes contraction of the myoepithelial cells that envelop the secretory alveoli of the mammary glands and thus enables the suckling infant to receive milk. Another action of AVP is to promote reabsorption of free water by the renal tubule and gives rise to its other name, anitdiuretic hormone. These two effects are mediated by two classes of receptors linked to separate transduction systems: V_1 receptors signal vascular muscle contraction by means of the phosphoinositol pathway, whereas V_2 receptors utilize the cyclic AMP system to produce the antidiuretic effect in renal tubules. Oxytocin appears to act through a single receptor that signals through the phosphoinositol pathway. The physiological actions of these hormones are considered further in Chapters 7 and 13.

Oxytocin and AVP are synthesized in separate neurons whose cell bodies are located in the *supraoptic* and *paraventricular nuclei* of the hypothalamus. They are formed as larger preprohormone molecules and packaged in secretory vesicles in the Golgi apparatus along with the enzymes that cleave them into their final secretory products. The secretory vesicles are then transported down the axons to the nerve terminals in the posterior gland where they are stored along with larger protein molecules called *neurophysins* which actually are the adjacent portions of the precursor molecules (Fig. 7). The neurophysins are co-secreted with AVP or oxytocin but have no known endocrine actions. The neurophysins, however, must play an important role in the posttranslational processing of the neurohypophyseal hormones because AVP is absent in rodents and humans that have mutations in the region of the gene that encodes the neurophysin component in the preprohormone.

Regulation of Posterior Pituitary Function

Because the hormones of the posterior pituitary gland are synthesized and stored in nerve cells, it should not be surprising that their secretion is controlled in the

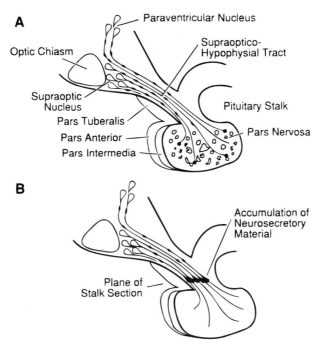

FIG. 7. Hypothalamic–neurohypophyseal relations showing the distribution of secretory granules before (**A**) and after (**B**) stalk section. From Scharrer, E. and Scharrer, B. (1954): *Recent Prog. Horm. Res.*, 10:193.

same way as that of more conventional neurotransmitters. Action potentials that arise from synaptic input to the cell bodies within the hypothalamus course down the axons in the pituitary stalk and release the contents of neurosecretory granules by triggering an influx of calcium into the nerve terminals. Either AVP or oxytocin are released along with their respective neurophysins, other segments of the precursor molecule, and presumably the enzymes responsible for cleavage of the precursor.

As discussed in Chapter 1, signals for the secretion of oxytocin originate in the periphery and are transmitted to the brain by sensory neurons. After appropriate processing in higher centers, cells in the supraoptic and paraventricular nuclei are signaled to release their hormone from nerve terminals in the posterior pituitary gland (Fig. 8). The importance of neural input to oxytocin secretion is underscored by the observation that it may also be secreted in a conditioned reflex. A nursing mother sometimes releases oxytocin in response to cries of her baby even before the infant begins to suckle.

Signals for AVP secretion in response to increased osmolality of the blood are thought to originate in hypothalamic neurons, though probably not in the AVP secretory cells. Osmoreceptor cells are exquisitely sensitive to small increases in osmolality and signal cells in the paraventricular and supraoptic nuclei to secrete AVP.

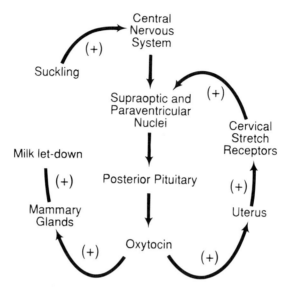

FIG. 8. Regulation of oxytocin secretion showing a positive feedback arrangement. Oxytocin stimulates the uterus to contract and causes the cervix to stretch. Increased cervical stretch is sensed by the neurons in the cervix and transmitted to the hypothalamus, which signals more oxytocin secretion. Oxytocin secreted in response to suckling forms an open-loop feedback system in which positive input is interrupted when the infant is satisfied and stops suckling. Further details are given in Chapter 13.

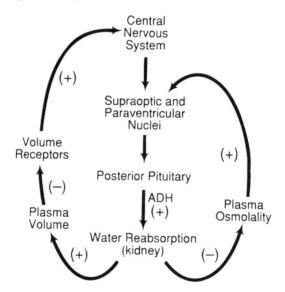

FIG. 9. Regulation of AVP secretion. Increased blood osmolality or decreased blood volume are sensed in the brain or thorax, respectively, and increase AVP secretion. Acting principally on the kidney, AVP produces changes that restore osmolality and volume, thereby shutting down further secretion in a negative feedback arrangement. Further details are given in Chapter 7. From Goodman H. (1980): In: *Medical Physiology*, 14th ed., edited by Mountcastle, Mosby, St. Louis.

Also AVP is secreted in response to decreased blood volume. Although the specific cells responsible for monitoring blood volume have not been identified, volume monitors appear to be located within the thorax and relay their information to the central nervous system in afferent neurons of the vagus nerves. The control of AVP secretion is shown in Fig. 9 and is discussed more fully in Chapter 7.

SUGGESTED READING

Conn, P. M., Staley, D., Harris C, Andrews, W. V., Gorospe, W. C., McArdle, C. A., Huckle, W. R., and Hansen, J. (1986): Mechanism of action of gonadotropin releasing hormone. *Annu. Rev. Physiol.*, 48:495–513.

Eipper, B. A., and Mains, R. E. (1980): Structure and biosynthesis of Pro-ACTH/endorphin and related peptides. *Endocr. Rev.*, 1:1–27.

Fiddes, J. C., and Talmadge, K. (1984): Structure, expression, and evolution of the genes for the human glycoprotein hormones. *Recent Prog. Horm. Res.*, 40:43–74.

Gershengorn, M. C. (1985): Thyrotropin-releasing hormone action: mechanism of calcium-mediated stimulation of prolactin secretion. *Recent Prog. Horm. Res.*, 41:607–646.

Ling, N., Zeytin, F., Böhlen, P., Esch, F., Brazeau, P., Wehrenberg, W. B., Baird, A., and Guillemin, R. (1985): Growth hormone releasing factors. *Annu. Rev. Biochem.*, 54:404–424.

Miller, W. L., and Eberhardt, N. L. (1983): Structure and evolution of the growth hormone gene family. *Endocr. Rev.*, 4:97–130.

Vale, W., Rivier, C., Brown, M. R., Spiess, J., Koob, G., Swanson, L., Bilezikjian, L., Bloom, F., and Rivier, J. (1984): Chemical and biological characterization of corticotropin releasing factor. *Recent Prog. Horm. Res.*, 40:245–270.

3

Thyroid Gland

OVERVIEW

In the adult human, normal operation of a variety of physiological processes affecting virtually every organ system requires appropriate amounts of thyroid hormone. Governing all of these processes, thyroid hormone acts as a modulator, or gain control, rather than an all-or-none signal that turns the process on or off. In the immature individual, thyroid hormone plays an indispensable role in growth and development. Its presence in optimal amounts at a critical time is an absolute requirement for normal development of the nervous system. In its role in growth and development too, its presence seems to be required for the normal unfolding of processes whose course it modulates but does not initiate. Because thyroid hormone affects virtually every system in the body in this way, it is difficult to give a simple, concise answer to the naive but profound question, ''What does thyroid hormone do?'' The response of most endocrinologists would be couched in terms of consequences of hormone excess or deficiency. Indeed, deranged function of the thyroid gland is among the most prevalent of endocrine diseases and may affect as many as 4% to 5% of the population in the United States. In regions of the world where the trace element iodine is scarce, the incidence of deranged thyroid function may be even higher.

MORPHOLOGY

The human thyroid gland is located at the base of the neck and wraps around the trachea just below the cricoid cartilage (Fig. 1). The two large lateral lobes that comprise the bulk of the gland lie on either side of the trachea and are connected by a thin isthmus. A third structure, the pyramidal lobe, which may be a remnant of the embryonic thyroglossal duct, is sometimes also seen as a finger-like projection extending headward from the isthmus. The thyroid gland in the normal human being weighs about 15 to 20 g but is capable of enormous growth, sometimes achieving a weight of several hundred grams when stimulated intensely over a long period of time. Such enlargement of the thyroid gland, which may be grossly obvious, is called a *goiter* and is one of the most common manifestations of thyroid disease.

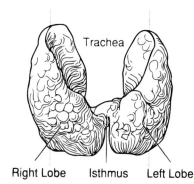

Right Lobe   Isthmus   Left Lobe

FIG. 1. A normal thyroid gland. From Anderson, J.E.(1972): *Grant's Atlas of Anatomy*, Williams & Wilkins, Baltimore, pp. 9–35.

The thyroid gland receives its blood supply through the inferior and superior thyroid arteries, which arise from the external carotid and subclavian arteries. Relative to its weight, the thyroid gland receives a greater flow of blood than most other tissues of the body. Venous drainage is through the paired superior, middle, and inferior thyroid veins into the internal jugular and innominate veins. The gland is also endowed with a rich lymphatic system that may play an important role in the delivery of hormone to the general circulation. The thyroid gland also has an abundant supply of sympathetic and parasympathetic nerves. Some studies suggest that sympathetic stimulation or infusion of epinephrine or norepinephrine may increase the secretion of thyroid hormone, but this mechanism is probably only of minor importance in the overall regulation of thyroid function.

The functional unit of the thyroid gland is the follicle, which is composed of epithelial cells arranged as hollow vesicles of various shapes ranging in size from 0.02 to 0.3 mm in diameter; it is filled with a glycoprotein colloid called thyroglobulin (Fig. 2). The epithelial cells lining each follicle may be cuboidal or columnar, depending on their functional state, with the height of the epithelium being greatest when its activity is highest. Each follicle is surrounded by a dense capillary network separated from the epithelial cells by a well-defined basement membrane. Groups of densely packed follicles are bound together by connective tissue septa to form lobules that receive their blood supply from a single small artery. The functional state of one lobule may differ widely from that of an adjacent lobule. The secretory cells of the thyroid gland are derived embryologically and phylogenetically from two sources. The follicular cells, which produce the classical thyroid hormones, thyroxine and triiodothyronine, arise from the endoderm of the primitive pharynx. The parafollicular, or C cells, are located on or between the follicles and produce the polypeptide hormone calcitonin, which is discussed in Chapter 8.

THYROID HORMONES

The thyroid hormones are α-amino acid derivatives of tyrosine (Fig. 3). The thyronine nucleus consists of two benzene rings in ether linkage, with an alanine

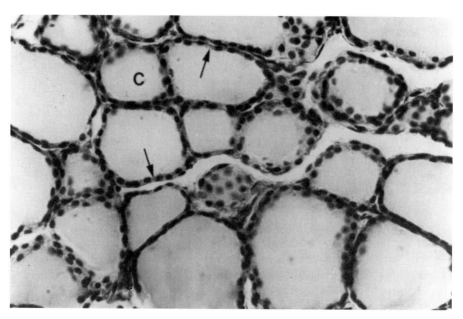

FIG. 2. Histology of the human thyroid. Simple cuboidal cells (*arrows*) make up the follicles. *C*, thyroid colloid (thyroglobulin), which fills the follicles. From Borysenko, M. and Beringer, T. (1979): *Functional Histology*, Little, Brown, Boston, p. 312.

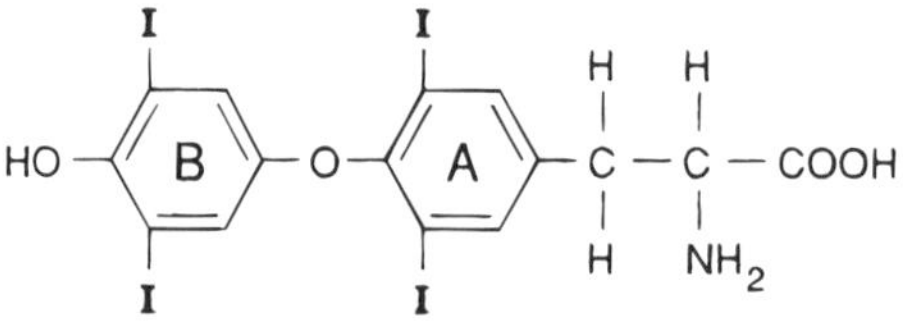

Thyroxine (3,5,3',5'-tetraiodo-L-thyronine)

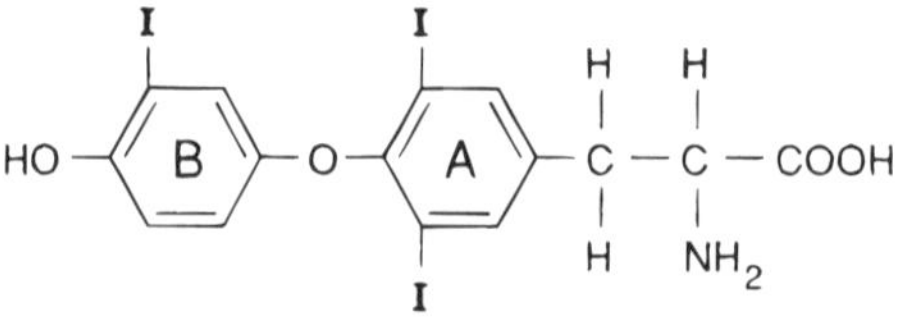

Triiodothyronine (3,5,3'-triiodo-L-thyronine)

FIG. 3. Thyroid hormones.

side chain in the *para* position on the A ring and a hydroxyl group in the *para* position in the B ring. Thyroxine was the first thyroid hormone to be isolated and characterized. Its name derives from *thyr*oid *oxy*indole, which describes the chemical structure erroneously assigned to it in 1914. Triiodothyronine, a considerably less abundant but more potent hormone, was not discovered until 1953. Both hormone molecules are exceptionally rich in iodine, which comprises more than one half of their molecular weight. Thyroxine, which contains four atoms of iodine, is abbreviated as T_4, and triiodothyronine, which has three atoms, as T_3. T_4 has two atoms of iodine on each of its phenolic rings, whereas T_3 has only one on the outer, or B, ring. The compound with the reverse configuration of iodines, two on the B ring and one on the A ring, is called reverse T_3 (rT_3), and although devoid of biological activity, it is nevertheless important as a major metabolite of T_4.

Biosynthesis

Several aspects of the production of thyroid hormone are unusual as follows:

1. Thyroid hormones contain large amounts of iodine. Biosynthesis of active hormone requires adequate amounts of this scarce element. This need is met by an efficient iodide pump that allows thyroid cells to take up and concentrate iodide. The thyroid gland is also the principal site of storage of this rare dietary constituent.
2. Thyroid hormones are partially synthesized extracellularly at the luminal surface of follicular cells and stored in an extracellular compartment, the follicular lumen.
3. The hormone therefore is doubly secreted, in that the precursor molecule, *thyroglobulin*, is released from apical surfaces of follicular cells into the follicular lumen, only to be taken up again by follicular cells and degraded to release T_4 and T_3, which are then secreted into the blood from the basal surfaces of follicular cells.
4. Thyroxine, the major secretory product, is probably not the biologically active form of the hormone, but must be transformed at extrathyroidal sites to T_3.

Biosynthesis of thyroid hormones can be considered as the sum of several discrete processes (Fig. 4).

Iodine Trapping

Thyroid follicular cells have an active iodide pump, which can concentrate iodide against a steep concentration gradient. Under normal circumstances, iodide within the thyroid gland is about 25 times more concentrated than it is in blood plasma, but during periods of active stimulation, the iodide concentration in follicular cells may be as high as 250 times that of plasma. Iodide uptake has all the characteristics of other active transport systems, i.e., it is specific, saturable, and energy dependent.

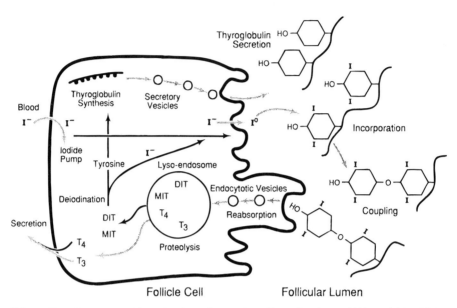

FIG. 4. Thyroid hormone biosynthesis and secretion. From Goodman, H.M. and Van Middlesworth, L. (1980): In: *Medical Physiology*, 14th ed., edited by Mountcastle, V.B. Mosby, St. Louis, pp. 1495–1518.

It can therefore be blocked by other anions that compete for sites on carrier molecules, e.g., perchlorate, pertechnetate, and thiocyanate. This property can be exploited for diagnostic or therapeutic purposes.

Thyroglobulin Precursor Synthesis

The other major component needed for the synthesis of T_4 and T_3 is thyroglobulin precursor, which is synthesized on polyribosomes as a high molecular weight ($>300,000$ Daltons) protein. Like other secretory proteins, thyroglobulin precursor enters the cisternae of the endoplasmic reticulum, is glycosylated, and is translocated to the Golgi apparatus, where it is packaged in secretory vesicles. Secretory vesicles carry the glycoprotein to the apical surface of follicular cells and discharge it into the lumen by a process of exocytosis. Little or no thyroglobulin precursor remains in follicular cells, which therefore do not have the extensive accumulation of secretory granules characteristic of protein-secreting cells. Iodination of the precursor to form mature thyroglobulin does not take place until either the glycoprotein is in the process of discharge into the lumen or perhaps just afterward.

Oxidation of Iodide

In order for iodide to be incorporated into tyrosine molecules, it must first be oxidized to some higher oxidation state, such as atomic iodine (I°) or I^{-3}. This step involves the action of a thyroid specific peroxidase, *thyroperoxidase*, located on the apical border, and probably spanning the plasma membrane of follicular cells. Thyroperoxidase is thought to catalyze the next two biosynthetic reactions as well.

Iodination

The addition of iodine molecules to tyrosine, a process called *organification*, also occurs at the apical surface of follicular cells. Iodine is added only to tyrosine molecules that are already incorporated in the high molecular weight thyroglobulin precursor. Thyroglobulin precursor is iodinated as it is extruded into the follicular lumen. Iodination of tyrosine residues is linked to thyroperoxidase activity and may occur spontaneously as soon as the I^o is formed. There is nothing special about the chemistry of thyroglobulin that makes it susceptible to iodination. Any number of proteins can also be iodinated in this way, which in fact, is quite analogous to laboratory methods devised for iodination of proteins for radioimmunoassay. Thyroglobulin is not unusually rich in tyrosine, which comprises only about 1 in 50 of its amino acids. Of these, fewer than 20% normally become iodinated. The initial products formed are *monoiodotyrosine* (MIT) and *diiodotyrosine* (DIT), and they remain in peptide linkage within the thyroid colloid. Normally, more DIT is formed than is MIT, but when iodine is scarce, there is less iodination and the ratio of MIT to DIT is reversed.

Coupling

The final stage of T_4 biosynthesis is the coupling of two molecules of DIT to form T_4 within the peptide chain. Only about 20% of iodinated tyrosine residues undergo coupling, with the rest remaining as MIT and DIT. After coupling is complete, each thyroglobulin molecule normally contains one to three molecules of T_4. T_3 is considerably scarcer, with one molecule being present in only 20% to 30% of thyroglobulin molecules. T_3 may be formed by deiodination of T_4 or coupling of one residue of DIT with one of MIT.

Exactly how coupling is achieved is not known. One possible mechanism involves joining two iodotyrosine residues that are in close proximity to each other either on two separate strands of thyroglobulin or adjacent folds of the same strand. Free radicals formed by the action of thyroperoxidase react to form the ether linkage at the heart of the thyronine nucleus, leaving behind in one of the peptide chains the serine or alanine residue that was once attached to the phenyl group that now comprises the B ring of T_4 (Fig. 5). An alternative mechanism involves coupling a free diiodophenylpyruvate (deaminated DIT) with a molecule of DIT in peptide linkage within the thyroglobulin molecule by a similar reaction sequence. Regardless of which model proves correct, it is sufficient to recognize the central importance of thyroperoxidase for formation of the thyronine nucleus as well as iodination of tyrosine residues. In addition, the mature hormone is formed while in peptide linkage

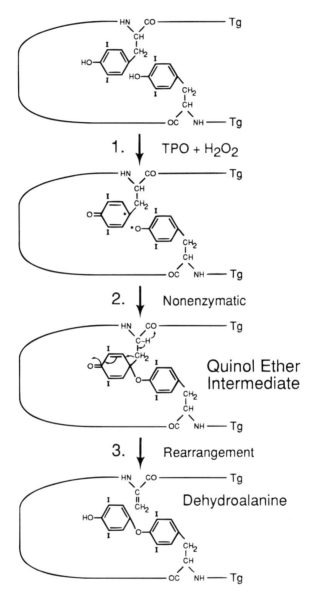

FIG. 5. Hypothetical coupling scheme for intramolecular formation of T$_4$ based on model reaction with purified thyroid peroxidase. From Taurog, A. (1986): Werner's *The Thyroid*, 5th ed., Ingbar and Braverman, p. 71.

within the thyroglobulin molecule, and remains a part of that large storage molecule until lysosomal enzymes set it free during the secretory process.

Hormone Storage

The thyroid is unique among endocrine glands in that it stores its product extracellularly in follicular lumens as large precursor molecules. In the normal individual, approximately 30% of the mass of the thyroid gland is thyroglobulin, which corresponds to about 2 to 3 months' supply of hormone. Mature thyroglobulin is a high molecular weight (660,000 Daltons) molecule, probably a dimer of the thyroglobulin precursor peptide, and contains about 10% carbohydrate and about 0.5% iodine. Its complete amino acid sequence and the positions of the tyrosine residues that are the principal loci for iodothyronine formation are known. Curiously, tyrosine residues that are just a few amino acids away from the carboxy and amino termini are the principal sites of iodothyronine formation. MIT and DIT at other sites in thyroglobulin comprise an important reservoir for iodine and constitute about 90% of the total pool of iodine in the body.

Secretion

Thyroglobulin stored within the follicular lumens is separated from extracellular fluid and the capillary endothelium by a virtually impenetrable layer of follicular cells. Under normal conditions, little or no thyroglobulin escapes into the circulation. In order for secretion to occur, thyroglobulin must be brought back into the follicular cells by a process of endocytosis. Upon acute stimulation with thyroid-stimulating hormone (TSH), long strands of protoplasm (pseudopodia) reach out from the apical surfaces of follicular cells to surround chunks of thyroglobulin, which are taken up in endocytic vesicles (Fig. 6). In chronic situations, uptake is probably less dramatic than that shown in Fig. 6, but nevertheless, it requires an ongoing endocytic process. The endocytic vesicles migrate toward the basal portion of the cells and fuse with lysosomes, which simultaneously migrate from the basal to the apical region of the cells to meet the incoming endocytic vesicles. As fused lysoendosomes migrate toward the basement membrane, thyroglobulin is completely degraded to free amino acids, including T_4, T_3, MIT, and DIT. Of these, only T_4 and T_3 are released into the blood stream, in a ratio of about 20:1, perhaps by a process of simple diffusion down a concentration gradient.

Free MIT and DIT cannot be utilized for synthesis of thyroglobulin and are rapidly deiodinated by a specific microsomal deiodinase. Virtually all of the iodide released from iodotyrosines is recycled into thyroglobulin. Deiodination of iodotyrosine provides about twice as much iodide for hormone synthesis as the iodide pump and is therefore of great significance in hormone biosynthesis. Patients who are genetically deficient in thyroid deiodinase readily suffer symptoms of iodine deficiency and

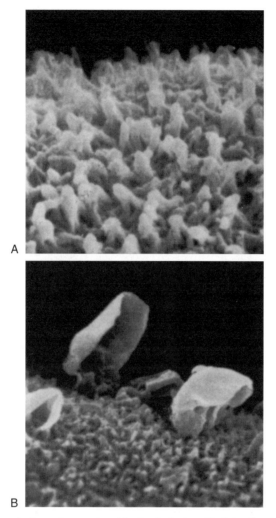

FIG. 6. Scanning electron micrographs of the luminal microvilli of dog thyroid follicular cells. **A:** TSH secretion suppressed by feeding thyroid hormone. **B:** At 1 hour after TSH. A, ×36,000; B, ×16,500. From Balasse, P.D., Rodesch, F.R., Neve, P.E., et al. Observations en microscopie a balayage de la surface apicale y de cellules folliculares thyroidiennes chez le chien. (1972): *C. R. Acad Sci [D] (Paris)*, 274:2332.

excrete MIT and DIT in their urine. Normally, virtually no thyroglobulin, MIT, or DIT escape from the gland.

Synthesis of thyroglobulin precursor and its export in vesicles into the follicular lumen is an ongoing process that takes place simultaneously with uptake of thyroglobulin in another set of vesicles moving in the opposite direction. These opposite processes, involving vesicles laden with thyroglobulin moving into and out of the cells are somehow regulated so that, under normal circumstances, thyroglobulin neither accumulates in the cells or follicular lumens nor is depleted. The physiological mechanisms for such traffic control are not yet understood.

REGULATION OF THYROID FUNCTION

Effects of TSH

Although the thyroid gland can carry out all the steps of hormone biosynthesis, storage, and secretion in the absence of any external signals, autonomous function is too sluggish to meet bodily needs for thyroid hormone. The principal regulator of thyroid function is TSH, which is secreted by the pituitary gland (see Chapter 2). In regulating the function of the thyroid gland, TSH acutely increases blood flow as well as hormone biosynthesis and secretion. Upon prolonged stimulation, TSH increases the height of the follicular epithelium (hypertrophy) by increasing the synthesis of ribonucleic acid (RNA) and cellular proteins and may promote the deoxyribonucleic acid (DNA) synthesis indicative of cell division (hyperplasia).

Thyroid-stimulating hormone binds to specific receptors that span the plasma membrane at the basal–lateral surfaces of thyroid follicular cells. It may be recalled that the α subunit of this glycoprotein hormone is common to TSH, follicle-stimulating hormone (FSH), and luteinizing hormone (LH, Chapter 2). The ß subunit is the part of the hormone that confers thyroid-stimulating activity, and hence, TSH receptors must recognize it. Because free ß subunits are inactive, however, receptors might also recognize some aspect of the α subunit, or the α subunit must somehow influence configuration of the ß subunit. It is of some interest that, just as the structures of the trophic hormones TSH and LH are closely related (see Chapter 2), so too are the amino acid sequences of their receptors. The TSH receptor belongs to the super-family of receptors whose signals are transduced by G proteins (see Chapter 1). Stimulation of TSH receptors results in the formation of cyclic adenosine monophosphate (AMP), which activates protein kinase A and the consequent phosphorylation of cellular proteins (see Chapter 1) that regulate hormone biosynthesis and secretion as well as a variety of metabolic functions of the follicular cell. Virtually all of the effects of TSH can be duplicated by cyclic AMP, including activation of genes for thyroglobulin, thyroperoxidase, and other proteins. Stimulation of thyroid follicular cells by TSH is a good example of a *pleiotropic* effect of a hormone in which there are multiple separate but complementary actions that summate to produce an overall response.

Each step of hormone biosynthesis, storage, and secretion appears to be directly stimulated by a cyclic AMP-dependent process that is accelerated independently of the preceding or following steps in the pathway. Thus, even when increased iodide transport is blocked with a drug that specifically affects the iodide pump, TSH nevertheless accelerates the remaining steps in the synthetic and secretory process. Similarly, when iodination of tyrosine is blocked by a drug specific for the organification process, TSH still stimulates iodide transport and thyroglobulin precursor synthesis.

Thyroid-stimulating hormone also produces a rapid and pronounced effect on phospholipid metabolism in thyroid follicular cells. Effects on phosphatidylinositol turnover and the accompanying production of inositol trisphosphate (IP_3) and diacylglycerol (DAG, Chapter 1) are particularly pronounced, but metabolism of other membrane phospholipids appears to be affected as well. Stimulation of phospholipid metabolism is not mediated by cyclic AMP and appears to reflect an additional signaling pathway that is activated when TSH binds to its receptor (see Chapter 1). Because TSH increases cyclic AMP production at much lower concentrations than are needed to increase phospholipid turnover, it is likely that IP_3 and DAG are redundant mediators that reinforce the effects of cyclic AMP at times of intense stimulation. In addition, increased turnover of phospholipid may be associated with release of arachidonic acid and the consequent increased production of prostaglandins that also follows TSH stimulation of the thyroid. It is of interest that prostaglandins, which increase the formation of cyclic AMP in thyroid follicular cells, also reproduce most of the effects of TSH.

Effects of the Thyroid-Stimulating Immunoglobulins

Overproduction of thyroid hormone, hyperthyroidism, which is also known as Graves' disease, is usually accompanied by extremely low concentrations of TSH in the blood plasma, yet the thyroid gland gives every indication of being under intense stimulation. This paradox was resolved when it was found that the blood plasma of affected individuals contains a substance that stimulates the thyroid gland to produce and secrete thyroid hormone. This substance is an immunoglobulin secreted by lymphocytes and is almost certainly an antibody to the TSH receptor. Thyroid-stimulating immunoglobulin can be found in the serum of virtually all patients with Graves's disease, suggesting an autoimmune etiology to this disorder. It is of interest to note that, when reacting with the TSH receptor, antibodies trigger the same sequence of responses that are produced when TSH interacts with the receptor. This fact indicates that all the information needed to produce the characteristic cellular response to TSH resides in the receptor rather than in the hormone. The role of the hormone therefore must be simply to activate the receptor at the cell surface. Similar effects have also been seen with antibodies to receptors for other hormones.

Effects of Iodine

When dietary iodide is in short supply, hormone biosynthesis is impaired, as might be expected, and hypothyroidism may result. When available in excess, however, iodide paradoxically inhibits thyroxine biosynthesis at the organification step. This effect of iodide depends on its being incorporated into some organic molecule and is thought to represent an autoregulatory phenomenon that protects against overproduction of T_4. Blockade of thyroid hormone production, however, is short lived, and the gland eventually "escapes" from the inhibitory effects of iodide. This effect of iodine has been exploited clinically.

THYROID HORMONES IN BLOOD

More than 99% of thyroid hormone circulating in blood is firmly bound to three plasma proteins. They are *thyroxine-binding globulin* (TBG), *thyroxine-binding prealbumin* (TBPA, which is also called *transthyretin*), and albumin. Of these, TBG is quantitatively the most important, accounting for more than 80% of the total protein-bound hormone (both T_4 and T_3). About 15% of circulating T_4 and less than 5% of circulating T_3 is bound to TBPA, with the bulk of the remainder bound to albumin. All three thyroid hormone binding proteins are large enough to escape filtration by the glomerulus. The less than 1% of hormone present in free solution is in equilibrium with bound hormone and is the only hormone that can escape from capillaries to produce biological activity or be acted on by tissue enzymes.

The total amount of thyroid hormone bound to plasma proteins represents about three times as much hormone as is secreted and degraded in the course of a single day. Thus, plasma proteins provide a substantial reservoir of extrathyroidal hormone. We should therefore not expect acute increases or decreases in the rate of secretion of thyroid hormones to bring about large or rapid changes in their circulating concentrations. For example, if the rate of thyroxine secretion were doubled for 1 day, we could expect its concentration in blood to increase by no more than 30%, even if there were no accompanying increase in the rate of hormone degradation. A tenfold increase in the rate of secretion lasting for 60 minutes would only give a 12% increase in total circulating T_4, and if T_4 secretion stopped completely for 1 hour, its concentration would decrease by only 1%. These considerations seem to rule out changes in thyroid hormone secretion as effectors of minute-to-minute regulation of any homeostatic process. On the other hand, because so much of the circulating hormone is bound to plasma binding proteins, we might expect that the total amount of T_4 and T_3 in the circulation would be affected significantly by decreases in the concentration of plasma binding proteins, as might occur with liver or kidney disease.

METABOLISM OF THYROID HORMONES

Because T_4 is bound much more tightly by plasma proteins then T_3, a greater fraction of T_3 is free to diffuse out of the vascular compartment and into cells where it can act or be degraded. Consequently, it is not surprising that the half-time for the disappearance of an administered dose of ^{125}I-labeled T_3 is only one sixth of that for T_4, or that the lag time needed to observe effects of T_3 is considerably shorter than that needed for T_4. However, because of the binding proteins, both T_4 and T_3 have unusually long half-lives in plasma, measured in days rather than in seconds

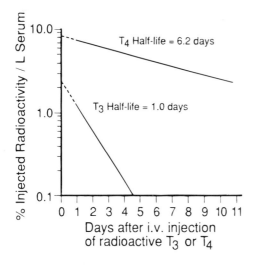

FIG. 7. Rate of loss of serum radioactivity after injection of labeled T_4 or T_3 into human subjects. Plotted from data of Nicoloff, J.T., Low, J.C., Dussault, J.H., et al. (1972): Simultaneous measurement of thyroxine and triiodothyronine peripheral turnover kinetics in man. *J. Clin. Invest.,* 51:473.

or minutes (Fig. 7). It is noteworthy that the half-lives of T_3 and T_4 are increased with thyroid deficiency and shortened with hyperthyroidism.

The normal human thyroid gland secretes about 80 to 100 μg of T_4 each day. Although a small amount (about 5%) of it is degraded by shortening of the alanine side chain to produce tetraiodothyroacetic acid (Tetrac) and subsequent deiodination products, the most important pathway for degradation is by stepwise deiodination of T_4 in peripheral tissues (Fig. 8). The liver and kidney are rich in an enzyme (deiodinase I) that removes iodine from either the outer ring (5' position) to yield T_3 or the inner ring (5 position) to yield reverse T_3 rT_3. Whereas rT_3 is devoid of

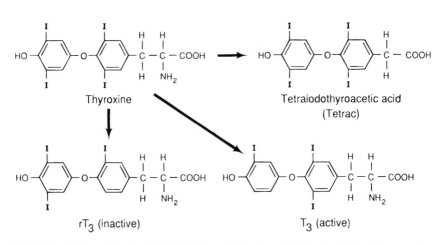

FIG. 8. Metabolism of T_4. About 90% of T_4 is metabolized by deiodination; the first step produces either an active or an inactive compound. Less than 10% of T_4 is metabolized by shortening the alanine side chain prior to deiodination.

biological activity, T_3 has three to five times the biological activity of T_4 in most assay systems and, in fact, is probably the biologically active form of thyroid hormone. Thus, the first step in the metabolic pathway for T_4 determines irreversibly whether an active or inactive hormone is formed. Deiodination of T_4 in liver and kidney provides about 80% of the T_3 in blood. Some tissues, notably brain and pituitary also produce their own T_3 from T_4 through the action of another enzyme, deiodinase II. Evidence that T_3 is actually formed extrathyroidally and can account for most of the biological activity of the thyroid gland includes the following observations.

1. Thyroidectomized subjects given pure T_4 in physiological amounts have normal amounts of T_3 in their circulation.
2. Studies of the rate of metabolism of T_3 indicate that about 30 μg is replaced daily. This amount compares with a release from the thyroid gland of only 5 μg. Thus, nearly 85% of the T_3 produced each day must be formed by deiodination of T_4 in extrathyroidal tissues. This extrathyroidal formation of T_3 consumes about 35% of the T_4 that is secreted each day.
3. Almost 90% of the thyroid hormone bound to receptors in responsive cells is T_3; T_4 comprises just over 10%.

Some evidence suggests that deiodination of T_4 to form either T_3 or rT_3 in extrathyroidal tissues is not random but, rather, is a carefully regulated process. Although mechanisms that regulate this process are not understood, available information indicates that some physiological circumstances favor production of T_3 over rT_3, whereas other circumstances favor formation of rT_3. Because formation of T_3 produces a highly active hormone and formation of rT_3 forms an inactive hormone, regulation of deiodination allows for substantial and rapid changes in the availability of active hormone despite the relatively unchanging large pool of T_4 in the circulation.

Thyroid hormones are also conjugated with glucuronic acid and excreted intact in the bile. Bacteria in the intestine can split the glucuronide bond, and some of the T_4 liberated can be taken up from the intestine and be returned to the general circulation. Thyroid hormones are among the few naturally occurring hormones that are sufficiently resistant to intestinal and hepatic destruction that they can readily be given by mouth. This cycle of excretion in bile and absorption from the intestine is called *enterohepatic circulation* and may be of importance in maintaining normal thyroid economy when thyroid function is marginal or dietary iodide is scarce.

PHYSIOLOGICAL EFFECTS OF THYROID HORMONES

Growth and Maturation

Skeletal System

One of the most striking effects of thyroid hormones is on bodily growth. Although fetal growth appears to be independent of the thyroid, attainment of normal adult stature requires optimal amounts of thyroid hormone. Because stature or height is determined by the length of the skeleton, we might anticipate an effect of thyroid hormone on the growth of bone. However, there is no evidence that T_3 acts directly on cartilage or bone cells to signal increased bone formation. Rather, at the level of bone formation, thyroid hormones appear to act permissively or synergistically with growth hormone, insulin-like growth factor (see Chapter 10), and other growth factors that promote bone formation. Thyroid hormones also promote bone growth indirectly by actions on the pituitary gland and hypothalamus. Thyroid hormone is required for normal growth hormone synthesis and secretion.

Skeletal maturation is distinct from skeletal growth. Maturation of bone results in the ossification and eventual fusion of the cartilaginous growth plates, which occurs with sufficient predictability in normal development that individuals can be assigned a specific "bone age" from radiological examination of ossification centers. Thyroid hormones profoundly affect skeletal maturation, perhaps by a direct action. Bone age is retarded relative to chronological age in children who are deficient in thyroid hormone and is advanced prematurely in hyperthyroid children. An uncorrected deficiency of thyroid hormone during childhood results in retardation of growth and in malformation of facial bones characteristic of juvenile hypothyroidism or *cretinism.*

Central Nervous System

The maturation of the nervous system during the perinatal period has an absolute dependence on thyroid hormone. During this critical period, thyroid hormone must be present for normal development of the brain. In rats made hypothyroid at birth, cerebral and cerebellar growth and nerve myelination are severely delayed. Overall size of the brain is reduced along with its vascularity, particularly at the capillary level. The decrease in size may be partially accounted for by a decrease in axonal density and dendritic branching. In human infants, the absence or deficiency of thyroid hormone during this period is catastrophic and results in permanent, irreversible mental retardation, even if large doses of hormone are given later in childhood (Fig. 9). If replacement therapy is instituted early in postnatal life, however, the tragic consequences of neonatal hypothyroidism can be averted. Mandatory neonatal screening for hypothyroidism has therefore been instituted in many states. Precisely what thyroid hormones do during the critical period, how they do it, and why the opportunity for intervention is so brief are subjects for future research.

The effects of T_3 and T_4 on the central nervous system are not limited to the perinatal period of life. In the adult, hyperthyroidism produces hyperexcitability, irritability, restlessness, and exaggerated responses to environmental stimuli. Emotional instability that can lead to full-blown psychosis may also occur. Conversely, decreased thyroid hormone results in listlessness, lack of energy, slowness of speech, decreased sensory capacity, impaired memory, and somnolence. Mental capacity is dulled, and psychosis (myxedema madness) may occur. Conduction velocity in

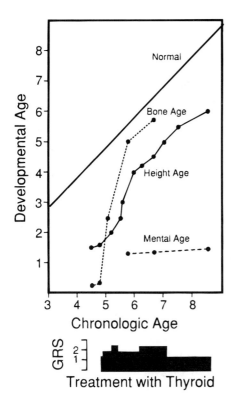

FIG. 9. Effects of thyroid therapy on growth and development of a child with no functional thyroid tissue. Treatment with 100 mg of thyroid daily began at 4.5 years of age. Bone age rapidly returned toward normal, and the rate of growth (height age) paralleled the normal curve. Mental development, however, remained infantile. From Wilkins (1965): *The Diagnosis and Treatment of Endocrine Disorders in Childhood and Adolescence*, Charles C. Thomas, Springfield, Illinois.

peripheral nerves is slowed, and reflex time is increased in hypothyroid individuals. The underlying mechanisms for these changes are not understood.

Autonomic Nervous System

Interactions between thyroid hormones and the autonomic nervous system, particularly the sympathetic branch, are important throughout life. Increased secretion of thyroid hormone exaggerates many of the responses regulated by sympathetic activity. In fact, many symptoms of hyperthyroidism, including tachycardia and increased cardiac output, resemble increased activity of the sympathetic nervous system. Some evidence suggests that thyroid hormones may increase the number of receptors for epinephrine and norepinephrine (ß-adrenergic receptors) in myocardium and other tissues. A substantial body of experimental evidence indicates that thyroid hormones exaggerate a variety of responses mediated by ß-adrenergic receptors; consequently, pharmacological blockade of these receptors is useful for treating hyperthyroidism. Conversely, the function of the sympathetic nervous system is compromised in hypothyroid states.

Metabolism

Oxidative Metabolism

Nearly a century has passed since it was recognized that the thyroid gland exerts profound effects on oxidative metabolism in humans. The so-called *basal metabolic rate* (BMR), which is a measure of oxygen consumption under defined resting conditions, is highly sensitive to thyroid status. A decrease in oxygen consumption results from a deficiency of thyroid hormones, and excessive thyroid hormone increases BMR. Oxygen consumption in all tissues except brain, testis, and spleen is sensitive to the thyroid status and increases in response to thyroid hormone (Fig. 10). Even though the dose of thyroid hormone given in the experiment shown in Fig. 10 was large, there was a delay of many hours before any effects were observable. In fact, the rate of oxygen consumption in the whole animal did not reach its maximum until 4 days after a single dose of hormone.

Oxygen consumption ultimately reflects activity of mitochondria and is coupled with formation of high-energy bonds in adenosine triphosphate (ATP). Splitting of ATP energizes cellular processes and, ultimately, results in heat production. Thyroid hormones are said to be calorigenic because they promote heat production. It is therefore not surprising that one of the classical signs of hypothyroidism is decreased tolerance to cold, whereas excessive heat production and sweating are seen in hyperthyroidism. Physiologically, oxygen consumption is proportional to energy utilization. Thus, if there is increased consumption of oxygen, there must be increased utilization of energy. We do not yet know which processes account for thyroid-sensitive oxygen consumption. About 20% of the energy consumed by the resting individual is thought to be used to maintain the ionic integrity of all cells by the sodium–potassium-dependent ATPase, or sodium pump, which constantly extrudes sodium from intracellular fluid in exchange for potassium. Some evidence suggests that a small portion of the calorigenic effect of T_3 may be related to increased energy consumption by the sodium pump and that T_3 increases the synthesis of the sodium–potassium-dependent ATPase. Other studies suggest that thyroid hormone increases oxygen consumption to provide energy used by calcium pumps in working muscles.

Carbohydrate Metabolism

Virtually all aspects of metabolism, including carbohydrate utilization, are accelerated by T_3. It increases glucose absorption from the digestive tract; glycogenolysis and gluconeogenesis in the hepatocytes; and glucose oxidation in the liver, fat, and muscle cells. No single or unique reaction in any pathway of carbohydrate metabolism has been identified as the rate-determining target of T_3 action. Rather, carbohydrate degradation appears to be driven by other factors, such as increased demand for ATP, the content of carbohydrate in the diet, or the nutritional state. Although

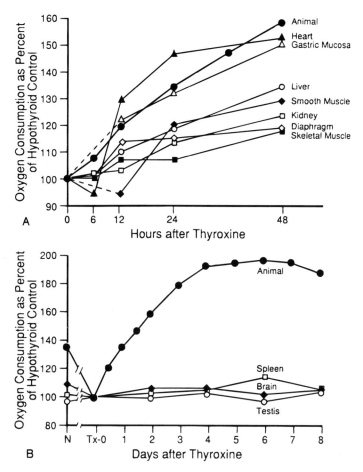

FIG. 10. Effects of T_4 on oxygen consumption by various tissues of thyroidectomized rats. Note in **A** the abscissa is in units of hours, and in **B**, the units are days. *N*, normal; *Tx−0*, thyroidectomized just prior to T_4. Redrawn from Barker, S.B. and Klitgaard, H.M. (1952): Metabolism of tissues excised from thyroxine-injected rats. *Am. J. Physiol.*, 170:81.

T_3 may induce the synthesis of specific enzymes of carbohydrate and lipid metabolism, e.g., the malic enzyme, glucose-6-phosphate dehydrogenase, and 6-phosphogluconate dehydrogenase, it appears principally to behave as an amplifier or gain control working in conjunction with other signals (Fig. 11). In the example shown, induction of the malic enzyme in hepatocytes was dependent on the concentration of glucose in the culture medium and on the concentration of T_3. However, T_3 had little effect on enzyme induction when there was no glucose but amplified the effectiveness of glucose as an inducer of genetic expression. This experiment provides a good example of how T_3 can amplify the readout of genetic information.

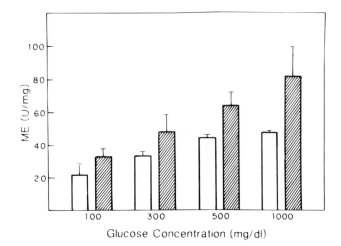

FIG. 11. The effects of glucose and T_3 on the induction of malic enzyme (*ME*) in isolated hepato-cyte cultures. Note that the amount of enzyme present in the tissues was increased by growing the cells in higher and higher concentrations of glucose. The *open bars* show effects of glucose in the presence of a low (10^{-10} M) concentration of T_3. The *crosshatched bars* indicate that the effects of glucose were exaggerated when the cells were grown in a high concentration of T_3 (10^{-8} M). From Mariash, G.N. and Oppenheimer, J.H. (1982): Thyroid hormone-carbohydrate interaction at the hepatic nuclear level. *Fed. Proc.*, 41:2674.

Lipid Metabolism

Because glucose is the major precursor for fatty acid synthesis in both liver and fat cells, it should not be surprising that optimal amounts of thyroid hormone are necessary for lipogenesis in these cells. Once again, the primary determinant of lipogenesis is not T_3 but, rather, the amount of available carbohydrate or insulin, with thyroid hormone acting as a gain control. Similarly, mobilization of fatty acids from storage depots in adipocytes is compromised in the thyroid-deficient subject and increased above normal when thyroid hormones are present in excess. Once again, T_3 amplifies physiological signals for fat mobilization without itself acting as such a signal.

Increased blood cholesterol (*hypercholesterolemia*) is typically found in hypothy-roidism. Thyroid hormones reduce cholesterol in the plasma of normal subjects and restore blood concentrations of cholesterol to normal in hypothyroid subjects. Hypercholesterolemia in hypothyroid subjects results from a decreased ability to excrete cholesterol in bile rather than an overproduction of cholesterol. In fact, cholesterol synthesis is impaired in the hypothyroid individual. T_3 may facilitate hepatic excretion of cholesterol by increasing the abundance of low density lipopro-tein (LDL) receptors in hepatocyte membranes, thereby enhancing the uptake of cholesterol from the blood.

Nitrogen Metabolism

Body proteins are constantly being degraded and resynthesized. Both synthesis and degradation are slowed in the absence of thyroid hormones, and conversely, both are accelerated by thyroid hormone. In the presence of excess T_4 or T_3, the effects of degradation predominate, and often, there is severe catabolism of muscle. In hyperthyroid subjects, body protein mass decreases. despite increased appetite and ingestion of dietary proteins. With thyroid deficiency, there is a characteristic accumulation of a mucus-like material consisting of protein complexed with hyaluronic acid and chondroitin sulfate in extracellular spaces, particularly in the skin. Because of its osmotic effect, this material causes water to accumulate in these spaces, giving rise to the edema typically seen in hypothyroid individuals and to the name *myxedema* for hypothyroidism.

THYROID AND TEMPERATURE REGULATION

The effects of thyroid hormone on oxidative metabolism are seen only in animals that maintain a constant body temperature, consistent with the idea that "calorigenic" effects may be related to thermoregulation. Thyroidectomized animals have a severely reduced ability to survive cold temperature, and hypothyroid individuals have a pronounced loss of tolerance to cold temperatures. Thyroid hormone contributes to both heat production and heat conservation.

Heat production by subjects exposed to a cold environment involves at least two mechanisms: shivering, which is a rapid increase in involuntary activity of skeletal muscle, and the so-called nonshivering thermogenesis seen in cold-acclimated individuals. The exact details of each of these mechanisms are still not understood. Thyroid hormone stimulates oxidative metabolism and heat production, but as we have seen, these effects have a long lag time and, hence, cannot be of much use for making rapid adjustments to cold temperatures. The role of T_3 in the shivering response is probably limited to its interactions with the sympathetic nervous system to maintain the sensitivity of tissues to sympathetic stimulation. In this context, we are dealing with indirect effects of T_3 that were produced before exposure to cold temperature. Maintenance of sensitivity to sympathetic stimulation is important for mobilizing the carbohydrate and fat needed to fuel the shivering response and to make circulatory adjustments for increased activity of skeletal muscle. It may be also recalled that the sympathetic nervous system regulates heat conservation by adjusting blood flow through the skin. Piloerection in animals increases the thickness of the insulating layer of fur. These responses are likely to be of importance in both acute and chronic responses to cold exposure.

Chronic nonshivering thermogenesis appears to require participation of the sympathetic nervous system acting in synergy with T_3, and this process may require increased production of T_3. Some data indicate that norepinephrine may increase the permeability of brown fat and skeletal muscle cells to sodium. Increased activity of the sodium pump could account for increased oxygen consumption and heat production in the cold-acclimatized individual. In muscles of cold-acclimated rats, the activity of the sodium–potassium ATPase is increased in a manner that appears to depend on thyroid hormone.

In some experimental animals, exposure to cold temperatures is an important stimulus for increased TSH secretion from the pituitary and the resultant increase in T_4 and T_3 secretion from the thyroid gland. Cold exposure does not increase TSH section in humans, except in the newborn. In humans and experimental animals, exposure to cold temperatures increases conversion of T_4 to T_3 by mechanisms that are still not understood.

MECHANISM OF THYROID HORMONE ACTION

As must already be obvious, virtually all cells appear to require optimal amounts of thyroid hormone for normal operation, even though different aspects of cellular function may be affected in different cells. Thyroid hormones affect cellular economy by amplifying or muting the readout of some of the genetic information that is expressed in each differentiated cell type. Thus, the different consequences produced in different cells by excesses or deficiencies may be determined by whatever regulates the expression or the accessibility of some genes and not others in the differentiated cell.

Both T_4 and T_3 enter cells by passive diffusion (because of their hydrophobic properties) and by active, stereospecific transport. Thyroxine is deiodinated to produce either T_3 or rT_3. The details of the processes that regulate how much T_4 is deiodinated to T_3 and how much to rT_3 have not yet been resolved. The T_3 formed in the target cell appears to mix freely with the T_3 taken up from the plasma and to enter the nucleus where it binds to specific receptors that are bound to chromatin. A small amount of T_4 may also bind to nuclear receptors, but all of the rT_3 appears to leave the cells and enter the circulation. Virtually all of the physiological effects of the thyroid hormones are mediated by nuclear receptors that regulate the expression of specific genes (see Chapter 1). There are at least three forms of the thyroid hormone receptor; $TR\alpha$ is encoded by a gene that resides on chromosome 17, while $TR\beta_1$ and $TR\beta_2$ are alternately spliced products of a gene that maps to chromosome 3. The $TR\alpha$ and $TR\beta_1$ are widely distributed, but $TR\beta_2$ appears to be expressed only in the pituitary. The significance of multiple forms of the thyroid hormone receptor is unknown. Mutations in the $TR\beta$ gene that decrease T_3 binding result in generalized resistance to thyroid hormone. Thyroid hormone receptors bind to specific response elements in susceptible genes whether or not T_3 is present, and in the absence of T_3, they inhibit expression of these genes. Binding of T_3 relieves the inhibition and allows these genes to be expressed. These cellular events are summarized in Fig. 12.

There are also extranuclear specific binding proteins for thyroid hormones in

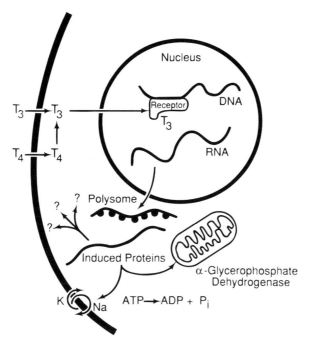

FIG. 12. The action of thyroid hormone. Both T_3 and T_4 enter the cell. T_4 is converted to T_3, which binds to a receptor that is an intrinsic protein of chromatin. T_3 modifies messenger RNA production and increases or decreases the synthesis of specific proteins, such as sodium–potassium ATPase and mitochondrial a-glycerophosphate dehydrogenase.

cytosol and mitochondria, but the function, if any, of these proteins is not known. In addition, some rapid effects that may not involve the genome have also been described.

REGULATION OF SECRETION

As already indicated, the secretion of thyroid hormones depends on stimulation of thyroid follicular cells by TSH. In the absence of TSH, thyroid cells are quiescent and atrophy, and as we have seen, administration of TSH increases both synthesis and secretion of T_4 and T_3. The secretion of TSH by the pituitary gland requires stimulation by the hypothalamic hormone thyrotropin-releasing hormone (TRH). Little TSH is produced by the pituitary gland when it is removed from contact with the hypothalamus and transplanted to some extrahypothalmic site. Positive input for thyroid hormone secretion thus originates in the central nervous system by way of TRH and the anterior pituitary gland. Constant levels of thyroid hormones in blood are achieved by negative feedback effects of T_4 and T_3, which inhibit secretion of TSH (Fig. 13). Administration of a small amount of T_4 or T_3 to an experimental

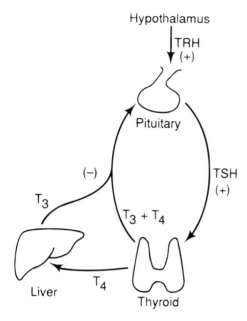

FIG. 13. Feedback regulation of thyroid hormone secretion. +, stimulation; −, inhibition.

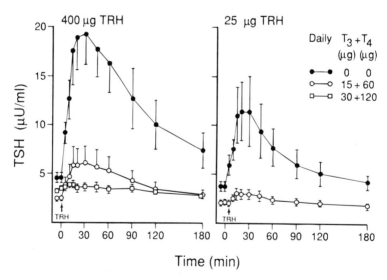

FIG. 14. The effect of treatment with thyroid hormones for 3 to 4 weeks on TSH secretion in normal young men in response to an intravenous injection of TRH. Eight subjects received 400 mg of TRH, and six received 25 mg. The values are expressed as the means ± the standard error of the mean. From Snyder, P.J. and Utiger, R.D. (1972): Inhibition of thyrotropin response to thyrotropin-releasing hormone by small quantities of thyroid hormones. *J. Clin. Invest.,* 52: 2077.

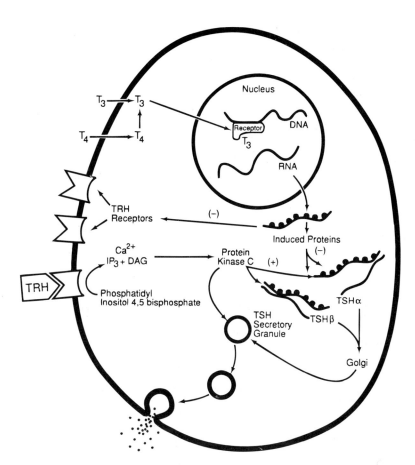

FIG. 15. The effects of TRH, T_3, and T_4 on the thyrotrope. T_3 decreases TRH receptors in the thyrotrope membrane through a transcription- and translation-dependent process. The TRH increases the synthesis and secretion of TSH. +, increase; −, decrease.

subject or a patient inhibits secretion of TSH to just the right extent to compensate for the amount of hormone given. Larger amounts of thyroid hormones shut off TSH secretion completely and, when given over time, produce atrophy of the thyroid gland.

Although negative feedback inhibition of TSH secretion may be accomplished by an action of thyroid hormones exerted at the level of either the hypothalamus or the pituitary, persuasive evidence indicates that thyroid hormones inhibit TSH secretion by a direct action on the thyrotropes. Both T_3 and T_4 inhibit the secretion of stored TSH and decrease its synthesis. In addition, they lower the sensitivity to TRH, probably by decreasing the synthesis of TRH receptors (Fig. 14). Although the secretion of TRH occurs in discrete pulses whose amplitude or frequency oscillates in a daily circadian rhythm, stimulatory input to the pituitary appears to be relatively constant, and the rate of TSH secretion reflects the inhibitory input from the free thyroid hormone in the blood.

The events thought to occur within the thyrotropes are illustrated in Fig. 15. After binding to specific receptors on the surface of thyrotropes TRH activates phospholipase C, which cleaves phosphatidylinositol 3,4,-bisphosphate into IP_3 and DAG. As discussed in Chapter 1, IP_3 promotes calcium mobilization, and DAG activates protein kinase C. Both the synthesis and secretion of TSH are stimulated through some calcium–calmodulin and phosphoprotein-mediated events. Meanwhile, both T_4 and T_3 enter the cell at a rate determined by their free concentrations in blood plasma, and deiodinase II converts the T_4 to T_3. The T_3 enters the nucleus, binds to its receptors, and through an event mediated by DNA transcription decreases the number of receptors for TRH and hence the sensitivity of the thyrotropes to TRH. It is likely that T_3 produces other effects as well, including the inhibition of TSH synthesis.

SUGGESTED READING

Brent, G. A., Moore, D. D., and Larsen P. R. (1991): Thyroid hormone regulation of gene expression. *Annu. Rev. Physiol.*, 53:17–35.

Chopra, I. J. (1991): Nature, sources and relative biological significance of circulating thyroid hormones. In: *Werner and Ingbar's The Thyroid*, 6th ed., edited by Braverman, L. E., and Utiger, R. D., pp. 126–143, Lippincott, Philadelphia.

Engler, D., and Burger, A. G. (1984): The deiodination of the iodothyronines and of their derivatives in man. *Endocr. Rev.*, 5:151–184.

Gershengorn, M. C. (1983): Thyroid hormone regulation of thyrotropin production and interaction with thyrotropin releasing hormone in thyrotropic cells in culture. In: *Molecular Basis of Thyroid Hormone Action*, edited by Oppenheimer, J. H., and Samuels, H. H., pp. 388–412, Academic Press, New York.

Nunez, J., and Pommier, J. (1986): Formation of thyroid hormones. *Vitam. Horm.*, 39:175–230.

Vassart, G., and Dumont, J. (1992): The thyrotropin receptor and the regulation of thyrocyte function and growth. *Endocr. Rev.*, 13:596–611.

4

Adrenal Glands

OVERVIEW

The adrenal glands are complex polyfunctional organs whose secretions are required for maintenance of life. Without them, deranged electrolyte or carbohydrate metabolism leads to circulatory collapse or hypoglycemic coma and death. The hormones of the outer region, or cortex, are steroids and act at the level of the genome to influence the operation of fundamental processes in virtually all cells. There are three major categories of adrenal steroid hormones: *mineralocorticoids,* whose actions defend the body content of sodium and potassium; *glucocorticoids,* whose actions affect body fuel metabolism, responses to injury, and general cell function; and *androgens*, whose actions are similar to the hormone of the male gonad. We focus on actions of these hormones on the limited number of processes that are most thoroughly studied, but it should be kept in mind that adrenal cortical hormones either directly or indirectly affect almost every physiological process and hence are central to the maintenance of homeostasis.

Secretion of mineralocorticoids is primarily controlled by the kidney through the secretion of *renin* and the consequent production of *angiotensin.* The secretion of glucocorticoids and androgens is controlled by the anterior pituitary gland through the secretion of corticotropin (ACTH). The inner region, the adrenal medulla, is actually a component of the sympathetic nervous system and participates in the wide array of regulatory responses that are characteristic of that branch of the nervous system.

The adrenal cortex and the medulla often behave as a functional unit, and together, they confer a remarkable capacity to cope with changes in the internal or external environment. Fast-acting medullary hormones are signals for physiological adjustments, and slower-acting cortical hormones maintain or increase the sensitivity of tissues to medullary hormones and other signals as well as maintain or enhance the capacity of tissues to respond to such signals. The cortical hormones thus tend to be modulators rather than initiators of responses.

MORPHOLOGY

The adrenal glands are bilateral structures situated above the kidneys. They are comprised of an outer region or cortex, which normally makes up more than three-

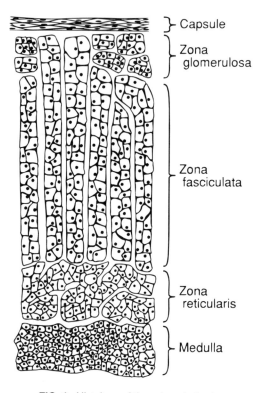

FIG. 1. Histology of the adrenal gland.

quarters of the adrenal mass, and an inner region or medulla (Fig. 1). The medulla is a modified sympathetic ganglion that, in response to signals reaching it through cholinergic preganglionic fibers, releases either or both of its two hormones, epinephrine and norepinephrine, into adrenal venous blood. The cortex arises from mesodermal tissue and produces a class of lipid-soluble hormones derived from cholesterol and called *steroids*. The cortex is subdivided histologically into three zones. Cells in the outer region, or *zona glomerulosa*, are arranged in clusters (glomeruli) and produce the hormone *aldosterone*. In the *zona fasciculata*, which comprises the bulk of the cortex, rows of lipid-laden cells are arranged radially in bundles of parallel cords (fasces). The inner region of the cortex consists of a tangled network of cells and is called the *zona reticularis*. The fasciculata and reticularis, which produce both *cortisol* and the adrenal androgens, are functionally separate from the zona glomerulosa.

The adrenal glands receive their blood supply from numerous small arteries that branch off the renal arteries or the lumbar portion of the aorta and its various major branches. These arteries penetrate the adrenal capsules and divide to form the subcapsular plexus from which small arterial branches pass centripetally toward the medulla. The subcapsular plexuses also give rise to long loops of capillaries that pass between the cords of fascicular cells and empty into sinusoids in the reticularis and medulla. Sinusoidal blood collects through venules into a single large central vein in each adrenal and drains into either the renal vein or the inferior vena cava.

ADRENAL CORTEX

In all species thus far studied, the adrenal cortex is essential for maintenance of life. Insufficiency of adrenal cortical hormones (Addison's disease) produced by pathological destruction or surgical removal of the adrenal cortices results in death within 1 to 2 weeks unless replacement therapy is instituted. Virtually every organ system goes awry with adrenal cortical insufficiency, but the most likely cause of death appears to be circulatory collapse secondary to sodium depletion. When food intake is inadequate, death may result instead from insufficient amounts of glucose in the blood (hypoglycemia).

The adrenal cortical hormones have been divided into two categories based on their ability to protect against these two causes of death. The so-called *mineralocorticoids* are necessary for the maintenance of sodium and potassium balance. Aldosterone is the physiologically important mineralocorticoid, although some deoxycorticosterone, another potent mineralocorticoid, is also produced by the normal adrenal gland (Fig. 2). Cortisol and, to a lesser extent, corticosterone are the physiologically

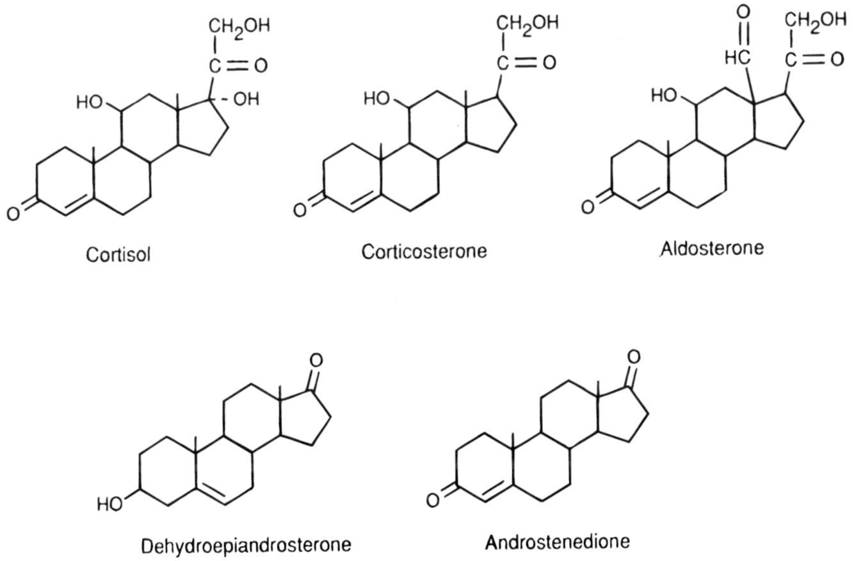

FIG. 2. Principal adrenal steroid hormones. Cortisol and corticosterone are glucocorticoids, aldosterone is a mineralocorticoid, and dehydroepiandrosterone and androstenedione are androgens.

important *glucocorticoids* and are so named for their ability to maintain carbohydrate reserves. Glucocorticoids have a variety of other effects as well. At high concentrations, aldosterone may exert glucocorticoid-like activity, and conversely, cortisol and corticosterone have some mineralocorticoid activity. The adrenal cortex also produces *androgens*, which as their name implies, have biological effects similar to those of the male gonadal hormones (see Chapter 11). Adrenal androgens mediate some of the changes that occur at puberty. Adrenal steroid hormones are closely related to the steroid hormones produced by the testis and ovary and are synthesized from common precursors. In some abnormal states, the adrenals may secrete any of the gonadal steroids.

Adrenocortical Hormones

All of the adrenal steroids are derivatives of the polycyclic phenanthrene nucleus, which is also present in cholesterol, ovarian and testicular steroids, bile acids, and precursors of vitamin D. Use of some of the standard conventions for naming the rings and the carbons facilitates discussion of the biosynthesis and metabolism of the steroid hormones. When drawing structures of steroid hormones, carbon atoms are indicated by junctions of lines that represent chemical bonds. The carbons are numbered and the rings are lettered as shown in Fig. 3. It should be remembered

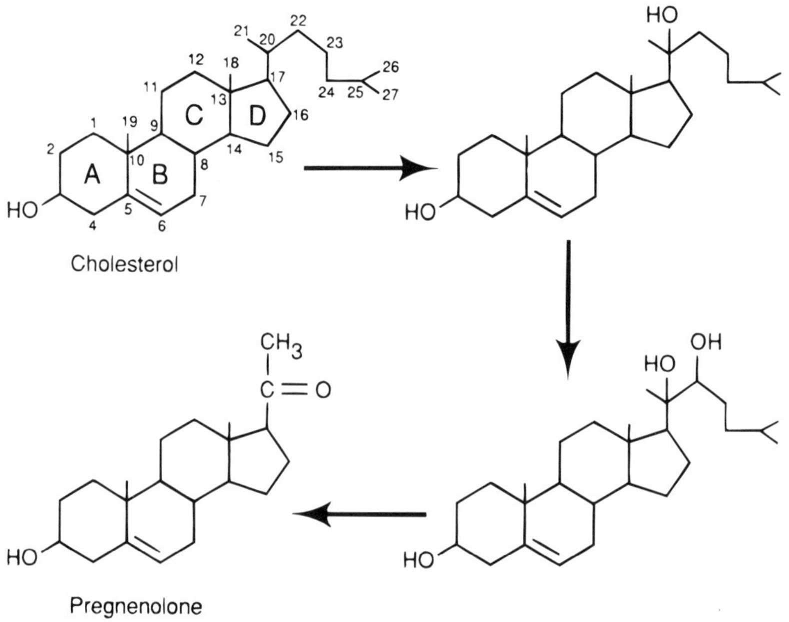

FIG. 3. Conversion of cholesterol to pregnenolone. Carbons 20 and 22 are sequentially oxidized (in either order) followed by enzymatic cleavage (desmolase reaction).

that steroid hormones have complex three-dimensional structures; they are not flat, two-dimensional molecules as we depict them for simplicity. Substituents on the steroid nucleus that project toward the reader are usually designated by the prefix ß. Those that project away from the reader are designated by α and are shown diagrammatically with dashed lines. The fully saturated 21-carbon molecule is called *pregnane*. When a double bond is present in any of the rings, the -*ane* in the ending is changed to -*ene* or to -*diene* when there are two double bonds, i.e., pregn*ene* or pregna*diene*. The location of the double bond is designated by the Greek letter Δ followed by one or more superscripts to indicate the location. The presence of a hydroxyl group (OH) is indicated by the ending -*ol*, and the presence of a keto group (O) by the ending -*one*. Thus, the important intermediate in the biosynthetic pathway for steroid hormones shown in Fig. 3 has a double bond in the B ring, a keto group on carbon 20, and a hydroxyl group on carbon 3, and hence is called Δ^5 pregnenolone.

The starting material for steroid hormone biosynthesis is cholesterol, most of which arrives at the adrenal cortex in the form of low density lipoproteins, which are avidly taken up from the blood by a process of receptor-mediated endocytosis. Adrenal cortical cells also synthesize cholesterol from carbohydrate or fatty acid precursors. Substantial amounts of cholesterol are stored in steroid hormone-producing cells, largely in the form of fatty acid esters.

The rate-limiting step of steroid hormone biosynthesis is the conversion of the 27-carbon cholesterol molecule to the 21-carbon pregnenolone molecule (Fig. 3). Hormone biosynthesis requires a complicated series of reactions that also involves (a) cleavage of the fatty acid ester bond, (b) transfer of cholesterol from its extramitochondrial storage sites into mitochondria, (c) cleavage of the side chain between C_{20} and C_{22} (desmolase reaction) to yield the 21-carbon compound pregnenolone, and (d) the subsequent transfer of pregnenolone to the cytoplasm. In the cytoplasm, the hydroxyl group at carbon 3 is oxidized, and the double bond is shifted from the B ring to the A ring. *A ketone group at carbon 3 is found in all biologically important adrenal steroids and appears necessary for physiological activity.*

Pregnenolone is the common precursor of all steroid hormones produced by the adrenals or the gonads. The specific hormone that is ultimately secreted once the cholesterol–pregnenolone roadblock has been passed is determined by the enzymatic makeup of the particular cells involved. For example, cells of the zona glomerulosa lack the enzyme needed to oxidize the carbon at position 17 (17α-hydroxylase) and, hence, can produce only corticosterone, aldosterone, and deoxycorticosterone. They are unique, however, in having the enzymes needed to oxidize the carbon at position 18 to an aldehyde. The abundance of these enzymes favors production of aldosterone from corticosterone. Cells of the fasciculata and reticularis can form cortisol because they have 17α-hydroxylase. Hydroxylation at the 17 position is also necessary for removal of the side chain (carbons 20 and 21) to convert the 21-carbon steroids to 19-carbon androgens. Hence, androgens are also produced by these cells but not by glomerulosa cells. Biosynthesis of the various steroid hormones involves oxygenation of carbons 21, 17, 11, and 18, as depicted in Fig. 4. The exact sequence of

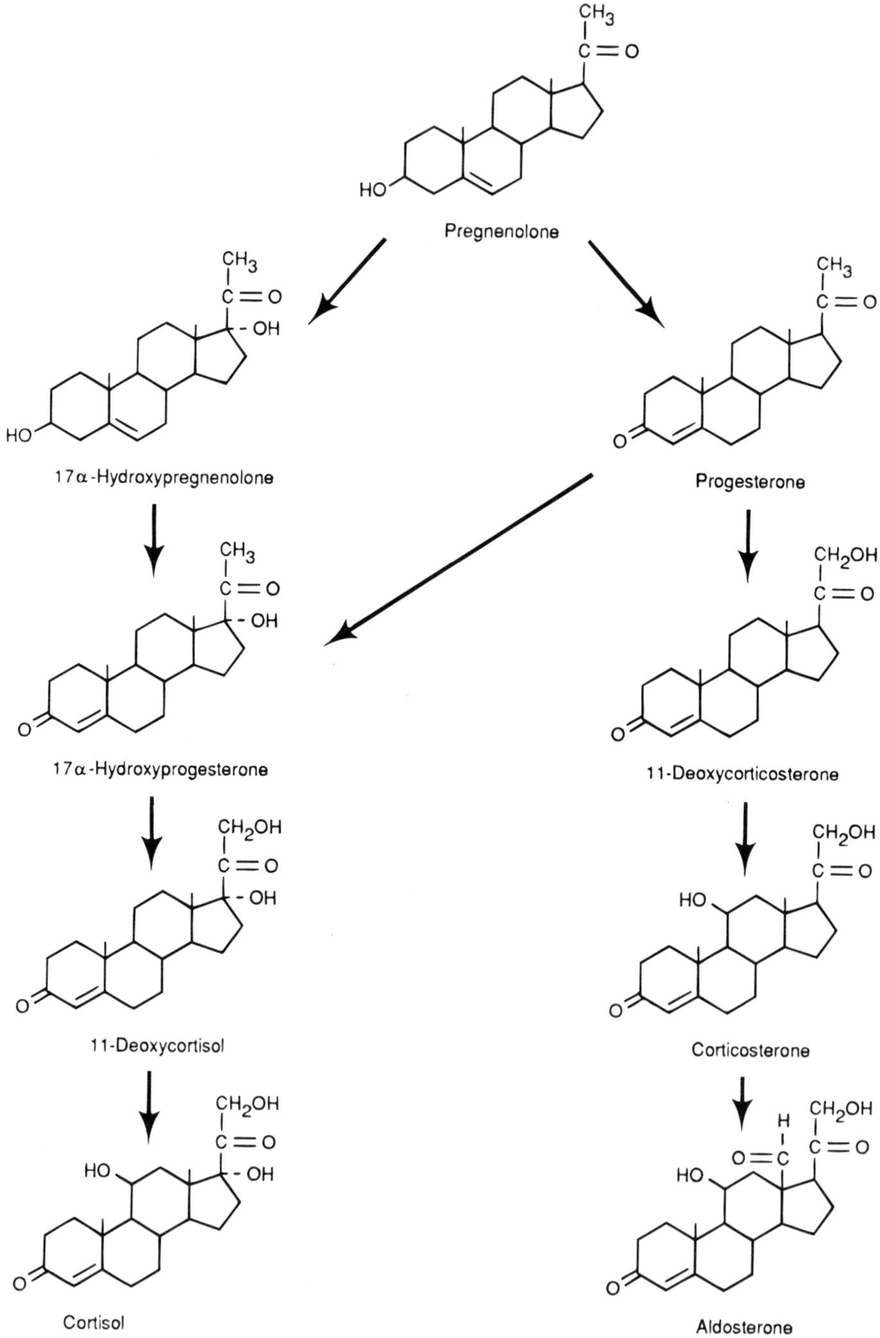

Pregnenolone

17α-Hydroxypregnenolone

Progesterone

17α-Hydroxyprogesterone

11-Deoxycorticosterone

11-Deoxycortisol

Corticosterone

Cortisol

Aldosterone

hydroxylations may vary, and some of the reactions may take place in a different order than that presented in the figure.

As is probably already apparent, steroid chemistry is complex and can be bewildering, but because these compounds are so important physiologically and therapeutically, some familiarity with their structures is required. We can simplify the task somewhat by noting that steroid hormones can be placed into three major categories: those that contain 21 carbon atoms, those that contain 19 carbon atoms, and those that contain 18 carbon atoms. In addition, there are relatively few sites where modification of the steroid nucleus determines its physiological activity.

The physiologically important steroid hormones of the *21-carbon series* are as follows:

1. *Progesterone*, which has the simplest structure, can serve as a precursor molecule for all of the other steroid hormones. Note that the only modifications to the basic carbon skeleton of the 21-carbon steroid nucleus are keto groups at positions 3 and 20. Normal adrenal cortical cells convert progesterone to other products so rapidly that none escapes into adrenal venous blood. Progesterone is a major secretory product of the ovaries and the placenta.

2. *Addition of a hydroxyl group to carbon 21 of progesterone is the minimal change required for adrenal corticoid activity.* This addition produces *deoxycorticosterone*, a potent mineralocorticoid that is virtually devoid of glucocorticoid activity. Deoxycorticosterone is only a minor secretory product of the normal adrenal gland but may become important in some disease states.

3. *An atom of oxygen at carbon 11 is found in all glucocorticoids.* Adding the hydroxyl group at carbon 11 confers glucocorticoid activity on deoxycorticosterone and reduces its mineralocorticoid activity tenfold. This compound is *corticosterone* and is produced in cells of all three zones of the adrenal cortex. Corticosterone is the major glucocorticoid in the rat but is of only secondary importance in humans.

4. Corticosterone is a precursor of *aldosterone*, which is produced in cells of the zona glomerulosa by adding an aldehyde to carbon 18. The oxygen at carbon 18 increases the mineralocorticoid potency of corticosterone by a factor of 200 and only slightly decreases its glucocorticoid activity.

5. *Cortisol* differs from corticosterone only by the presence of a hydroxyl group at carbon 17. Cortisol is the most potent of the naturally occurring glucocorticoids. It has ten times as much glucocorticoid activity as aldosterone but less than 0.25% of aldosterone's mineralocorticoid activity. Synthetic glucocorticoids with even greater potency than cortisol are available for therapeutic use.

FIG. 4. Biosynthesis of adrenal cortical hormones. The pathway on the *left* is the principal sequence followed in the zona fasciculata and zona reticularis. Hydroxylation at carbon 17 usually precedes hydroxylation at carbon 11. However, because the zona fasciculata and zona reticularis also produce some corticosterone, some hydroxylation of carbon 21 must occur without previous hydroxylation at carbon 17. The pathway on the *right* represents that found in the zona glomerulosa.

6. *Cortisone*, a minor secretory product, differs from cortisol only in that the substituent on carbon 11 is a keto group rather than a hydroxyl group.

Steroids in the *19-carbon series* usually have androgenic activity and are precursors of the estrogens (female hormones). Hydroxylation of either pregnenolone or progesterone at carbon 17 is the critical prerequisite for cleavage of the $C_{20,21}$ side chain to yield the adrenal androgens *dehydroepiandrosterone* or *androstenedione* (Fig. 5). These compounds, are also called *17-ketosteroids*. The principal testicular androgen is *testosterone*, which has a hydroxyl group rather than a keto group at carbon 17.

Steroids of the *18-carbon series* usually have estrogenic activity. *Estrogens* characteristically have an unsaturated A ring. Oxidation of the A ring (a process called *aromatization*) results in the loss of the methyl carbon at position 19. This reaction, which takes place principally in the ovaries and placenta, can also occur in a variety of nonendocrine tissues where aromatization of the A ring of either testicular or adrenal androgens comprises the principal source of estrogens in men and postmenopausal women.

Effects of ACTH

Adrenocorticotropic hormone maintains normal secretory activity of the inner zones of the adrenal cortex. After removal of the pituitary gland, little or no steroidogenesis occurs in the zona fasciculata or reticularis, but the zona glomerulosa continues to function. In cells of all three zones, ACTH interacts with a specific membrane receptor and triggers production of cyclic adenosine monophosphate (AMP) by activating adenylyl cyclase (see Chapter 1). Cyclic AMP activates protein kinase A, which catalyzes the phosphorylation of a variety of proteins and thereby modifies their activity. Although detailed information is still lacking, the critical consequence of increased cyclic AMP production in the adrenal cortical cell is that pregnenolone is formed from cholesterol. Once pregnenolone is formed, the remaining steps in steroid biosynthesis can proceed without further intervention from ACTH, although some evidence suggests that ACTH may also speed up some later reactions in the biosynthetic sequence (Fig. 6). The finding that inhibitors of protein synthesis block stimulation of steroidogenesis by ACTH has led to the suggestion that formation of pregnenolone may depend on synthesis of some rapidly turning over protein that is needed for transfer of cholesterol into mitochondria.

In most species, ACTH is not an important regulator of aldosterone production, although it is required for optimal secretion. *Angiotensin II,* an octapeptide whose production is regulated by the kidney (see the following and Chapter 7) is the hormonal signal for increased production of aldosterone (Fig. 7). Like ACTH, angiotensin II reacts with specific membrane receptors on cells of the zona glomerulosa, but it does not use cyclic AMP as its second messenger. Instead, it acts through inositol 1,4,5 trisphosphate (IP_3) and calcium to promote the formation of pregnenolone

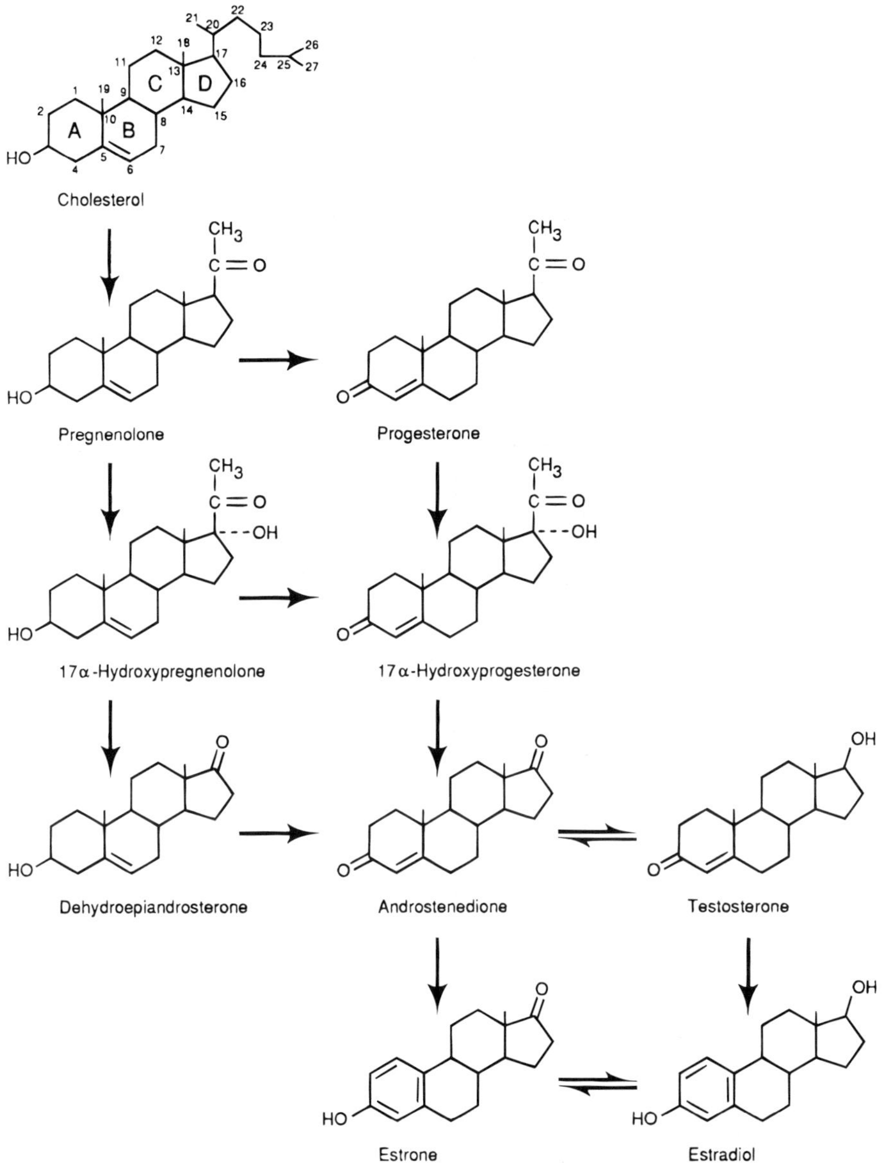

FIG. 5. Biosynthetic pathway for androgens and estrogens. In the adrenal gland, the sequence does not usually proceed all the way to testosterone and the estrogens, which are the gonadal hormones. Because the cells of the zona glomerulosa lack 17α-hydroxylase, these reactions can occur only in the inner zones.

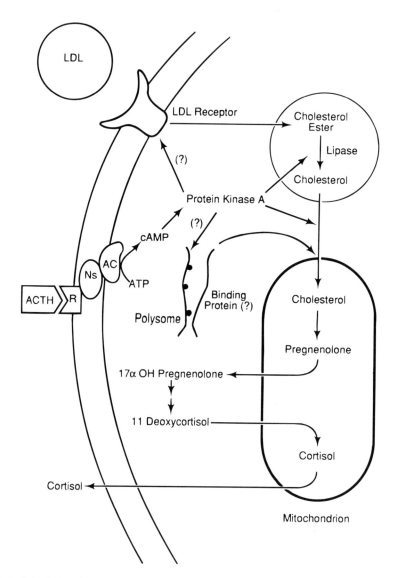

FIG. 6. Stimulation of steroidogenesis in adrenal cortical cells by ACTH. The rate-determining reaction lies between cholesterol in its storage droplet and pregnenolone in the mitochondrion but has not been more closely identified. The stimulation of the conversion of cholesterol to pregnenolone by ACTH requires ongoing protein synthesis, but it is not known with any certainty that protein kinase affects the synthesis of the critical protein(s). ACTH may increase cholesterol uptake by increasing the number or affinity of low density lipoprotein (*LDL*) receptors. *R,* ACTH receptor; *N*ₛ, stimulatory guanine nucleotide-binding protein; *AC,* adenylyl cyclase.

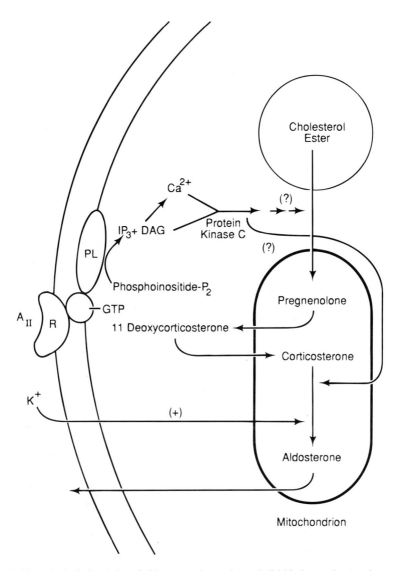

FIG. 7. Hypothetical stimulation of aldosterone by angiotensin II (A_{II}). A_{II} accelerates the conversion of cholesterol to pregnenolone and corticosterone to aldosterone. *R*, receptor; *GTP*, guanosine binding protein (probably G_i or G_q); *PL*, phospholipase C. High concentrations of potassium (K^+) in blood also accelerate corticosterone conversion to aldosterone.

from cholesterol and, to a lesser extent, to stimulate conversion of corticosterone to aldosterone by enhancing the oxidation of carbon 18.

Although it is generally agreed that ACTH controls the synthesis of androgens as well as glucocorticoids, in some physiological conditions, androgens are produced in disproportionately greater amounts than glucocorticoids. For example, the arrival of puberty is heralded by increased production of adrenal androgens, which are responsible for growth of pubic and axillary hair. This and other findings have led some investigators to propose separate control of androgen production, possibly by another, as yet unidentified pituitary factor.

The effects of ACTH on adrenal steroidogenesis are not limited to accelerating the rate-determining step in steroid hormone production. In addition, ACTH enhances storage of cholesterol by promoting uptake of low density lipoproteins, which are rich in cholesterol, and activates an esterase that liberates cholesterol from its storage form. This action makes free cholesterol available to enter the biosynthetic sequence. Either directly or indirectly, ACTH also increases blood flow to the adrenal glands and thereby provides, not only the needed oxygen and metabolic fuels, but also an increased capacity to deliver newly secreted hormone to the general circulation. Finally, ACTH maintains the functional integrity of the inner zones of the adrenal cortex. Chronic stimulation increases their mass, and conversely, the absence of ACTH leads to atrophy of these two zones. Similarly, increased stimulation of the zona glomerulosa cells with angiotensin produces hypertrophy of these cells, while conditions that inhibit angiotensin production result in atrophy of the glomerulosa.

Stimulation with ACTH increases steroid hormone secretion within 1 to 2 minutes, and peak rates of secretion are seen in about 15 minutes. Unlike other glandular cells, steroid-producing cells do not store hormones, and hence, biosynthesis and secretion are components of a single process regulated at the step of cholesterol conversion to pregnenolone. Because steroid hormones are lipid soluble, they can diffuse through the plasma membrane and probably enter the circulation through simple diffusion down a concentration gradient. It is not surprising therefore that biosynthetic intermediates may escape into the circulation during intense stimulation. Human adrenal glands normally produce about 20 mg of cortisol, about 2 mg of corticosterone, and about 250 μg of aldosterone each day, but with sustained stimulation, they can increase this output many fold.

Adrenal Steroid Hormones in Blood

Adrenal cortical hormones are transported in blood bound to a specific plasma protein, called *transcortin* or *corticosteroid binding globulin* (CBG), and to a lesser extent to albumin. Like albumin, CBG is synthesized and secreted by the liver, but its concentration in plasma (10^{-7} M) is only about 1,000th that of albumin. It is a glycoprotein with a molecular weight of about 50,000 Daltons and has a single steroid hormone binding site whose affinity for glucocorticoids is about five times higher than for aldosterone. About 95% of the glucocorticoids and about 60% of the aldosterone in blood are bound to protein. Probably because they circulate bound to plasma proteins, adrenal steroids have a relatively long half-life in blood, i.e., about 90 minutes for cortisol and about 30 minutes for aldosterone.

Metabolism and Excretion of Adrenal Cortical Hormones

Because mammals cannot degrade the steroid nucleus, elimination of steroid hormones is achieved by inactivation through metabolic changes that make them unrecognizable to their receptors. Inactivation of glucocorticoids occurs mainly in the liver and is achieved primarily by reduction of the A ring and its keto group at position 3. Conjugation of the resulting hydroxyl group on carbon 3 with glucuronic acid or sulfate increases water solubility and decreases binding to CBG so the steroid can now pass through renal glomerular capillaries and be excreted in the urine. The major urinary products of steroid hormone degradation are glucuronide esters of 17-hydroxycorticosteroids derived from cortisol and 17-ketosteroids derived from glucocorticoids and androgens. Because recognizable hormonal products can be identified in the urine, it is possible to estimate the daily secretory rate of steroid hormones by the noninvasive technique of analyzing urinary excretory products.

Physiology of the Mineralocorticoids

Although many naturally occurring adrenal cortical hormones, including glucocorticoids, can produce mineralocorticoid effects, aldosterone is by far the most, and perhaps the only, physiologically important mineralocorticoid. In its absence, there is a progressive loss of sodium, which results secondarily in a loss of extracellular fluid (see Chapter 7). With a severe loss of blood volume (*hypovolemia*), water is retained in an effort to restore volume, and the concentration of sodium in blood plasma may gradually fall (*hyponatremia*) from the normal value of 140 mEq/liter to as low as 100 mEq/liter in extreme cases. With the decrease in concentration of sodium, the principal cation of extracellular fluid, there is a net transfer of water from the extracellular to the intracellular space, further aggravating hypovolemia. Diarrhea frequently occurs, and it too worsens hypovolemia. Loss of plasma volume increases the hematocrit and viscosity of blood (*hemoconcentration*). Simultaneous with the loss of sodium, the ability to excrete potassium is impaired. With continued dietary intake, plasma concentrations of potassium may increase from the normal value of 4 mEq/liter to 8 to 10 mEq/liter (*hyperkalemia*). Increased concentrations of potassium in blood, and therefore in extracellular fluid, result in partial depolarization of plasma membranes of all cells, leading to cardiac arrhythmia and weakness of muscles, including the heart. Blood pressure falls from the combined effects of decreased vascular volume, decreased cardiac contractility, and decreased responsiveness of vascular smooth muscle to vasoconstrictor agents caused by hyponatremia. Mild acidosis is seen with mineralocorticoid deficiency, partly as a result of deranged potassium balance and partly from direct effects on hydrogen ion excretion.

All of these life-threatening changes can be reversed by administration of aldosterone and can be traced to the ability of aldosterone to promote inward transport of sodium across epithelial cells of kidney tubules, sweat glands, the colon, and the salivary glands. At the same time, aldosterone promotes the transport of potassium and hydrogen ions in the opposite direction. Of these target tissues, the kidney is by far the most important. It has been estimated that aldosterone is required for the reabsorption of only about 2% of the sodium filtered at the glomerulus; even in its absence, about 98% of the filtered sodium is reabsorbed. However, 2% of the sodium filtered each day corresponds to the amount present in about 3.5 liters of extracellular fluid.

Effects of Aldosterone on the Kidney

Initial insights into the action of aldosterone on the kidney were obtained from observations of the effects of hormone deprivation or administration on the composition of the urine. Mineralocorticoids decrease the ratio of urinary sodium to potassium concentrations; in the absence of mineralocorticoids, the ratio increases. However, although aldosterone promotes sodium conservation and potassium excretion, the two effects are not tightly coupled, and sodium is not simply exchanged for potassium. Indeed, the same amount of aldosterone that increased both sodium retention and potassium excretion when given to adrenalectomized dogs stimulated only potassium excretion in normal, sodium-replete dogs. Similarly, when normal human subjects were given aldosterone for 25 days, the sodium-retaining effects lasted only for the first 15 days, but increased excretion of potassium persisted for as long as the hormone was given (Fig. 8). The underlying mechanism for this so-called escape from the sodium-conserving effects of aldosterone is not known. However, renal handling of sodium and potassium is complex, and compensatory mechanisms exerted at some aldosterone-insensitive locus within the kidney might well offset sustained effects of aldosterone on sodium absorption when measured in the intact subject (see Chapter 7).

The principal site of action of aldosterone in the nephron is the cortical collecting duct, where it promotes the transfer of sodium from the tubular fluid to the interstitium and, ultimately, to the blood through the activity of an electrogenic sodium pump. This action of aldosterone requires a lag period of at least 30 minutes, is sensitive to inhibitors of ribonucleic acid (RNA) and protein synthesis, and appears to be initiated by the same sequence of events seen for other steroid hormones (see Chapter 1). That is, after binding to its receptor, the aldosterone–receptor complex binds to hormone response elements near the promoters of certain genes and activates their transcription.

Reabsorption of sodium in the cortical collecting duct depends on the activity of the sodium–potassium-dependent ATPase that is located in the basolateral mem-

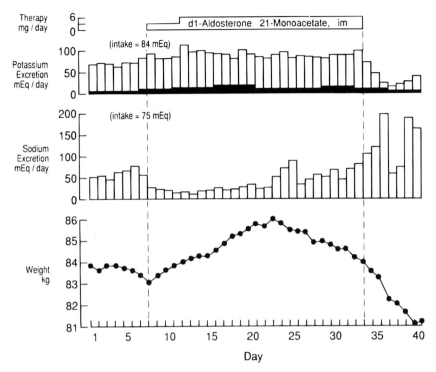

FIG. 8. Effects of continuous administration of aldosterone to a normal man. Aldosterone (3 to 6 mg/day) increased potassium excretion and sodium retention, represented here as a decrease in urinary sodium. The increased retention of sodium, which continued for 2 weeks, caused fluid retention and hence an increase in body weight. The subject "escaped" from the sodium-retaining effects but continued to excrete increased amounts of potassium for as long as aldosterone was given. From August, J.T, Nelson, D.H. and Thorn, G.W. (1958): Response of normal subjects to large amounts of aldosterone. *J. Clin. Invest.*, 37:1549.

branes of tubular cells. This enzyme pumps out as much sodium as enters by diffusion across the luminal surface of tubular epithelial cells (Fig. 9). Aldosterone is thought to increase the availability of two substrates to this enzyme: sodium ions and adenosine triphosphate (ATP). Aldosterone appears to increase sodium permeability of the luminal membrane by increasing the number of channels through which sodium can diffuse. Proteins induced by aldosterone may be the sodium channels themselves, or they may be cytoskeletal elements that insert "spare," preexisting channels into the luminal membrane. Simultaneously, aldosterone increases energy generation, perhaps by promoting synthesis of some mitochondrial enzymes. Some evidence also suggests that aldosterone may increase synthesis of the sodium–potassium ATPase itself.

The actions of aldosterone on potassium excretion are not fully understood. Some of the increased potassium loss is probably a direct consequence of sodium retention; some potassium may be driven across the luminal membrane into tubular fluid by

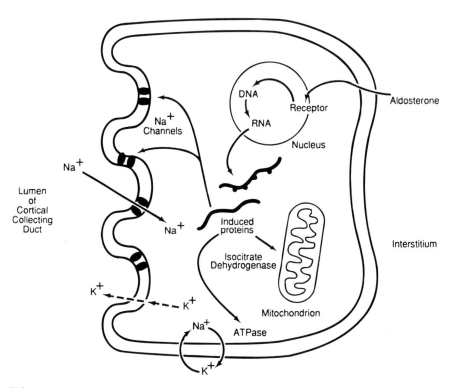

FIG. 9. Proposed mechanisms for sodium retention by aldosterone. Aldosterone induces the transcription and translation of new proteins. The new proteins may be sodium channels in the luminal membrane, mitochondrial enzymes (such as isocitrate dehydrogenase), or sodium–potassium-dependent ATPase, which pumps sodium out of the tubular cells into the interstitium. Note that increased entry of sodium and increased activity of the sodium–potassium ATPase must inevitably drive out potassium even if the membrane permeability to potassium is unchanged.

the increased electrochemical gradient produced by sodium resorption. However, other factors, some of which may be indirect, must also be operative to explain the slower onset of the kaliuretic (potassium-losing) effects than the antinatriuretic (sodium-conserving) effects and the finding that aldosterone promotes potassium loss by actions that may be independent of RNA synthesis. Aldosterone promotes hydrogen ion excretion by actions that are independent of sodium transport and that are probably exerted on different cells further down in the medullary portion of the collecting ducts. The underlying mechanisms for the effects of aldosterone on hydrogen ion transport are not understood.

Aldosterone also decreases the ratio of sodium to potassium concentrations in sweat and salivary secretions. The formation of these fluids is analogous to the formation of urine. The initial secretions are ultrafiltrates of blood plasma whose ionic composition is modified by epithelial cells of the duct that carries the fluid from its site of generation to its site of release. Under the influence of aldosterone, sodium is reabsorbed, probably in exchange for potassium and probably by the same cellular mechanism as described for the cells of the cortical collecting duct. The effect of aldosterone on these secretions is not subject to the escape phenomenon. Because perspiration can be an important avenue for sodium loss, the action of aldosterone on sweat glands is physiologically significant. Persons suffering from adrenal insufficiency are especially sensitive to extended exposure to a hot environment and may become severely dehydrated. The importance of the effects of aldosterone on the ionic composition of saliva is not apparent, as virtually all of the saliva is swallowed.

The mineralocorticoid receptor that mediates the effects of aldosterone binds cortisol with comparable affinity, and when purified and studied in cell-free preparations cannot distinguish between the two classes of steroid hormones. However, despite the considerably greater abundance of cortisol than of aldosterone, mineralocorticoid responses reflect the availability of aldosterone. Mineralocoid specificity is conferred by the action of an enzyme, 11ß-hydroxysteroid dehydrogenase, that converts cortisol to cortisone, which is not recognized by the receptor. Persons with a genetic defect in this enzyme suffer from symptoms of mineralocorticoid excess (hypertension and hypokalemia) as a result of overstimulation of the mineralocorticoid receptor by cortisol. An acquired form of the same ailment is seen after ingestion of excessive amounts of licorice, which contains an inhibitor of 11ß-hydroxysteroid dehydrogenase.

Regulation of Aldosterone Secretion

Angiotensin II is the most important signal for aldosterone secretion. Angiotensin II is an octapeptide formed in blood by a two step process:

$$\text{Angiotensinogen} \rightarrow \text{angiotensin I} \rightarrow \text{angiotensin II}$$

Angiotensinogen, an α_2-globulin, is secreted by the liver in sufficient quantity to maintain virtually constant concentrations in the blood. Angiotensin I is a decapeptide formed from angiotensinogen by proteolytic cleavage catalyzed by the enzyme *renin*, which is secreted by the kidneys. Angiotensin I is biologically inactive and is converted to angiotensin II by the converting enzyme, which removes two amino acids from the carboxy terminus, mainly as it passes through the pulmonary circulation, but some angiotensin II is also formed in glomerular capillaries. Converting enzyme is widely distributed in vascular epithelium. The rate-determining reaction for angiotensin II formation is cleavage of angiotensinogen to angiotensin I. Thus *the secretion of aldosterone is regulated by the secretion of renin by the kidneys.*

Renin is synthesized and secreted into the blood by the *juxtaglomerular cells,* which are modified smooth muscle cells in the walls of the afferent glomerular arteriole. These cells and cells of the *macula densa*, which are located in the wall of the distal convoluted tubule of the nephron where it loops back to come in contact

Glomerulus

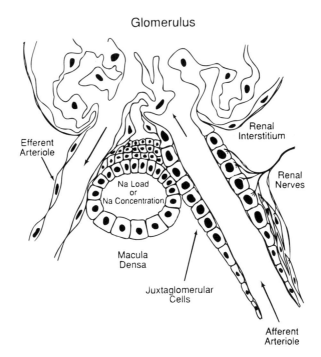

FIG. 10. Juxtaglomerular apparatus. The distal convoluted tubule is shown in the center in cross section and runs perpendicular to the page. From Davis, J.O. (1975): Regulation of aldosterone secretion. In: *Handbook of Physiology, Sect. 7: Endocrinology,* edited by Greep, R.O., Astwood, E.B., Blaschko, H., et al., American Physiological Society, Washington, DC.

with its own glomerulus, make up the *juxtaglomerular apparatus* (Fig. 10). Juxtag-lomerular cells secrete renin in response to decreased pressure in the afferent glomer-ular arterioles as well as in response to decreased sodium in tubular fluid, which is sensed by cells of the macula densa. Juxtaglomerular cells are richly innervated and also secrete renin in response to sympathetic stimulation. All of these stimuli are related to a decrease in blood volume, which is the physiological parameter defended by the renin–angiotensin–aldosterone system (see Chapter 7).

Aldosterone secretion is regulated by negative feedback, but the concentration of aldosterone *per se* is not the controlled variable. Increased blood volume, which is the ultimate result of sodium retention, provides the negative feedback signal for regulation of renin and aldosterone secretion (Fig. 11). Although preservation of body sodium is the central theme of aldosterone physiology, the concentration of sodium in blood does not appear to be monitored directly, and fluctuations in plasma concentrations have little direct effect on the secretory activity of the adrenal cortex. However, a large decrease in sodium concentration, on the order of 10 to 20 mEq/ liter, may directly stimulate glomerulosa cells to secrete aldosterone, but such a change is generally outside of the physiological range. In contrast, increased concen-trations of potassium of as little as 0.1 mEq/liter directly stimulate cells of the zona

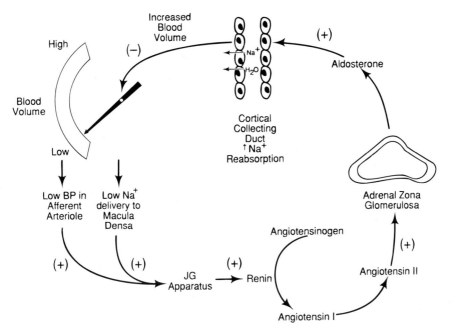

FIG. 11. Negative feedback control of aldosterone secretion. The monitored variable is blood volume. +, stimulates; −, inhibits.

glomerulosa to secrete aldosterone. Increased potassium also sensitizes these cells to angiotensin.

Physiology of the Glucocorticoids

Although named for their critical role in maintaining carbohydrate reserves, glucocorticoids produce a number of diverse physiological actions, many of which are still not well understood and, therefore, can be considered only phenomenologically. Virtually every tissue of the body is affected by an excess or deficiency of glucocorticoids (Table 1). If any simple phrase could describe the role of glucocorticoids, it would be *"coping with adversity."* Even if sodium balance could be preserved and carbohydrate intake were adequate to meet energy needs, individuals suffering from adrenal insufficiency would still teeter on the brink of disaster when faced with a threatening environment. We shall consider here only the most thoroughly studied actions of glucocorticoids.

Effects on Energy Metabolism

The ability to maintain and draw on metabolic fuel reserves is ensured by actions and interactions of many hormones and is critically dependent on normal function

TABLE 1. *Some effects of glucocorticoids*

Tissue	Effects
Central nervous system	Taste, hearing, and smell ↑ in acuity with adrenal cortical insufficiency and ↓ in Cushing's disease ↓corticotropin-releasing hormone (see text); ↓ADH secretion
Cardiovascular system	Maintain sensitivity to epinephrine and norepinephrine, ↑sensitivity to vasoconstrictor agents, maintain microcirculation
Gastrointestinal tract	↑Gastric acid secretion, ↓gastric mucosal cell proliferation
Liver	↑Gluconeogenesis
Lungs	↑Maturation and surfactant production during fetal development
Pituitary	↓ACTH secretion (acute) and synthesis (chronic)
Kidney	↑GFR, needed to excrete dilute urine
Bone	↑Resorption, ↓formation
Muscle	↓Fatigue (probably secondary to cardiovascular actions), ↑protein catabolism, ↓glucose oxidation, ↓insulin sensitivity, ↓protein synthesis
Immune system (see text)	↓Mass of thymus and lymph nodes; ↓blood concentrations of eosinophils, basophils, and lymphocytes; ↓cellular immunity
Connective tissue	↓Activity of fibroblasts, ↓collagen synthesis

ADH, antidiuretic hormone; ACTH, adrenocorticotropic hormone; 6FR, glomerular filtration rate.

of the adrenal cortex (Fig. 12). Although we speak of maintaining carbohydrate reserves as the hallmark of glucocorticoid activity, it must be understood that metabolism of carbohydrate, protein, and lipid are inseparable components of overall energy balance. This complex topic is considered further in Chapter 9.

In the absence of adrenal function, even relatively short periods of fasting may produce a catastrophic decrease in blood sugar (*hypoglycemia*) accompanied by depletion of muscle and liver glycogen. A drastically compromised ability to produce sugar from nonglucose precursors (*gluconeogenesis*) forces these individuals to rely almost exclusively on dietary sugars to meet their carbohydrate needs. Their metabolic problems are further complicated by a decreased ability to utilize alternative substrates, such as fatty acids and protein. Glucocorticoids promote gluconeogenesis by complementary mechanisms.

1. *Extrahepatic actions provide substrate*. Glucocorticoids promote proteolysis and inhibit protein synthesis in muscle and lymphoid tissues, thereby causing amino acids to be released into the blood. In addition, they increase blood glycerol concentrations by acting with other hormones to increase lipolysis in adipose tissue.

2. *Hepatic actions enhance the flow of glucose precursors through existing enzymatic machinery and induce the synthesis of additional gluconeogenic and glycogen-forming enzymes along with the enzymes needed to convert amino acids to usable precursors of carbohydrate.*

Nitrogen excretion during fasting is lower than normal in persons with adrenal insufficiency, reflecting decreased conversion of amino acids to glucose. High concentrations of glucocorticoids, as seen in states of adrenal hyperfunction, inhibit

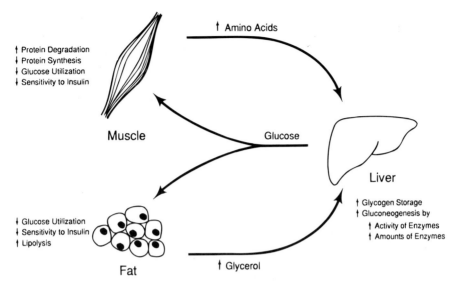

FIG. 12. Principal effects of glucocorticoids on the metabolism of body fuels. ↑, increased; ↓, decreased.

protein synthesis and promote rapid breakdown of muscle and lymphoid tissues that serve as repositories for stored protein. These effects result in increased blood urea nitrogen and enhanced nitrogen excretion. Individuals with hyperfunction of the adrenal cortex (Cushing's disease) characteristically have spindly arms and legs, reflecting increased breakdown of their muscle protein. Protein wasting in these patients may also extend to skin and connective tissue, and it contributes to their propensity to bruise easily.

Glucocorticoids defend against hypoglycemia in yet another way. In experimental animals, glucocorticoids decrease the utilization of glucose by muscle and adipose tissue and lower the sensitivity of these tissues to insulin. Prolonged exposure to high levels of glucocorticoids often leads to diabetes mellitus (Chapter 5). About 20% of patients with Cushing's disease are also diabetic, and virtually all of the remainder have some milder impairment of glucose metabolism. Despite the relative decrease in insulin sensitivity and increased tendency for fat mobilization seen in experimental animals, patients with Cushing's disease paradoxically accumulate fat in the face (moon face), between the shoulders (buffalo hump), and in the abdomen (truncal obesity). As yet, there is no explanation for this redistribution of body fat.

Water Balance

In the absence of the adrenal glands, renal plasma flow and glomerular filtration are reduced, and it is difficult to produce either concentrated or dilute urine. One of the diagnostic tests for adrenal cortical insufficiency is the rapidity with which a water load can be excreted. Glucocorticoids facilitate excretion of free water and are more important in this regard than mineralocorticoids. The mechanism for this effect is still debated. It has been suggested that glucocorticoids may maintain normal rates of glomerular filtration by acting directly on glomeruli or glomerular blood flow, or indirectly by facilitating the action or production of the atrial natriuretic hormone (see Chapter 7). In addition, in the absence of glucocorticoids, antidiuretic hormone (vasopressin, AVP) secretion is increased.

Glucocorticoids and Responses to Injury

One of the most remarkable effects of glucocorticoids was discovered almost by chance during the late 1940s when it was observed that cortisone dramatically reduced the severity of disease in patients suffering from rheumatoid arthritis. This observation, in addition to leading to the award of a Nobel Prize, called attention to the antiinflammatory effects of glucocorticoids, which are still not fully understood and are dismissed by some as pharmacological side effects because supraphysiological concentrations of glucocorticoids are required to produce these effects. As more is learned of the antiinflammatory actions, however, it is becoming increasingly apparent that they are indeed important physiological actions that are expressed through the glucocorticoid receptor by the same cellular mechanisms as other steroid hormone responses. Some evidence suggests that partial proteolysis of CBG by enzymes released from activated mononuclear leukocytes may produce a localized increase in free cortisol concentration at the site of inflammation. As might be anticipated, glucocorticoids and related compounds devised by the pharmaceutical industry are exceedingly important therapeutic agents for treating such diverse conditions as poison ivy, asthma, a host of inflammatory conditions, and various autoimmune diseases. The latter reflects their related ability to diminish the immune response.

Antiinflammatory Effects

Inflammation is the term used to encompass the various responses of tissues to injury. It is characterized by redness, heat, swelling, pain, and loss of function. Redness and heat are manifestations of increased blood flow resulting from vasodilation. Swelling is due to formation of a protein-rich exudate that collects because capillaries and venules become leaky to proteins. Pain is caused by chemical products of cellular injury and sometimes by mechanical injury to nerve endings. Loss of function may be a direct consequence of injury or secondary to the pain and swelling that injury evokes. An intimately related component of the early response to tissue injury is the migration of white blood cells to the injured area and the subsequent recruitment of the immune system.

The initial pattern of the inflammatory response is independent of the injurious agent or causal event. This response is presumably defensive and may be a necessary antecedent of the repair process. Increased blood flow accelerates delivery of the white blood cells that combat invading foreign substances or organisms and clean up the debris of injured and dead cells. Increased blood flow also facilitates dissemination of chemoattractants to white blood cells and promotes their migration to the site of injury. In addition, increased blood flow provides more oxygen and nutrients to cells at the site of damage and facilitates removal of toxins and wastes. Increased permeability of the microvasculature allows fluid to accumulate in the extravascular space in the vicinity of the injury and thus dilute noxious agents.

Although we are accustomed to thinking of physiological responses as having beneficial effects, it is apparent that some aspects of inflammation may actually cause or magnify tissue damage. Lysosomal hydrolases released during phagocytosis of cellular debris or invading organisms may damage nearby cells that were not harmed by the initial insult. Loss of fluid from the microvasculature at the site of the injury may increase the viscosity of the blood, slowing its flow, and even leaving some capillaries clogged with stagnant red blood cells. Decreased perfusion may cause further cell damage. In addition, massive disseminated fluid loss into the extravascular space sometimes compromises cardiovascular function.

Inflammation is triggered and sustained by the release of a large number of chemical mediators derived from multiple sources. Prostaglandins and leukotrienes are released principally from vascular endothelial cells and macrophages, but virtually all cell types can produce and release them. Histamine and serotonin are released from mast cells and platelets. Macrophages and possibly other cells also release interleukin-1 (IL-1) whose effects are discussed subsequently. Enzymes and superoxides released from dead or dying cells or from cells that remove debris by phagocytosis contribute directly and indirectly to the spread of inflammation by activating other mediators (e.g., bradykinin) that arise from humoral precursors associated with the immune and clotting systems.

We are still far from understanding the physiological importance of glucocorticoids in the response to tissue injury and in the manner by which they temper the inflammatory response. New information is being generated at an astounding rate, however, and some general unifying hypotheses are likely to emerge in the near future. Several actions of glucocorticoids that may explain at least some aspects of their role in inflammation warrant some consideration.

Glucocorticoids and the Metabolites of Arachidonic Acid

Prostaglandins and the closely related leukotrienes are derived from the 20-carbon polyunsaturated essential fatty acid arachidonic acid (Fig. 13). These compounds play a central role in the inflammatory response. They generally act locally on cells in the immediate vicinity of their production, including the cells that produced them, but some also survive in blood long enough to act on distant tissues. Prostaglandins act directly on blood vessels to cause vasodilation and indirectly increase vascular

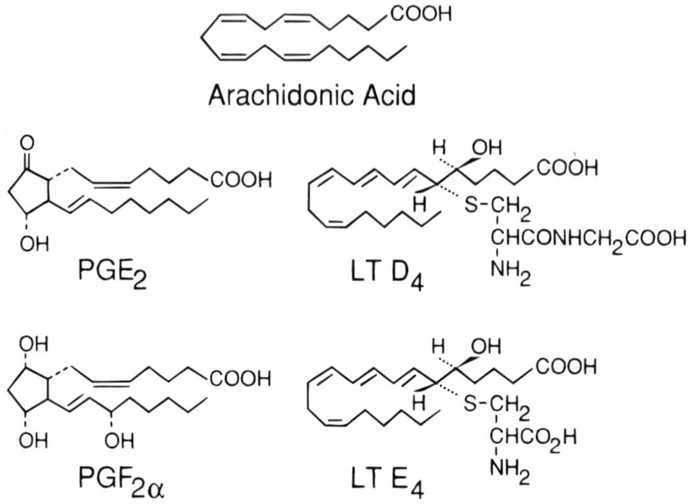

FIG. 13. Structures of arachidonic acid and some of its metabolites. *PG,* prostaglandin; *LT,* leukotriene. The designations E_2 or $F_{2\alpha}$ refer to substituents on the ring structure of the PG. The designations D_4 and E_4 refer to glutathione derivatives in a thioester linkage at carbon 6 of LT. Redrawn from Simmet and Peskar (1986): *Rev. Physiol. Biochem. Pharmacol.,* 104:1.

permeability by potentiating the actions of histamine and bradykinin. Prostaglandins sensitize nerve endings of pain fibers to other mediators of inflammation, such as histamine, serotonin, bradykinin, and substance P, thereby producing increased sensitivity to touch (hyperalgesia). The leukotrienes act directly on the microvasculature to increase permeability. Leukotrienes also attract white blood cells to the site of the injury and increase their stickiness to vascular endothelium. The physiology of arachidonate metabolites is complex, and a thorough discussion is not possible here. There are a large number of these compounds with different biological activities. Some have actions that are antiinflammatory; these compounds may play a counterregulatory role in limiting the overall response. On balance, however, the evidence is overwhelming that arachidonic acid derivatives are major contributors to inflammation.

Arachidonic acid is released from membrane phospholipids by phospholipase A_2, which is activated by injury, phagocytosis, or a variety of other stimuli in responsive cells. The first step in the production of prostaglandins from arachidonate is catalyzed by the cytosolic enzyme, cyclooxygenase. Glucocorticoids suppress the formation of prostaglandins by inhibiting the synthesis of cyclooxygenase and probably also by interfering with the activation of phospholipase A_2. Nonsteroidal antiinflammatory drugs, such as indomethacin and aspirin, also block the cyclooxygenase reaction.

Glucocorticoids and the Release of Other Inflammatory Mediators

Granulocytes, mast cells, and macrophages contain vesicles filled with serotonin, histamine, or degradative enzymes, all of which contribute to the inflammatory

response. These mediators and lysosomal enzymes are released in response to arachidonate metabolites, cellular injury, reaction with antibodies, or during phagocytosis.
Glucocorticoids protect against the release of all these compounds by inhibiting
cellular degranulation. It has been suggested that glucocorticoids inhibit histamine
formation and stabilize lysosomal membranes, but the molecular mechanisms for
these effects are unknown.

Glucocorticoids and Cytokines

Cytokines are peptides secreted by the various cells of the immune system, and
they coordinate the immune response. It is not clear just how many of these hormone-
like molecules are produced. At present, they number in the teens and include the
interleukins, the interferons, colony-stimulating factor, tumor necrosis factor, and
transforming growth factor. Two of these factors, IL-1 and IL-2, are particularly
noteworthy, but it is clear that these two compounds do not account for all of the
various responses that are signaled by the immune system.

A protein with a molecular weight of about 15,000 Daltons, IL-1 is produced
primarily by macrophages and to a lesser extent by other connective tissue elements,
skin, and endothelial cells. Its release from macrophages is stimulated by interaction
with immune complexes, activated lymphocytes, and metabolites of arachidonic
acid. It is not stored in its cells of origin but is synthesized and secreted within hours
of stimulation in a response mediated by calcium and protein kinase C (see Chapter
1). IL-1 acts on many cells to produce a variety of responses, all of which are
components of the inflammatory and immune response (Fig. 14). Many of the consequences of these actions can be recognized from personal experience as nonspecific
symptoms of viral infection.

Glucocorticoids antagonize the release of IL-1 and many, if not all, of its actions.
Although the underlying molecular mechanisms are still not known, it is noteworthy
that many of the responses to IL-1 may be mediated by prostaglandins or other
arachidonate metabolites. For example, IL-1, which is identical with what was once
called endogenous pyrogen, may cause fever by inducing the formation of prostaglandins in the thermoregulatory center of the hypothalamus. Glucocorticoids might
therefore exert their antipyretic effect at two levels, i.e., at the level of the macro-
phage by inhibiting IL-1 production and at the level of the hypothalamus by blocking
prostaglandin synthesis. It is possible that inhibition of arachidonate metabolism
accounts for many of the actions of glucocorticoids.

One of the most important effects of IL-1 is stimulation of T (thymus-derived)
lymphocytes to produce IL-2, which promotes cell division in T lymphocytes that
have been activated by their specific antigens. Only certain clones of T cells are
stimulated to divide because there are no receptors for IL-2 on the surface membranes
of T lymphocytes until they interact with their specific antigen. Antigenic stimulation
triggers the temporary expression of IL-2 receptors only in those T cells that recognize the antigen. Glucocorticoids block the production, but probably not the response,
to IL-2 and thereby inhibit the proliferation of T lymphocytes.

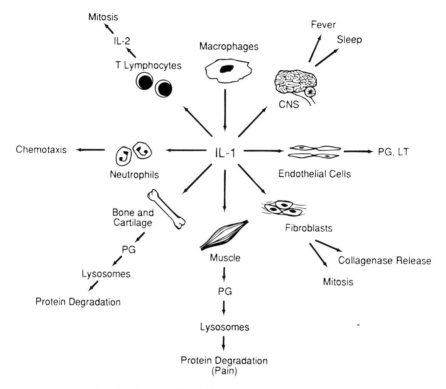

FIG. 14. Effects of IL-1. *PG,* prostaglandin; *LT,* leukotriene.

Interleukin-2 not only stimulates T cells to proliferate but also causes them to produce interferon, which plays a role in the destruction of virus-infected or tumor cells. Interferon also activates macrophages and stimulates production of IL-1. Glucocorticoids suppress the formation of interferon by T lymphocytes. Macrophages, T lymphocytes, and secretory products are arranged in a positive feedback relationship (Fig. 15) and produce a self-amplifying cascade of responses. The cycle is broken only when the foreign antigen is completely removed. Glucocorticoids restrain the cycle by suppressing production of each of the mediators. Curiously, in high concentrations, prostaglandins may also inhibit lymphocyte activity, which may be another example of a counterregulatory role for some prostaglandins.

Glucocorticoids and the Immune Response

The immune system, whose function is destruction and elimination of foreign substances or organisms, has two major components. Humoral immunity is the province of B lymphocytes which, upon differentiation into plasma cells, are responsible for production of antibodies. In mammals, B cells are formed in bone marrow and develop in liver or spleen. Large numbers circulate in blood or reside in lymph

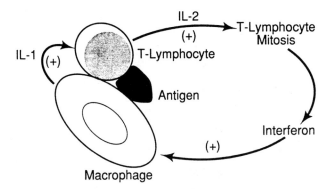

FIG. 15. Positive feedback stimulation of IL-1 secretion. +, stimulates.

nodes. The reaction of a B cell with an antigen stimulates it to divide and produce a clone of cells capable of recognizing the antigen and producing antibodies to it. Such proliferation depends on cytokines (B cell growth factors) released from the macrophages and helper T cells. Antibodies, which are circulating immunoglobulins, bind to foreign substances and thus mark them for destruction. High concentrations of glucocorticoids eventually interfere with antibody production and reduce circulating concentrations of immunoglobulins. Corticosteroids inhibit cytokine production by macrophages and T cells and thus decrease the normal proliferation of B cells. They may also act directly on B cells to inhibit antibody synthesis and, in high concentrations, may even kill B cells.

T cells are responsible for cellular immunity, and participate in destruction of cells that express foreign surface antigens as might follow viral infection or transformation into tumor cells. Glucocorticoids suppress cellular immunity by blocking cytokine production, and they may also kill T cells. The physiological implications of the suppressive effects of glucocorticoids on humoral and cellular immunity are not understood, but it has been suggested that suppression of the immune response might prevent the development of autoimmunity that might otherwise follow from the release of fragments of injured cells. It must be pointed out that much of the immunosuppression by glucocorticoids requires concentrations that may never be reached under physiological conditions. Nevertheless, this property of glucocorticoids is immensely important therapeutically, and high doses of glucocorticoids are often administered to combat rejection of transplanted tissues and to suppress various immune and allergic responses. On the down side, however, high doses of glucocorticoids can so impair immune responses that relatively innocuous infections with some organisms can become overwhelming and cause death.

Other Effects of Glucocorticoids on Lymphoid Tissues

Sustained high concentrations of glucocorticoids produce a dramatic reduction in the mass of all lymphoid tissues including the thymus, spleen, and lymph nodes.

The thymus contains germinal centers for lymphocytes, and large numbers of T lymphocytes are formed and mature within it. Lymph nodes contain large numbers of both T and B lymphocytes. Immature lymphocytes of both lineages have glucocorticoid receptors and respond to hormonal stimulation by the same series of events as seen in other steroid-responsive cells except that the DNA transcribed contains the program for cellular destruction. Although the physiological significance is not known, we have the unique situation of a hormone acting as a cytotoxic agent. Loss in mass of the thymus and lymph nodes can be accounted for by the destruction of lymphocytes rather than the stromal or supporting elements. Mature lymphocytes and germinal centers seem to be unresponsive to this action of glucocorticoids.

Glucocorticoids also decrease circulating levels of lymphocytes and particularly a class of white blood cells known as eosinophils (for their cytological staining properties). This decrease is partly due to the cytolytic effects described previously and partly to sequestration in the spleen and lungs. Curiously, the total white blood cell count does not decrease because glucocorticoids also induce a substantial mobilization of neutrophils from bone marrow.

Maintenance of Vascular Responsiveness to Catecholamines

A final action of glucocorticoids relevant to inflammation and the response to injury is maintenance of sensitivity of vascular smooth muscle to vasoconstrictor effects of norepinephrine released from autonomic nerve endings or the adrenal medulla. By counteracting local vasodilator effects of inflammatory mediators, norepinephrine decreases blood flow and limits the availability of fluid to form the inflammatory exudate. In addition, arteriolar constriction decreases capillary and venular pressure and favors reabsorption of extracellular fluid, thereby reducing swelling. The vasoconstrictor action of norepinephrine is compromised in the absence of glucocorticoids. The mechanism for this action is not known, but at high concentrations, glucocorticoids may block inactivation of norepinephrine.

Adrenal Cortical Function During Stress

During the mid-1930s, the Canadian endocrinologist Hans Selye observed that animals respond to a variety of seemingly unrelated threatening or noxious circumstances with a characteristic pattern of changes that include an increase in size of the adrenal glands, involution of the thymus, and a decrease in the mass of all lymphoid tissues. He inferred that the adrenal glands are stimulated whenever an animal is exposed to any of a number of unfavorable circumstances he called "stress." Stress does not directly affect adrenal cortical function, but rather, it increases the output of ACTH from the pituitary gland (discussed subsequently). In fact, stress is now defined operationally by endocrinologists as any of the variety of conditions that increase ACTH secretion.

Although it is clear that relatively benign changes in the internal or external environment may become lethal in the absence of the adrenal glands, we know little more than Selye did about what cortisol might be doing to protect against stress. The favored experimental model used to investigate this problem was the adrenalectomized animal, which might have further complicated an already complex experimental question.

It appears that many cellular functions require glucocorticoids either directly or indirectly for their maintenance, suggesting that these steroid hormones govern some process that is fundamental to the normal operation of most cells. Consequently, without replacement therapy, many systems are functioning only marginally even before the imposition of stress. Any insult may therefore prove overwhelming. It further became apparent that glucocorticoids are required for normal responses to other hormones or to drugs, even though steroids themselves do not initiate similar responses in the absence of these agents.

Treatment of adrenalectomized animals with a constant basal amount of glucocorticoid prior to and during a stressful incident prevented the devastating effects of stress and permitted expression of expected responses to stimuli. This finding introduced the idea that glucocorticoids act in a normalizing, or *permissive,* way. That is, by maintaining normal operation of cells, glucocorticoids permit normal regulatory mechanisms to act. Because it was not necessary to increase the amounts of adrenal corticoids to ensure survival of stressed adrenalectomized animals, it was concluded that increased secretion of glucocorticoids was not required to combat stress. However, this conclusion is not consistent with clinical experience. Persons suffering from pituitary insufficiency or who have undergone hypophysectomy have severe difficulty withstanding stressful situations, even though at other times, they get along reasonably well on the small amounts of glucocorticoids produced by their adrenals in the absence of ACTH. Patients suffering from adrenal insufficiency are routinely given increased doses of glucocorticoids before undergoing surgery or other stressful procedures. We have already seen that glucocorticoids suppress the inflammatory response. It is also known that these hormones increase the sensitivity of various tissues to epinephrine and norepinephrine, which are also secreted in response to stress (see subsequent text). Although we still do not understand the role of increased concentrations of glucocorticoids in the physiological response to stress, it appears likely that they are beneficial. The question remains open, however, and will not be resolved until a better understanding of glucocorticoid actions is obtained.

Mechanism of Action of Glucocorticoids

With the exception of rapid feedback effects (see the following discussion), virtually all known physiological actions of the glucocorticoid hormones fit the general pattern of steroid hormone action described in Chapter 1. There is a lag period of at least 30 minutes during which specific genes are transcribed and translated. These events require binding of cortisol to specific glucocorticoid receptors, which activates and releases them from associated proteins and allows them to bind to glucocorticoid response elements in the promoter region of responsive genes. (Although their structures are quite similar, the glucocorticoid and mineralocorticoid receptors are separate entities.) As we have seen, glucocorticoids produce a wide range of effects in a great variety of cells. Different responses presumably reflect a differing accessibility of glucocorticoid-responsive genes to the activated glucocorticoid receptor in each differentiated cell type. In addition, it is possible that the diversity of responses may result from differences in the substrates on which glucocorticoid-sensitive gene products act in different cell types.

Regulation of Glucocorticoid Secretion

Secretion of glucocorticoids is regulated by the anterior pituitary gland through the hormone ACTH, whose effects on the inner zones of the adrenal cortex have already been described. In the absence of ACTH, the concentration of cortisol in blood decreases to low values, and the inner zones of the adrenal cortex atrophy. The secretion of ACTH requires vascular contact between the hypothalamus and the anterior lobe of the pituitary gland and is driven primarily by corticotropin-releasing hormone (CRH). The CRH-containing neurons are widely distributed in the forebrain and brainstem but are heavily concentrated in the paraventricular nuclei in close association with AVP-secreting neurons. They stimulate the pituitary to secrete ACTH by releasing CRH into the hypophyseal portal capillaries (Chapter 2). After binding to membrane receptors on corticotropes CRH increases secretion of stored ACTH and transcription of the pro-opiomelanocortin (POMC) gene. These effects are secondary to activation of adenylyl cyclase, cyclic AMP production, and activation of protein kinase A (Chapter 1). Vasopressin also exerts an important influence on ACTH secretion, principally by augmenting the response to CRH. Under some circumstance, AVP is co-secreted with CRH. It binds to specific membrane receptors on corticotropes and exerts its actions by way of IP_3 and DAG.

Upon stimulation with ACTH, the adrenal cortex secretes cortisol, which inhibits further secretion of ACTH in a typical negative feedback arrangement (Fig. 16). Cortisol exerts its inhibitory effects both on CRH neurons in the hypothalamus and on corticotropes in the anterior pituitary. The initial actions of glucocorticoids suppress secretion of CRH and ACTH from storage granules. The subsequent actions of glucocorticoids result from inhibition of transcription of the genes for CRH and POMC in hypothalamic neurons and corticotropes. This feedback system closely resembles the one described earlier for regulation of thyroid hormone secretion even though the adrenal–ACTH system is much more dynamic and subject to episodic changes.

It was pointed out earlier that negative feedback systems ensure constancy of the controlled variable. However, even in the absence of stress, ACTH and cortisol concentrations in blood plasma are not constant but oscillate with a 24-hour periodicity. This so-called *circadian rhythm* is sensitive to the daily pattern of physical activity. For all but those who work the night shift, hormone levels are highest in

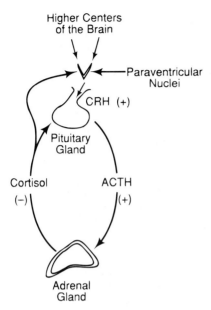

FIG. 16. Negative feedback control of glucocorticoid secretion. +, stimulates; −, inhibits.

the early morning hours just before arousal and lowest in the evening (Fig. 17). Rhythmic secretion can be explained in terms of the negative feedback model shown in Fig. 16. In the negative feedback system, the positive limb (CRH and ACTH secretion) is inhibited when the negative limb (cortisol concentration in blood) reaches some set point. For basal ACTH secretion, the set point of the CRH-secreting cells is thought to vary in its sensitivity to cortisol. Decreased sensitivity to inhibitory

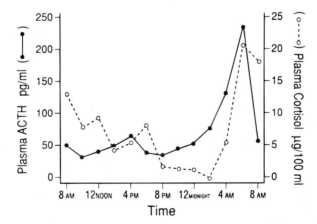

FIG. 17. Variations in plasma concentrations of ACTH and cortisol at different times of day. From Matsukura, et al. (1971): *J. Lab. Clin. Med.*, 77:490.

effects of cortisol in the early morning results in increased output of CRH, ACTH, and cortisol. As the day progresses, sensitivity to cortisol increases, and there is a decrease in the output of CRH and, consequently, of ACTH and cortisol. The mechanism for periodic increases and decreases in sensitivity of CRH-secreting neurons is not understood. Two points emerge from this discussion as follows: (a) *the secretion of ACTH, and therefore cortisol, is driven by changes in the rate of CRH secretion*, and (b) *although they vary with time of day, cortisol concentrations in blood are precisely controlled throughout the day.*

Negative feedback also governs the response of the pituitary–adrenal axis to most stressful stimuli. Different mechanisms appear to apply at different stages of the response. With the imposition of a stressful stimulus, there is a sharp increase in ACTH secretion driven by CRH and AVP. The rate of ACTH secretion is determined by both the intensity of the stimulus to CRH-secreting neurons and the negative feedback influence of cortisol. In the initial moments of the stress response, pituitary corticotropes and CRH neurons monitor the rate of change rather than the absolute concentration of cortisol and decrease their output accordingly. After about 2 hours, negative feedback seems to be proportional to the total amount of cortisol secreted during the stressful episode. With chronic stress, a new steady state is reached, and the negative feedback system again seems to monitor the concentration of cortisol in blood, but with the set point readjusted at a higher level.

Each phase of negative feedback involves different cellular mechanisms. During the first few minutes, inhibitory effects of cortisol occur without a lag period and are expressed too rapidly to be mediated by altered genomic expression. Indeed, the rapid inhibitory action of cortisol is unaffected by inhibitors of protein synthesis. Its molecular basis is unknown, but receptors for steroids in neuronal membranes have been described. The negative feedback effect of cortisol in the subsequent interval occurs after a lag period and seems to require RNA and protein synthesis typical of the steroid actions discussed earlier. In this phase, cortisol restrains secretion of CRH and ACTH but not their synthesis. At this time, corticotropes are less sensitive to CRH. With chronic administration of glucocorticoids or with chronic stress, negative feedback is also exerted at the level of POMC messenger RNA and ACTH synthesis.

Major features of the regulation of ACTH secretion include:

1. Basal secretion of ACTH follows a diurnal rhythm driven by CRH.
2. Stress increases CRH secretion through neural pathways.
3. Secretion of ACTH is subject to negative feedback control under basal conditions and during the response to most stressful stimuli.
4. Cortisol inhibits the secretion of both CRH and ACTH.

Some observations suggest that cytokines produced by cells of the immune system may directly affect the secretion of ACTH and cortisol. In particular, IL-1, IL-2, and IL-6 stimulate CRH secretion and may also act directly on the pituitary. Also, IL-2 may stimulate cortisol secretion by a direct action on the adrenal gland. In addition, lymphocytes express ACTH and related products of the POMC gene and are responsive to the stimulatory effects of CRH and the inhibitory effects of gluco-corticoids. Because glucocorticoids inhibit cytokine production, there may be some "cross talk" between the immune system and the adrenals. Neither the quantitative importance nor the significance of such cross talk for overall regulation of adrenal cortical function have been established.

In our discussion of the regulation of cortisol and ACTH secretion, we have ignored other members of the ACTH family that reside in the same secretory granule and are released along with ACTH. Endocrinologists have focused their attention on the physiological implications of increased secretion of ACTH and glucocorticoids in response to stress but as yet have not shown much concern about the other peptides, such as ß-endorphin, whose concentration in blood increases in parallel with that of ACTH. No hormonal role for these peptides has been established, although ß-endorphin may have inhibitory effects on the immune system.

Understanding the negative feedback relationship between the adrenal and pitui-tary glands has important diagnostic and therapeutic applications. Normal adrenocor-tical function can be suppressed by injection of large doses of glucocorticoids. For these tests, a potent synthetic glucocorticoid, usually dexamethasone, is adminis-tered, and at a predetermined time later, the natural steroids or their metabolites are measured in blood or urine. If the hypothalamus–pituitary–adrenal system is intact, production of cortisol is suppressed, and its concentrations in blood is low. On the other hand, if cortisol concentrations remain high, an autonomous adrenal or ACTH-producing tumor may be present.

Another clinical application is the treatment of adrenogenital syndrome. As pointed out earlier, adrenal glands produce androgenic steroids by extension of the synthetic pathway for glucocorticoids (Fig. 5). Defects in the production of glucocor-ticoids, particularly in enzymes responsible for hydroxylation of carbons 21 or 11, may lead to increased production of adrenal androgens. Overproduction of androgens in female patients leads to masculinization, which is manifest, for example, by en-largement of the clitoris, increased muscular development, and growth of facial hair. Severe defects may lead to masculinization of the genitalia of female infants and, in male babies, may produce the supermasculinized "infant Hercules." Milder de-fects may show up simply as the growth of excessive facial hair (hirsutism) in women. Overproduction of androgens occurs in the following way.

Stimulation of the adrenal cortex by ACTH increases pregnenolone production, most of which is normally converted to cortisol, which exerts negative feedback inhibition of ACTH secretion. With a partial block in cortisol production, much of the pregnenolone is diverted to androgens, which have no inhibitory effect on ACTH secretion. Therefore, ACTH secretion remains high, stimulates more pregnenolone production, and causes adrenal hyperplasia (Fig. 18). Eventually, the hyperactive adrenals produce enough cortisol for negative feedback to be operative but at the expense of maintaining a high rate of androgen production. The whole system can be brought into proper balance by giving sufficient glucocorticoids to decrease ACTH secretion and therefore remove the stimulus for androgen production.

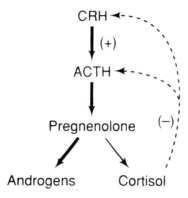

FIG. 18. Consequences of a partial block of cortisol production by defects in either 11- or 21-hydroxylase. Pregnenolone is diverted to androgens, which exert no feedback activity on ACTH secretion. The thickness of the *arrows* connotes relative amounts. *Broken arrows* indicate impairment is in the inhibitory limb of the feedback system. The administration of glucocorticoids shuts down androgen production by inhibiting ACTH secretion.

ADRENAL MEDULLA

The adrenal medulla accounts for about 10% of the mass of the adrenal gland and is embryologically and physiologically distinct from the cortex, although cortical and medullary hormones often act in a complementary manner. The cells of the adrenal medulla have an affinity for chromium salts in histological preparations and, hence, are called *chromaffin cells*. They arise from neuroectoderm and are innervated by neurons whose cell bodies lie in the intermediolateral cell column in the thoracolumbar portion of the spinal cord. Axons of these cells pass through the paravertebral sympathetic ganglia to form the splanchnic nerves. Chromaffin cells are thus modified postganglionic neurons. Their principal secretory products, epinephrine and norepinephrine, are derivatives of the amino acid tyrosine and belong to a class of compounds called *catecholamines*. About 5 to 6 mg of catecholamines are stored in membrane-bound granules within chromaffin cells. Epinephrine is about five times as abundant in the human adrenal medulla as is norepinephrine, but only norepinephrine is found in postganglionic sympathetic neurons and extraadrenal chromaffin tissue. Although medullary hormones affect virtually every tissue of the body and play a crucial role in the acute response to stress, the adrenal medulla is not required for survival so long as the rest of the sympathetic nervous system is intact.

Biosynthesis of the Medullary Hormones

The biosynthetic pathway for epinephrine and norepinephrine is shown in Fig. 19. Hydroxylation of tyrosine to form dihydroxyphenylalanine (DOPA) is the rate-determining reaction and is catalyzed by the enzyme tyrosine hydroxylase. The

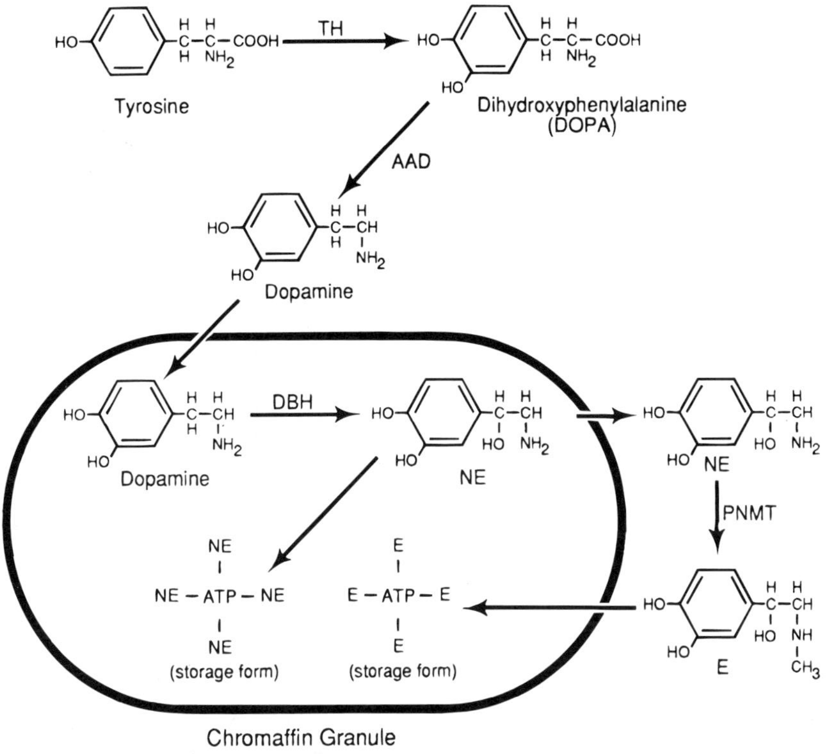

FIG. 19. Biosynthetic sequence for epinephrine (*E*) and norepinephrine (*N*) in adrenal medullary cells. *TH*, tyrosine hydroxylase; *AAD*, aromatic L-amino acid decarboxylase (also called DOPA decarboxylase); *DBH*, dopamine beta-hydroxylase; *PNMT*, phenylethanolamine-*N*-methyltransferase.

activity of this enzyme is inhibited by catecholamines (product inhibition) and stimulated by phosphorylation. In this way, regulatory adjustments are made rapidly and are closely tied to bursts of secretion. A protracted increase in secretory activity induces synthesis of additional enzyme after a lag time of about 12 hours.

Tyrosine hydroxylase and DOPA decarboxylase are cytosolic enzymes, but the enzyme that catalyzes the ß-hydroxylation of dopamine to form norepinephrine resides within the secretory granule. Dopamine is pumped into the granule by an energy-dependent, stereospecific process. For sympathetic nerve endings and those adrenomedullary cells that produce norepinephrine, synthesis is complete with the formation of norepinephrine, and the hormone remains in the granule until it is secreted. The synthesis of epinephrine, however, requires that norepinephrine reenter the cytosol for the final methylation reaction. The enzyme required for this reaction, phenylethanolamine-*N*-methyltransferase, is at least partly inducible by glucocorticoids. Induction requires concentrations of cortisol that are considerably higher than those found in peripheral blood. The vascular arrangement in the adrenals is such that interstitial fluid surrounding cells of the medulla can equilibrate with venous blood that drains the cortex and therefore has a much higher content of glucocorticoids than arterial blood. Glucocorticoids may thus determine the ratio of epinephrine to norepinephrine production. Once methylated, epinephrine is pumped back into the storage granule, whose membrane protects stored catecholamines from oxidation by cytosolic enzymes.

Storage, Release, and Metabolism

Catecholamines are stored in secretory granules in close association with ATP and at a molar ratio of 4:1, suggesting some hydrostatic interaction between the positively charged amines and the four negative charges on ATP. Some opioid peptides, including the enkephalins, ß-endorphin, and their precursors, are also found in these granules. Acetylcholine released during neuronal stimulation increases sodium conductance of the chromaffin cell membrane. The resulting influx of sodium ions depolarizes the plasma membrane, leading to an influx of calcium through voltage-sensitive channels. Calcium is required for catecholamine secretion. Increased cytosolic concentrations of calcium promote phosphorylation of microtubules and the consequent translocation of secretory granules to the cell surface. Secretion occurs when membranes of the chromaffin granules fuse with the plasma membranes and the granular contents are extruded into the extracellular space. Fusion of the granular membrane with the cell membrane may also require calcium. Then, ATP, opioid peptides, and other contents of the granules are released along with epinephrine and norepinephrine. As yet, the physiological significance of opioid secretion by the adrenals is not known, but it has been suggested that the analgesic effects of these compounds may be of importance in the stress response.

All the epinephrine in blood originates in the adrenal glands. However, norepinephrine may reach the blood by either adrenal secretion or diffusion from sympathetic synapses. The half-lives of the medullary hormones in the peripheral circulation have been estimated to be less than 10 seconds for epinephrine and less than 15 seconds for norepinephrine. Up to 90% of the catecholamines are removed in a single passage through most capillary beds. Clearance from the blood requires uptake by both neuronal and nonneuronal tissues. Significant amounts of norepinephrine are taken up by sympathetic nerve endings and incorporated into secretory granules for release at a later time. Epinephrine and norepinephrine that is taken up in excess of storage capacity are degraded in neuronal cytosol, principally by the enzyme monoamine oxidase. This enzyme catalyzes the oxidative deamination of epinephrine, norepinephrine, and other biologically important amines (Fig. 20). Catecholamines taken up by the endothelium, heart, liver, and other tissues are also inactivated enzymatically, principally by catechol-O-methyl-transferase, which catalyzes the transfer of a methyl group from S-adenosyl methionine to one of the hydroxyl groups. Both of these enzymes are widely distributed and can act sequentially in either order

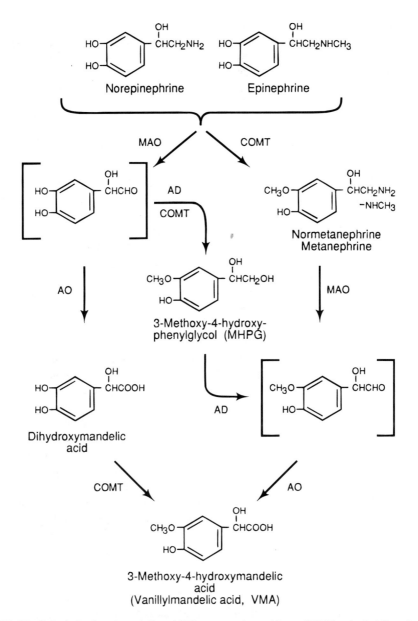

FIG. 20. Catecholamine degradation. *MAO*, monoamine oxidase; *COMT*, catechol-O-methyltransferase; *AD*, alcohol dehydrogenase; *AO*, aldehyde oxidase. From Cryer, P. (1987): Disease of the sympathochromaffin system. In: *Endocrinology and Metabolism*, 2nd ed., edited by Felig, P., Baxter, J.D., Broadus, A.E., et al., McGraw Hill, New York.

on both epinephrine and norepinephrine. A number of pharmaceutical agents have been developed to modify the actions of these enzymes and, thus, modify sympathetic responses. Inactivated catecholamines, chiefly vanillylmandelic acid and 3-methoxy-4-hydroxyphenylglycol, are conjugated with sulfate or glucuronide and excreted in the urine. As with steroid hormones, measurement of urinary metabolites of catecholamines is a useful, noninvasive source of diagnostic information.

Physiological Actions of Medullary Hormones

The sympathetic nervous system and adrenal medullary hormones, like the cortical hormones, act on a wide variety of tissues to maintain the integrity of the internal environment, both at rest and in the face of internal and external challenges. Catecholamines enable us to cope with emergencies and equip us for what Cannon called "fright, fight, or flight." Responsive tissues make no distinctions between blood-borne catecholamines and those released locally from nerve endings. In contrast to adrenal cortical hormones, the effects of catecholamines are expressed within seconds and dissipate as rapidly when the hormone is removed. The medullary hormones are thus ideally suited for making the rapid short-term adjustments demanded by a changing environment, whereas cortical hormones, which act only after a lag period of at least 30 minutes, are of little use at the onset of stress. The cortex and medulla together, however, provide an effective "one–two punch," with cortical hormones maintaining and even amplifying the effectiveness of medullary hormones.

Cells in virtually all tissues of the body have receptors for epinephrine and norepinephrine on their surface membranes. These so-called adrenergic receptors were originally divided into two categories, α and ß, based on their activation or inhibition by various drugs. Subsequently, the α and ß receptors were further subdivided into α_1, α_2, $ß_1$, and $ß_2$ receptors. All these receptors recognize both epinephrine and norepinephrine (at least to some extent), and a given cell may have more than one class of adrenergic receptor. Not surprisingly, these receptors are closely related proteins whose single chain is woven through the plasma membrane seven times such that the amino terminal tail and three loops are on the extracellular surface and the carboxyl terminal tail and three loops dangle into the cytosol. Interaction with catecholamines involves the extracellular loops, while interaction with G proteins involves the intracellular loops (Fig. 21).

The biochemical mechanisms of signal transduction follow the pharmacological subdivisions of the adrenergic receptors. Stimulation of either $ß_1$ or $ß_2$ receptors activates adenylyl cyclase. Beta-adrenergic responses typically result from increased production of cyclic AMP. From a physiological perspective, the only difference between $ß_1$ and $ß_2$ receptors is the low sensitivity of the $ß_2$ receptors to norepinephrine. Stimulation of α_2 receptors inhibits adenylyl cyclase and may block the increase in cyclic AMP produced by other agents. For the ß effects, the receptor communicates with adenylyl cyclase through the stimulatory guanosine binding protein, Gs (see Chapter 1). For α_2 effects, the receptor communicates with adenylyl cyclase through

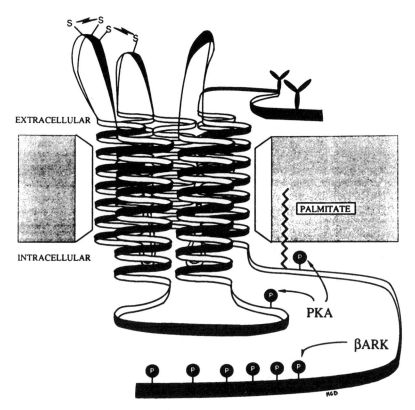

FIG. 21. Schematic model of the ß₂ adrenergic receptor. The receptors in this superfamily contain seven alpha helices clustered in the membrane to form a pocket in which the hormone binds. There are two N-linked carbohydrate complexes on the extracellular portion near the amino terminus (shown as Y-shaped structures). The disulfide bridges linking adjacent loops are also shown (*S–S*). The long intracellular loop and the carboxyl tail contain sites of interaction with G proteins. The *palmitate* molecule (shown as a *zigzag line*) may stabilize the receptor in the membrane. Receptor activity is modulated by phosphorylation (*P*) catalyzed by either protein kinase A (*PKA*) or the ß-adrenergic receptor kinase (*ßARK*). From Collins, S., Lohse, M.J., O'Down, B., et al. (1991): Structure and regulation of G protein-coupled receptors: the ß₂-adrenergic receptor as a model. *Vitam. Horm.*, 46:1.

the inhibitory G protein, Gi. Responses initiated by the α_1 receptor are mediated by the IP₃–DAG mechanism (see Chapter 1).

Some of the physiological effects of catecholamines are listed in Table 2. Although these actions may seem diverse, in actuality, they constitute a magnificently coordinated set of responses that Cannon aptly called ''the wisdom of the body.'' When producing their effects, catecholamines maximize the contributions of each of the various tissues to resolve the challenges to survival. On the whole, the cardiovascular effects maximize cardiac output and ensure perfusion of the brain and working muscles. The metabolic effects ensure an adequate supply of energy-rich substrate.

TABLE 2. *Typical responses to stimulation of the adrenal medulla*

Target	Responses	Receptor
Cardiovascular system		
Heart	↑Frequency and rate of contraction	
	↑Conduction	β
	↑Blood flow (dilation of coronary arterioles)	β
	↑Glycogenolysis	α
Arterioles		
Skin	Constriction	α
Mucosae	Constriction	α
Skeletal muscle	Constriction	α
	Dilation	β
Metabolism		
Fat	↑Lipolyis	β
	↑Blood FFA and glycerol	β
Liver	↑Glycogenolysis and gluconeogenesis	β and $α_1$
	↑Blood sugar	β and $α_1$
Muscle	↑Glycogenolysis	β
	↑Lactate and pyruvate release	β
Bronchial muscle	Relaxation	β
Stomach and intestines	↑Motility	β
	↑Sphincter contraction	α
Urinary bladder	↑Sphincter contraction	α
Skin	↑Sweating	α
Eyes	Contraction of radial muscle of the iris	α
Salivary gland	↑Amylase secretion	α
	↑Watery secretion	α
Kidney	↑Renin secretion	β
Skeletal muscle	↑Tension generation	β
	↑Neuromuscular transmission (defatiguing effect)	β

FFA, free fatty acids.

The relaxation of bronchial muscles facilitates pulmonary ventilation. The ocular effects increase visual acuity. The effects on skeletal muscle and transmitter release from motor neurons increase muscular performance, and the quiescence of the gut permits diversion of blood flow, oxygen, and fuel to reinforce these effects.

Regulation of Adrenal Medullary Function

The sympathetic nervous system, including its adrenal medullary component, is activated by any actual or threatened change in the internal or external environment. It responds to physical changes, emotional inputs, and anticipation of increased physical activity. Input reaches the adrenal medulla through its sympathetic innervation. Signals arising in the hypothalamus and other integrating centers activate both the neural and hormonal components of the sympathetic nervous system but not necessarily in an all-or-none fashion. Activation may be general or may be selectively limited to discrete targets. The adrenals can be preferentially stimulated, and it is even possible that norepinephrine- or epinephrine-secreting cells may be selectively

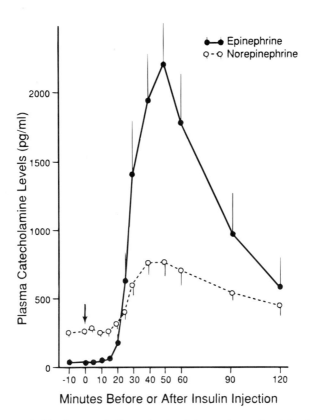

FIG. 22. Changes in blood concentrations of epinephrine and norepinephrine in response to hypoglycemia. Insulin, which produces hypoglycemia, was injected at the time indicated by the *arrow*. From Garber, A.J., Cryer, P.E., Santiago, J.V., et al. (1976): The role of adrenergic mechanisms in the substrate and hormonal response to insulin-induced hypoglycemia in man. *J. Clin. Invest.*, 58:7.

activated, as shown in Fig. 22. In response to hypoglycemia detected by glucose-monitoring cells in the central nervous system, the concentration of norepinephrine in blood increased threefold, whereas that of epinephrine, which tends to be a more effective hyperglycemic agent, increased 50-fold. The metabolic actions of epinephrine are discussed further in Chapter 9.

SUGGESTED READING

Bateman, A., Singh, A., Kral, T., and Solomon, S. (1989): The immune-hypothalamic-pituitary adrenal axis. *Endocr. Rev.*, 10:92–112.

Davies, A. O., and Lefkowitz, R. J. (1984): Regulation of ß-adrenergic receptors by steroid hormones. *Annu. Rev. Physiol.*, 46:119–130.

Funder, J. W. (1991): Steroids, receptors, and response elements: the limits of signal specificity. *Recent Prog. Horm. Res.*, 47:191–210.

Hall, P. F. (1985): Trophic stimulation of steroidogenesis: in search of the elusive trigger. *Recent Prog. Horm. Res.*, 41:1–31.

Keller-Wood, M. E., and Dallman, M. F. (1984): Corticosteroid inhibition of ACTH secretion. *Endocr. Rev.*, 5:1–24.

Morris, D. J. (1981): The metabolism and mechanism of action of aldosterone. *Endocr. Rev.*, 2:234–247.

Munck, A., McGuyre, P. M., and Holbrook, N. J. (1984): Physiological functions of glucocorticoids in stress and their relation to pharmacological actions. *Endocr. Rev.*, 5:25–44.

Needleman, P., Turk, J., Jakschik, B. A., Morrison, A. R., and Lefkowith, J. B. (1986): Arachidonic acid metabolism. *Annu. Rev. Biochem.*, 55:69–102.

Orth, D.N. (1992): Corticotropin-releasing hormone in humans. *Endocr. Rev.*, 13:164–191.

Ungar, A., and Phillips, J. H. (1983): Regulation of the adrenal medulla. *Physiol. Rev.*, 63:787–843.

5

Islets of Langerhans

OVERVIEW

The principal pancreatic hormones are *insulin* and *glucagon*, whose opposing effects on the liver regulate hepatic storage, production, and release of energy-rich fuels. Insulin is an anabolic hormone that promotes sequestration of carbohydrate, fat, and protein in storage depots throughout the body. Its powerful actions are exerted principally on skeletal muscle, liver, and adipose tissue, whereas those of glucagon are restricted to the liver, which responds by forming and secreting energy-rich water-soluble fuels: glucose, acetoacetic acid, and β-hydroxybutyric acid. The interplay of these two hormones contributes to constancy in the availability of metabolic fuels to all cells. *Somatostatin* is a third islet hormone, but a physiological role for pancreatic somatostatin has not been established. A fourth substance, *pancreatic polypeptide*, is even less understood. Glucagon acts in concert with other fuel-mobilizing hormones to counterbalance the fuel-storing effects of insulin. Because compensatory changes in the secretion of all of these hormones are readily made, states of glucagon excess or deficiency rarely lead to overt human disease. Insulin, on the other hand, acts alone, and survival beyond a few days or perhaps weeks is not possible in its absence. An inadequacy of insulin due either to insufficient production (*diabetes mellitus type I*) or end-organ unresponsiveness (*diabetes mellitus type II*) results in one of the most common of the endocrine diseases that affects about 3% of the American population.

MORPHOLOGY OF THE ENDOCRINE PANCREAS

The one to two million islets of the human pancreas average about 300 μm in diameter and collectively comprise only 1% to 2% of the pancreatic mass. They are highly vascular, with each cell seemingly in direct contact with a capillary. Blood is supplied by the pancreatic artery and drains into the portal vein, which thus delivers the entire output of pancreatic hormones to the liver. The islets are also richly innervated with both sympathetic and parasympathetic fibers that terminate on or near the secretory cells.

113

Histologically, the islets consist of three cell types. The beta cells, which synthesize and secrete insulin, make up about 60% to 75% of a typical islet. The alpha cells are the source of glucagon and comprise perhaps as much as 20% of islet tissue. The delta cells, which are considerably less abundant, produce somatostatin, and an occasional cell might also produce gastrin. An additional but rarer cell type, the PP cell, may also appear in the exocrine part of the pancreas. It contains and secretes a compound of unknown function called pancreatic polypeptide.

The beta cells occupy the central region of the islet, whereas the alpha cells occupy the outer rim. The delta cells are interposed between them and are thus in contact with both types (Fig. 1). Gap junctions link alpha cells to each other, beta cells to each other, and alpha cells to beta cells. Although experimental proof is lacking, this arrangement may account for synchronous secretory activity. There are also tight junctions between various islet cells. These sites of close apposition or actual fusion of plasma membranes of adjacent cells may affect diffusion of substances into or out of intercellular spaces. This arrangement could either facilitate or hinder paracrine communication between alpha, beta, and delta cells. Blood flows through an anastomosing network of capillaries from the center of the islet toward the periphery. This arrangement favors intraislet delivery of insulin from the centrally located beta cells to the peripherally located alpha cells. The physiological consequences of these complex anatomical specializations are not understood.

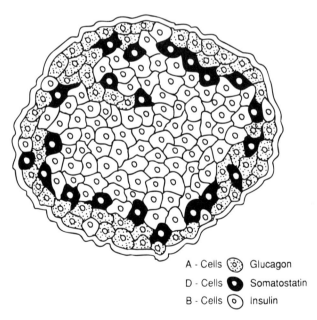

A - Cells   Glucagon
D - Cells   Somatostatin
B - Cells   Insulin

FIG. 1. Arrangement of cells in a typical islet. From Orci, L. and Unger, R.H. (1975): Functional subdivision of islets of langerhans and possible role of D cells. *Lancet*, 2:1243.

GLUCAGON

Chemistry, Secretion, and Metabolism

Glucagon is a simple unbranched peptide chain that consists of 29 amino acids and has a molecular weight of about 3,500 Daltons. Its amino acid sequence has been remarkably preserved throughout evolution of the vertebrates and is identical in all mammalian species. As for other peptide hormones, the gene product is considerably larger than the final secretory product, and occasionally, larger precursors of 9,000 to 12,000 Daltons are secreted. Based on homologies in amino acid sequence, glucagon is a member of the family of gastrointestinal hormones that also includes secretin, vasoactive inhibitory peptide (VIP), gastric inhibitory peptide (GIP), and a larger molecule of unknown function called enteric glucagon. Glucagon is packaged, stored in membrane-bound granules, and secreted like other peptide hormones (see Chapter 1).

Glucagon circulates without binding to carrier proteins and has a half-life in blood of only 3 to 4 minutes. Both liver and kidney are important sites of degradation. Glucagon concentrations in peripheral blood are considerably lower than those in portal venous blood. This difference reflects, not only greater dilution in the general circulation, but also the fact that some glucagon is destroyed during passage through the liver.

Physiological Actions of Glucagon

The physiological role of glucagon is to stimulate hepatic production and secretion of metabolic fuels. Under normal circumstances, the liver and possibly pancreatic beta cells are the only targets of glucagon action. Experimentally, glucagon can also stimulate adipose tissue and the heart, but the concentrations needed are about 1,000 times higher than those found in peripheral blood. Glucagon produces a prompt increase in blood glucose concentration. Glucose that is released from the liver in response to glucagon is obtained from the breakdown of stored glycogen (*glycogenolysis*) and new synthesis (*gluconeogenesis*). Because the principal precursors for gluconeogenesis are amino acids, especially alanine, glucagon also increases hepatic production of urea (*ureogenesis*). Glucagon also increases production of ketone bodies (*ketogenesis*) by directing the metabolism of long-chain fatty acids toward oxidation and away from esterification and export as lipoproteins. Concomitantly, glucagon may also promote the breakdown of hepatic triglycerides to yield long-chain fatty acids which, along with the fatty acids that reach the liver from peripheral fat depots, provide the substrate for ketogenesis. Most of the effects of glucagon are mediated by cyclic adenosine monophosphate (AMP, see Chapter 1). In fact, it was studies of the glycogenolytic action of glucagon that led to the discovery of cyclic AMP and its role as a second messenger. Glucagon may also activate the inositol trisphosphate (IP_3)–diacylglycerol (DAG) messenger system to mobilize calcium and increase protein kinase C activity (see Chapter 1).

Glucose Production

To understand how glucagon stimulates the hepatocyte to release glucose, we must first consider some of the biochemical reactions that govern glucose metabolism in the liver. The biochemical pathways that link these reactions are illustrated in Fig. 2. It is important to recognize that not all enzymatic reactions are freely reversible under conditions that prevail in living cells. Phosphorylation and dephosphorylation of substrate usually require separate enzymes. This sets up substrate cycles that would spin futilely in the absence of some regulatory influence exerted on either or both opposing reactions. These reactions are often strategically situated at or near

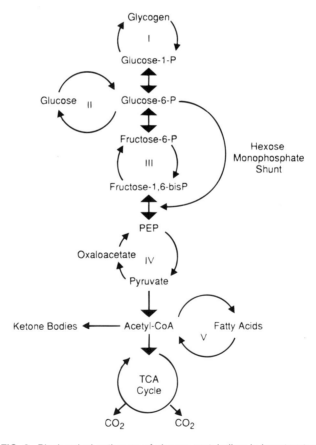

FIG. 2. Biochemical pathways of glucose metabolism in hepatocytes.

branch points in metabolic pathways and can therefore direct the flow of substrates toward one fate or another. Regulation is achieved both by modulating the activity of enzymes already present in cells and by increasing or decreasing rates of enzyme synthesis and therefore the amounts of enzyme molecules. Enzyme activity can be regulated by substrates, cofactors, or phosphorylation and dephosphorylation of the enzymes themselves. Changing the activity of an enzyme requires only seconds, whereas minutes or hours are needed to change the amount of an enzyme.

Glycogenolysis

Cyclic AMP formed in response to the interaction of glucagon with its receptors on the surface of the hepatocyte (see Chapter 1) activates protein kinase A, which catalyzes the phosphorylation, and hence activation, of an enzyme called *phosphorylase kinase* (Fig. 3). This enzyme, in turn, catalyzes the phosphorylation of another enzyme, *glycogen phosphorylase*, which cleaves glycogen stepwise to form glucose-1-phosphate. Glucose-1-phosphate is the substrate for *glycogen synthetase*, which catalyzes the incorporation of glucose into glycogen. Glycogen synthetase is inactivated when phosphorylated by protein kinase A. Thus, by increasing the formation of cyclic AMP, glucagon simultaneously promotes glycogen breakdown and prevents recycling of glucose to glycogen. Cyclic AMP-dependent phosphorylation of enzymes that regulate the glycolytic and shunt pathways at the level of phosphofructokinase and acetyl coenzyme A (CoA) carboxylase (see subsequent discussion) pre-

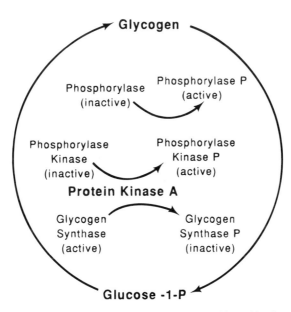

FIG. 3. Role of protein kinase A (cyclic AMP-dependent protein kinase) in glycogen metabolism.

vents consumption of glucose by the hepatocyte itself, leaving dephosphorylation and diffusion into the blood as the only pathway open to newly depolymerized glucose.

Gluconeogenesis

Precursors of glucose enter the gluconeogenic pathway as three- or four-carbon compounds. Glucagon directs their conversion into glucose by accelerating their condensation to fructose phosphate while simultaneously blocking their escape from the gluconeogenic pathway (cycles III and IV in Fig. 2). Cyclic AMP controls the production of a potent regulator of metabolism called *fructose-2,6-bisphosphate*. This compound, when present even in tiny amounts, activates *phosphofructokinase* and inhibits fructose-1,6-bisphosphatase, thereby directing the flow of substrates toward glucose breakdown rather than glucose formation (Fig. 4). Fructose-2,6-bisphosphate, which should not be confused with fructose-1,6-bisphosphate, is formed from fructose-6-phosphate by the action of an unusual bifunctional enzyme that catalyzes either phosphorylation of fructose-6-phosphate to fructose-2,6-bisphosphate or dephosphorylation of fructose-2,6-bisphosphate to fructose-6-phosphate, depending on its own state of phosphorylation. This enzyme is a substrate for protein

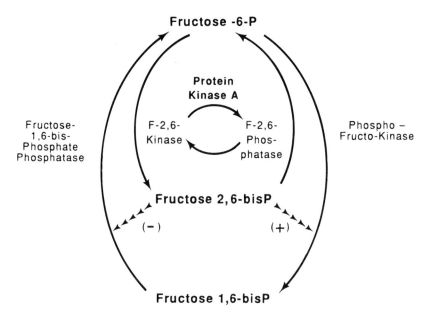

FIG. 4. Regulation of fructose-1,6-bisphosphate metabolism by protein kinase A (cyclic AMP-dependent protein kinase) and fructose-2,6-bisphosphate. Fructose-2,6-bisphosphate, whose formation depends on protein kinase A, activates (+) phosphofructokinase and inhibits (−) fructose-1,6-bisphosphatase.

kinase A and behaves as a kinase when it is in its dephosphorylated form and as a phosphatase when it is phosphorylated. Its activity in the presence of cyclic AMP rapidly depletes the hepatocyte of fructose-2,6-bisphosphate, and substrate therefore flows toward glucose production.

The other important regulatory step in gluconeogenesis is phosphorylation and dephosphorylation of pyruvate (cycle IV in Fig. 2). It is here that three- and four-carbon fragments enter or escape from the gluconeogenic pathway. The cytosolic enzyme that catalyzes dephosphorylation of phosphoenol pyruvate (PEP) was inappropriately named *pyruvate kinase* before it was recognized that direct phosphorylation of pyruvate does not occur under physiological conditions and that this enzyme acts only in the direction of dephosphorylation (Fig. 5). The regulation of this enzyme is complex. Pyruvate kinase is another substrate for protein kinase A and is powerfully inhibited when phosphorylated, but the inhibition can be overcome by fructose-1,6-bisphosphate. Thus, activation of protein kinase A has the duel effect of decreasing pyruvate kinase activity directly and of decreasing the abundance of its activator, fructose-1,6-bisphosphate, by the reactions shown in Fig. 4. Inhibiting pyruvate kinase may be the single most important effect of glucagon on the gluconeogenic pathway.

Phosphorylation of pyruvate requires a complex series of reactions in which pyruvate must first enter the mitochondria where it is carboxylated to form oxaloacetate, which is subsequently converted to cytosolic PEP by the catalytic activity of *PEP carboxykinase*. Synthesis of this enzyme is accelerated by cyclic AMP. Cyclic AMP may also indirectly accelerate the pyruvate carboxylase reaction somewhat.

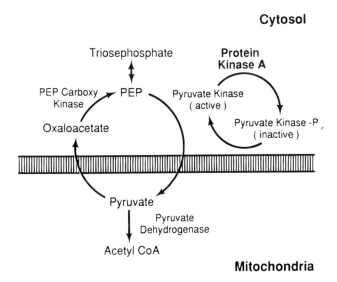

FIG. 5. Regulation of PEP formation by protein kinase A (cyclic AMP-dependent protein kinase). Protein kinase A catalyzes the phosphorylation and, hence, inactivation of pyruvate kinase whose activity limits the conversion of PEP to pyruvate.

Lipogenesis and Ketogenesis

The alternate fate of pyruvate is decarboxylation to form acetyl CoA (Fig. 5). This two-carbon acetyl unit is the building block of fatty acids and eventually finds its way back to the cytosol where fatty acid synthesis (*lipogenesis*) takes place. Lipogenesis is the principal competitor of gluconeogenesis for three-carbon precursors. The first committed step in fatty acid synthesis is the carboxylation of acetyl CoA to form malonyl CoA. *Acetyl CoA carboxylase*, the enzyme that catalyzes this reaction, is yet another substrate for protein kinase A and is powerfully inhibited when phosphorylated. Inhibition of fatty acid synthesis not only preserves the substrate for gluconeogenesis but also prevents oxidation of glucose by the hexose monophosphate shunt pathway (Fig. 2). Nicotinamide adenine dinucleotide phosphate (NADP), which is required for shunt activity, is reduced in the initial reactions of this pathway and can be regenerated only by transferring protons to the elongating fatty acid chain.

Fatty acid synthesis and oxidation constitute another substrate cycle and another regulatory site for cyclic AMP action. The same reaction that inhibits fatty acid synthesis promotes fatty acid oxidation and consequently *ketogenesis* (ketone body formation, Fig. 6). Long-chain fatty acid molecules that reach the liver can either be oxidized or esterified and exported to adipose tissue as the triglyceride component of low density lipoproteins. To be esterified, fatty acids remain in the cytosol, and to be oxidized they must enter the mitochondria. Long-chain fatty acids can cross

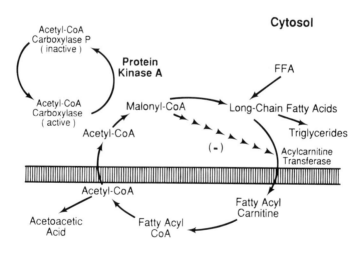

FIG. 6. Protein kinase A (cyclic AMP-dependent protein kinase) indirectly stimulates ketogenesis by decreasing the formation of malonyl CoA, thus removing a restriction on the accessibility of fatty acids to intramitochondrial oxidative enzymes.

the mitochondrial membrane only when linked to carnitine. *Carnitine acyl transferase*, the enzyme that catalyzes this linkage, is powerfully inhibited by malonyl CoA. Thus, when malonyl CoA concentrations are high, coincident with fatty acid synthesis, fatty acid oxidation is inhibited. Conversely, when the formation of malonyl CoA is blocked, fatty acids readily enter mitochondria and are oxidized to acetyl CoA. Because long-chain fatty acids typically contain 16 or 18 carbons, each molecule that is oxidized yields eight or nine molecules of acetyl CoA. The ketone bodies, β-hydroxybutyrate and acetoacetate, are formed from the condensation of two molecules of acetyl CoA.

By reducing the concentration of malonyl CoA, glucagon sets the stage for ketogenesis, but the actual amount of ketone production is determined by the amount of long-chain fatty acids available for oxidation. Most fatty acids oxidized in liver originate in adipose tissue, but glucagon, through cyclic AMP, may also activate a lipase and thereby provide fatty acids from breakdown of hepatic triglycerides.

Ureogenesis

Whenever the carbon chains of amino acids are used as substrate for gluconeogenesis, the amino groups must be disposed of in the form of urea, which thus becomes a byproduct of gluconeogenesis. By promoting gluconeogenesis, therefore, glucagon also increases the formation of urea (*ureogenesis*). The carbon skeletons of most amino acids can be converted to glucose, but because of peculiarities of peripheral metabolism, alanine is quantitatively the most important glucogenic amino acid. By accelerating conversion of pyruvate to glucose (see the preceding discussion), glucagon indirectly accelerates transamination of alanine to pyruvate. Glucagon also accelerates ureogenesis by increasing the transport of amino acids across hepatocyte plasma membranes by an action that requires the synthesis of new ribonucleic acid (RNA) and protein. In addition, glucagon also promotes the synthesis of some urea cycle enzymes.

Regulation of Glucagon Secretion

The concentration of glucose in blood is the most important determinant of glucagon secretion in normal individuals. When the plasma glucose concentration exceeds 200 mg/dl, glucagon secretion is maximally inhibited. The inhibitory effects of glucose are proportionately less at lower concentrations and disappear below 50 mg/dl. Except immediately after a meal rich in carbohydrate, the blood glucose concentration remains constant at around 90 mg/dl. The set point for glucose concentration thus falls well within the range over which glucagon secretion is regulated, and alpha cells can respond to changes in blood glucose with either an increase or a decrease in glucagon output. We do not yet understand how the alpha cell monitors blood glucose concentration and translates that information into an appropriate rate of glucagon secretion.

Low blood glucose (*hypoglycemia*) not only relieves the inhibition of glucagon secretion, but this life-threatening circumstance stimulates the central nervous system to signal both parasympathetic and sympathetic nerve endings within the islet to release their neurotransmitters. Alpha cells have receptors for acetylcholine and norepinephrine, and they secrete glucagon in response to both parasympathetic and sympathetic stimulation. Some sympathetic fibers may also release vasoactive intestinal peptide (VIP) as a stimulatory neurotransmitter. The sympathetic response to hypoglycemia also involves secretion of epinephrine and norepinephrine from the adrenal medulla (see Chapter 4). Adrenomedullary hormones further stimulate alpha cells to secrete glucagon and reinforce its actions on the hepatocyte.

Glucagon secretion is evoked by a meal rich in amino acids. The alpha cells respond directly to increased blood levels of certain amino acids, particularly arginine. In addition, the digestion of protein-rich foods triggers the release of *cholecystokinin-pancreazymin* from cells in the duodenal mucosa. This gastrointestinal hormone is a secretagogue for islet hormones as well as pancreatic enzymes and may alert the alpha cells to an impending influx of amino acids. Increased secretion of glucagon in response to a protein meal not only prepares the liver to dispose of excess amino acids by gluconeogenesis but also signals the liver to release glucose. Thus, increased secretion of glucagon counteracts the hypoglycemic effects of insulin, whose secretion is simultaneously increased by amino acids (see subsequent discussion).

Inhibitory influences on glucagon secretion include insulin, somatostatin, and free fatty acids (FFA) as well as glucose (Fig. 7). Insulin, which may reach the alpha cells by either the endocrine or paracrine route, directly inhibits glucagon secretion and is required for expression of the inhibitory effects of glucose. In fact, it has been

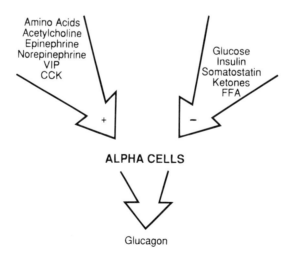

FIG. 7. Stimulatory and inhibitory signals for glucagon secretion.

suggested that glucose may inhibit glucagon secretion indirectly through increased secretion of insulin. In persons suffering from insulin deficiency (see following discussion), glucagon secretion is brisk despite high blood glucose concentrations.

INSULIN

Chemistry, Secretion, and Metabolism

Insulin is composed of two unbranched peptide chains joined together by two disulfide bridges (Fig. 8). The two chains of insulin and their disulfide cross bridges are formed as a single-chain proinsulin molecule from which the connecting peptide is excised by a trypsin-like enzyme. The conversion of proinsulin to insulin takes place slowly within storage granules, which contain the necessary endopeptidase. The connecting peptide therefore accumulates within the granules in equimolar amounts with insulin. Insulin is secreted by exocytosis (see Chapter 1). The entire contents of the storage granules are disgorged into extracellular fluid. Consequently, the connecting peptide, and any remaining proinsulin are released into the circulation whenever insulin is secreted. When secretion is rapid, proinsulin may comprise as much as 20% of the circulating peptides detected by insulin antibodies, but it contrib-

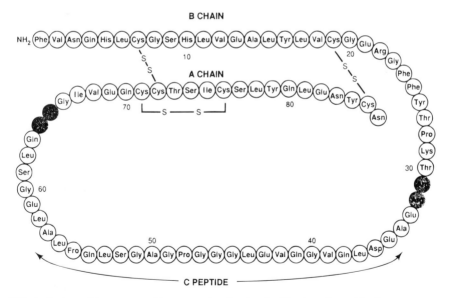

FIG. 8. Amino acid sequence of human proinsulin. A pair of basic amino acids shown as *open circles* at both ends of the connecting peptide are removed during the cleavage process which separates the A chain of insulin (amino acids 1 to 30) from the B chain (amino acids 66 to 86). From Oyer, P.E., Cho, S., Peterson, J.D., et al. (1971): Studies on human proinsulin. *J. Biol. Chem.*, 246:1375.

utes little biological activity. The connecting peptide has no known biological activity, but its presence in blood is useful for estimating beta cell function in patients who are receiving injections of insulin.

The insulin storage granule contains a variety of proteins that are also released into the extracellular space whenever insulin is secreted. In addition to insulin processing, these proteins are thought to maintain optimal conditions for storage and processing of insulin. Their fate and actions, if any, are largely unknown. One such protein, however, called *amylin*, may contribute to the accumulation of amyloid that is found in and around the beta cells in states of insulin hypersecretion and may contribute to islet pathology. In some experiments, amylin also antagonized peripheral actions of insulin.

Insulin is cleared rapidly from the circulation with a half-life of less than 10 minutes, and it is destroyed by a specific enzyme system, insulinase, that is present in liver, muscle, kidney, and other tissues. Proinsulin has a half-life that is at least twice as long and is not converted to insulin outside the pancreas. The liver may inactivate as much as 40% of the insulin that reaches it in hepatic portal blood and thus has the potential for regulating the amount of insulin that enters the systemic circulation. Normally, little or no insulin is found in urine.

Physiological Actions of Insulin

Effects of Insulin Deficiency

In many areas of endocrinology, basic insights into the physiological role of a hormone can be gained from examining the consequences of its absence. In such studies, secondary or tertiary effects may overshadow the primary cellular lesion but, nevertheless, ultimately broaden our understanding of cellular responses in the context of the whole organism. Insights into the physiology of insulin and the physiological processes it affects directly and indirectly were originally gained from clinical observation. Consideration of some of the classic signs of this disease therefore provides a good starting point for discussing the physiology of insulin.

Hyperglycemia

In the normal individual, the concentration of glucose in blood is maintained at around 90 mg/dl of plasma. Blood glucose concentrations may be 300 to 400 mg/dl and even reach 1,000 mg/dl on occasion in people with inadequate insulin secretion. These people have particular difficulty removing excess glucose from their blood. Normally, after ingestion of a meal rich in carbohydrate, there is only a small and transient increase in the concentration of blood glucose, and excess glucose disappears rapidly from the plasma. The diabetic, however, is ''intolerant'' of glucose, and the ability to remove it from plasma is severely impaired.

Oral glucose tolerance tests, which assess the ability to dispose of a glucose load,

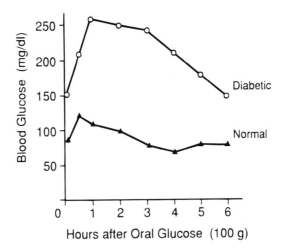

FIG. 9. Idealized glucose tolerance tests in normal and diabetic subjects.

are used diagnostically to evaluate existing or impending diabetic conditions. A standard load of glucose is given by mouth, and the blood glucose concentration is measured periodically over the course of the subsequent 4 hours. In normal subjects, the blood glucose concentrations return to baseline values within 2 hours, and the peak value does not rise above 180 mg/dl. In the diabetic or ''prediabetic'' subject, blood glucose values rise much higher and take a longer time to return to basal levels (Fig. 9).

Glycosuria

Normally, the renal tubule has adequate capacity to transport and reabsorb all the glucose filtered at the glomerulus so that little or none escapes into the urine. Because of hyperglycemia, however, the concentration of glucose in the glomerular filtrate is so high that it exceeds the capacity for reabsorption and ''spills'' into the urine, causing *glycosuria* (excretion of glucose in urine).

Polyuria

Polyuria is defined as excessive production of urine. Because more glucose is present in the glomerular filtrate than can be reabsorbed by the proximal tubules, it remains in the tubular lumen and exerts an osmotic hindrance to water and salt reabsorption in this portion of the nephron, which normally reabsorbs about two thirds of the glomerular filtrate. The abnormally high volume of fluid that remains cannot be reabsorbed by the more distal portions of the nephron, with the result that water excretion is increased (*osmotic diuresis*). Increased flow through the nephron increases urinary loss of sodium and potassium as well.

Polydipsia

Dehydration results from the copious flow of urine and stimulates thirst, a condition called polydipsia, or excessive drinking. The untreated diabetic person is characteristically thirsty and consumes large volumes of water to compensate for water lost in the urine. Polydipsia is often the first symptom that is noticed by the patient or parents of a diabetic child.

Polyphagia

By mechanisms that are not yet understood, appetite is increased in what seems to be an effort to compensate for urinary loss of glucose. The condition is called *polyphagia* (excessive food consumption).

Weight Loss

Despite increased appetite and food intake, however, insulin deficiency reduces all anabolic processes and accelerates catabolic processes. Accelerated protein degradation, particularly in muscle, provides a substrate for gluconeogenesis. Increased mobilization and utilization of stored fats indirectly leads to increased triglyceride concentrations in plasma and often results in *lipemia* (high concentration of lipids in blood). Fatty acid oxidation by the liver results in increased production of ketone bodies (*ketosis*), which are released into the blood and cause *ketonemia*. Because ketone bodies are small, readily filtrable molecules that are actively reabsorbed by a renal mechanism of limited capacity, high blood levels may result in loss of ketone bodies in the urine (*ketonuria*). Ketone bodies are organic acids and produce acidosis, which may be aggravated by excessive washout of sodium and potassium in the urine. Plasma pH may become so low that acidotic coma and death may follow unless insulin therapy is instituted.

The hyperglycemia that causes this whole sequence of events arises from an "*underutilization*" of glucose by muscle and adipose tissue and an "*overproduction*" of glucose by the liver. Gluconeogenesis is increased at the expense of muscle protein, which is the chief source of the amino acid substrate. Consequently, there is marked wasting of muscle along with depletion of body fat stores. Other less obviously related complications, including lesions in the microvasculature of the retina and kidneys and in peripheral nerves, result from prolonged hyperglycemia and complete the clinical picture.

The net effect of insulin lack is a severe reduction in the ability to store glycogen, fat, and protein. Conversely, *the physiological role of insulin is to promote storage of metabolic fuel.* Insulin has many effects on different cells. Even within a single cell, it produces multiple effects that, at present, cannot be attributed to an initial primary action. Insulin acts on adipose tissue, skeletal muscle, and liver to defend and expand reserves of triglyceride, glycogen, and protein. Within a few minutes after an intravenous injection of insulin, there is a striking decrease in the plasma concentrations of glucose, amino acids, FFA, ketone bodies, and potassium. If the dose of insulin is large enough, the blood glucose concentration may fall too low to meet the needs of the central nervous system, and *hypoglycemic coma* may occur. Insulin lowers blood glucose in two ways: (a) it increases uptake by muscle and adipose tissue and (b) it decreases output by liver. It lowers the concentration of amino acids by stimulating their uptake by muscle and reducing their release. Insulin lowers the concentration of FFA by blocking their release from adipocytes, and this action in turn lowers the blood ketone level. The decrease in potassium, though not well understood, results in hyperpolarization of plasma membranes of muscle, liver, and fat cells.

Effects on Adipose Tissue

Storage of fat in adipose tissue depends on multiple insulin-sensitive reactions, including: (a) synthesis of long-chain fatty acids from glucose, (b) synthesis of triglycerides from fatty acids and glycerol (*esterification*), (c) breakdown of triglycerides to release glycerol and long-chain fatty acids (*lipolysis*), and (d) uptake of fat from the lipoproteins of blood. The relevant biochemical pathways are shown in Fig. 10.

Lipolysis and esterification are central events in the physiology of the adipocyte. The rate of lipolysis depends on the activity of triglyceride lipase. Lipolysis proceeds at a basal rate in the absence of hormonal stimulation but increases dramatically when cyclic AMP is increased. The hormone-sensitive lipase catalyzes the breakdown of triglycerides into fatty acids and glycerol. Fatty acids can either escape from the adipocyte and become the FFA of the blood or be reesterified into triglycerides. Fatty acid esterification requires a source of glycerol that is phosphorylated in its α carbon; free glycerol cannot be used. Because adipose tissue lacks the enzyme needed to phosphorylate it, all of the free glycerol that was produced by lipolysis is unusable and escapes into the blood. The α-glycerol phosphate needed for esterification is derived from phosphorylated three-carbon intermediates formed from oxidation of glucose (Fig. 10).

As its name implies, the *hormone-sensitive lipase* is activated by lipolytic hormones, which promote its phosphorylation by protein kinase A. Insulin interferes with the activation of lipase by inhibiting the formation of cyclic AMP and accelerating its degradation. Simultaneously, insulin increases the rate of fatty acid esterification by increasing the availability of α-glycerol phosphate. The net result of these actions is the preservation of triglyceride stores at the expense of FFA, whose concentration in blood plasma promptly falls.

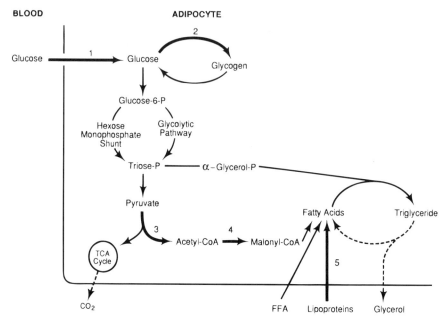

FIG. 10. Carbohydrate and lipid metabolism in adipose tissue. Reactions enhanced by insulin (*heavy arrows*) are as follows: (*1*) transport of glucose into adipose cell, (*2*) conversion of excess glucose to glycogen, (*3*) decarboxylation of pyruvate, (*4*) initiation of fatty acid synthesis, and (*5*) uptake of fatty acids from circulating lipoproteins. Breakdown of triglycerides is inhibited by insulin (*broken arrow*).

Because glucose does not readily diffuse across the plasma membrane, its entry into adipocytes and most other cells depends on carrier-mediated transport. Insulin increases cellular uptake and metabolism of glucose by accelerating transmembrane transport of glucose and structurally related sugars. This action depends upon the availability of glucose transporters (abbreviated GLUT) in the plasma membrane. These transporters are large proteins that weave in and out of the membrane 12 times to form stereospecific channels through which glucose can diffuse down its concentration gradient. There are at least five isoforms of GLUT expressed in various cell types. In addition to GLUT 1, which is present in the plasma membrane of most cells, insulin-sensitive cells, such as adipocytes, contain pools of intracellular membrane vesicles that are rich in GLUT 4. Insulin increases the number of glucose carriers on the adipocyte surface by stimulating the translocation and fusion of GLUT 4-containing vesicles with the adipocyte plasma membrane (Fig. 11).

Insulin accelerates the synthesis of fatty acids by increasing the uptake of glucose and by activating at least two enzymes that direct the flow of glucose-derived carbons into fatty acids. It increases conversion of pyruvate to acetyl CoA, which is the immediate precursor of long-chain fatty acids, and stimulates the carboxylation of acetyl CoA to malonyl CoA, which is the rate-determining reaction in fatty acid

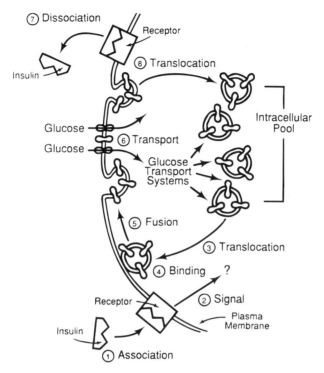

FIG. 11. Hypothetical model of insulin's action on glucose transport. Upon associating with its receptors in the cell membrane, insulin signals the translocation of glucose transport systems to the plasma membrane. From Karnieli, E., Zarnowski, M.J., Hissin, P.J., et al. (1981): Insulin-stimulated translocation of glucose transport systems in the isolated rat adipose cell. *J. Biol. Chem.*, 256:4772.

synthesis. In humans, adipose tissue is relatively unimportant as a site of fatty acid synthesis, particularly in Western cultures where the diet is rich in fat.

Dietary fat and triglycerides synthesized in the liver are packaged as lipoproteins and exported to adipose tissue for storage. Uptake of the lipid portion by adipocytes depends on cleavage of ester bonds to release fatty acids. This reaction occurs at the fat cell surface or within the capillaries. Insulin promotes the synthesis of the required *lipoprotein lipase*.

Effects on Muscle

Insulin increases the uptake of glucose by muscle and directs its intracellular metabolism toward the formation of glycogen (Fig. 12). It activates glycogen synthesis by a mechanism that is independent of cyclic AMP but that may involve some other second messenger. Because it comprises about 50% of body mass, uptake by

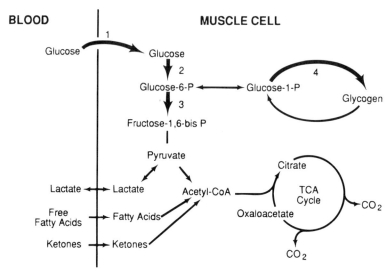

FIG. 12. Metabolism of carbohydrate and lipid in muscle. Rate-limiting reactions accelerated by insulin (*heavy arrows*) are as follows: (*1*) transport of glucose into muscle cells, (*2*) phosphoryla-tion of glucose by hexokinase, (*3*) addition of the second phosphate by phosphofructokinase, and (*4*) storage of glucose as glycogen.

muscle accounts for a major fraction of the glucose that disappears from the blood after an injection of insulin. As in adipocytes, glucose utilization in muscle is limited by the permeability of the plasma membrane. Insulin accelerates the entry of glucose into muscle by mobilizing GLUT 4-containing vesicles by the same mechanism as is operative in adipocytes.

In order to be metabolized, glucose must be converted to glucose-6-phosphate in a reaction catalyzed by the enzyme *hexokinase*. In the basal state, glucose is phosphorylated as rapidly as it enters the cell, and hence, the intracellular concentra-tion of free glucose is virtually nil. When fatty acid oxidation is rapid, however, phosphorylation may diminish because products of fatty acid oxidation inhibit the enzyme *phosphofructokinase* (see Chapter 9). Glucose-6-phosphate, which accumu-lates as a result, powerfully inhibits hexokinase, allowing intracellular free glucose to accumulate and diminish the transmembrane concentration gradient needed for further uptake of glucose. Insulin indirectly accelerates phosphorylation of glucose in muscle by limiting the release of fatty acids from adipose tissue. This indirect effect of insulin on hexokinase activity requires a longer time frame (minutes to hours) than does the acceleration of glucose transport (seconds). On an even longer time scale, insulin increases the synthesis of hexokinase.

Protein synthesis and degradation are ongoing processes in all tissues and, in the nongrowing individual, are completely balanced so that, on average, there is no net increase or decrease in body protein. Insulin increases protein synthesis and decreases

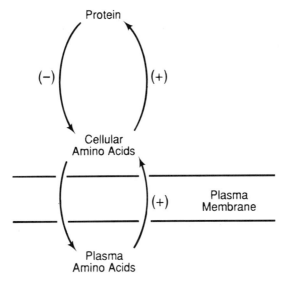

FIG. 13. Effects of insulin on protein turnover in muscle. Insulin (*1*) stimulates (+) amino acid transport across the cell membrane, (*2*) stimulates protein synthesis, and (*3*) inhibits (−) protein breakdown.

protein degradation (Fig. 13). In its absence, there is net loss of muscle protein and muscle becomes a net exporter of amino acids, which serve as substrate for gluconeogenesis and ureogenesis in the liver. As with its effects on carbohydrate and fat metabolism, insulin intercedes in protein synthesis at several levels in the reaction sequence. It increases uptake of amino acids from blood by stimulating their transport across the plasma membrane and their incorporation into proteins. Under the influence of insulin, the attachment of messenger RNA to ribosomes is enhanced, as reflected by the higher content of polysomes compared to monosomes. In addition, insulin increases the total RNA in muscle. We do not yet understand how insulin decreases protein degradation.

Effects on Liver

Insulin reduces outflow of glucose from the liver and promotes storage of glycogen. It inhibits glycogenolysis, gluconeogenesis, ureogenesis, and ketogenesis, and it stimulates the synthesis of fatty acids and proteins. These effects are accomplished by a combination of actions that change the activity of some hepatic enzymes and the rates of synthesis of other enzymes. Hence, not all the effects of insulin occur on the same time scale. In addition, all these effects are reinforced indirectly by actions of insulin on muscle and fat to reduce the influx of substrates for gluconeogenesis and ketogenesis.

Glucose Production

In general, the liver takes up glucose when the circulating concentration is high and releases it when the blood level is low. Glucose transport in hepatocytes depends upon an insulin-insensitive isoform of the glucose transporter (GLUT 2), and net uptake or release of glucose depends upon whether the concentration of free glucose is higher in extracellular or intracellular fluid. The intracellular concentration of free glucose depends on the balance between phosphorylation and dephosphorylation of glucose (Fig. 2, cycle II). The two enzymes that catalyze phosphorylation are *hexokinase*, which has a high affinity for glucose and other six-carbon sugars, and *glucokinase*, which is specific for glucose. Glucokinase is active only when glucose concentrations are relatively high. Dephosphorylation requires the activity of *glucose-6-phosphatase*. Insulin suppresses the synthesis of glucose-6-phosphatase and increases the synthesis of glucokinase, thereby decreasing net output of glucose while promoting net uptake. This response to insulin is relatively sluggish and does not contribute to minute-to-minute regulation.

Most of the hepatic actions of insulin are opposite to those of glucagon, discussed earlier, and can be traced to inhibition of cyclic AMP accumulation and action. These effects largely affect the activity of enzymes already present in hepatocytes and, thus, are rapid. Insulin decreases the formation of cyclic AMP, activates the enzyme that degrades it, and interferes with its ability to activate protein kinase A. The immediate consequences can be seen in Fig. 14. Glycogen synthesis is favored over glycogen breakdown. There is increased formation of fructose-2,6-bisphosphate, which accelerates the formation of glucose-1,6-bisphosphate, which in turn, gives rise to triose phosphates. Pyruvate kinase and acetyl CoA carboxylase are freed from inhibition. Consequently, glucose phosphate is consumed within the hepatocyte and is not available for export as glucose.

Lipogenesis and Ketogenesis

Insulin affects several enzymes in the PEP substrate cycle (Fig. 2 cycle IV) and, in so doing, directs substrate flow away from gluconeogenesis and toward lipogenesis (Fig. 15). With relief of inhibition of pyruvate kinase, PEP can be converted to pyruvate, which then enters mitochondria. Insulin stimulates the mitochondrial enzyme that catalyzes decarboxylation of pyruvate to acetyl CoA and, thus, irreversibly removes it from the gluconeogenic pathway. Acetyl CoA must get to the cytoplasm where lipogenesis occurs. This roundabout process requires condensation of acetyl CoA with oxaloacetate to form citrate, which is transported across the mitochondrial membrane. Once in the cytosol, citrate is cleaved to release acetyl CoA and oxaloacetate. It might be recalled from our earlier discussion that oxaloacetate is a crucial intermediate in gluconeogenesis and is converted to PEP by PEP carboxykinase. Insulin bars the flow of this lipogenic substrate into the gluconeogenic pool

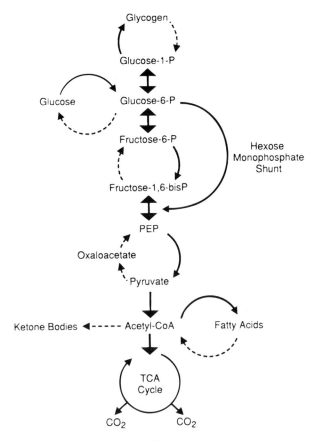

FIG. 14. Effects of insulin on glucose metabolism in hepatocytes. *Heavy arrows* indicate reactions that are increased, and *broken arrows* indicate reactions that are decreased.

by inhibiting the synthesis of *PEP carboxykinase*. The only fate left to cytosolic oxaloacetate is decarboxylation to pyruvate.

Finally, insulin increases the activity of *acetyl CoA carboxylase*, which catalyzes the rate-determining reaction in fatty acid synthesis. Activation is accomplished in part by relieving the cyclic AMP-dependent inhibition and in part by promoting the polymerization of inactive subunits of the enzyme into an active complex. The resulting malonyl CoA not only condenses to form long-chain fatty acids but also prevents oxidation of newly formed fatty acids by blocking their entry into mitochondria (Fig. 6).

It may be noted that hepatic oxidation of either glucose or fatty acids increases the delivery of acetyl CoA to the cytosol, but ketogenesis results only from the oxidation of fatty acids. The primary reason is that lipogenesis usually accompanies glucose utilization and provides an alternate pathway for disposal of acetyl CoA.

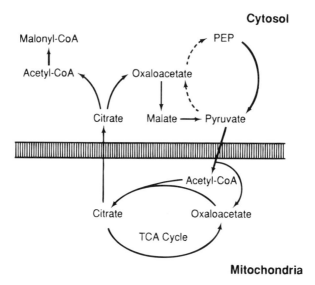

FIG. 15. Effects of insulin on lipogenesis in hepatocytes. *Heavy arrows* indicate reactions that are increased, and *broken arrows* indicate reactions that are decreased.

There is also a quantitative difference in the rate of acetyl CoA production from the two substrates: 1 mole of glucose yields only 2 moles of acetyl CoA compared to 8 or 9 moles for each mole of fatty acids.

Although we have used the terms "block" and "inhibit" to describe the actions of insulin, it is important to remember that these verbs are used in the relative and not the absolute sense. Rarely would inhibition of an enzymatic transformation be absolute. Physiologically, both insulin and glucagon are present simultaneously, and the direction that metabolic pathways assume depends on the relative influences of both of these hormones (and others). The rates of secretion of both insulin and glucagon are dictated by physiological demand. Because of their antagonistic influences on hepatic function, however, it is the ratio, rather than the absolute concentrations, of these two hormones that determines the overall hepatic response.

Mechanism of Insulin Action

The many changes that insulin produces at the molecular level—membrane transport, enzyme activation, and enzyme synthesis—have been described. The molecular events that link these changes with the interaction of insulin and its receptor in the plasma membrane have not yet been identified. It is possible that one or more second messengers are involved, but the weight of available evidence favors the idea that enzymatic activity of the receptor itself initiates a cascade of phosphorylation and dephosphorylation reactions that regulate the activity of enzymes and transcription factors.

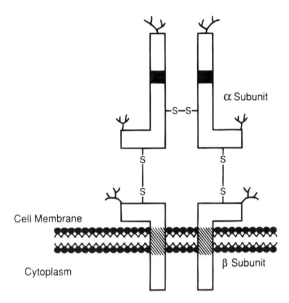

FIG. 16. Current model of the insulin receptor. Two α subunits, which recognize and bind insulin, are linked to each other by a disulfide bond, and each a subunit is also linked to a β subunit. The α subunits are entirely on the external surface of the cell, but the β subunits span the membrane. The *crosshatched areas* on the α subunits represent areas rich in the amino acid cysteine. The *branched lines* represent carbohydrate components. From Goldfine, I.D. (1987): The insulin receptor: molecular biology and transmembrane signaling. *Endocr. Rev.*, 8:235.

The insulin receptor is a tetramer composed of two α and two β glycoprotein subunits that are held together by disulfide bonds (Fig. 16). In contrast to the pituitary glycoprotein hormones (Chapter 2), the α and β subunits of insulin are encoded in the same gene. The α subunit is completely extracellular and contains the insulin-binding domain. The β subunit spans the plasma membrane and contains *tyrosine kinase* activity in its cytosolic domain. Binding to insulin is thought to produce a conformational change that relieves the β subunit from the inhibitory effects of the α subunit, allowing it to phosphorylate itself and other proteins at tyrosine residues. Autophosphorylation prolongs kinase activity after insulin dissociates from the receptor. Although the target proteins for the insulin receptor kinase have not been identified, they are likely to be other kinases that phosphorylate other proteins on serine or threonine residues and, thereby, start a chain reaction of successive phosphorylations and dephosphorylations. The insulin receptor is also a substrate for protein kinases A and C, and when it is phosphorylated at specific serine residues, such properties as the affinity for insulin are changed.

Insulin which is bound to its receptor enters target cells by a process of receptor-mediated endocytosis, but such internalization is more likely related to hormone degradation than to an intracellular site of insulin action. Some internalized receptors recycle to the cell surface. Internalization of insulin-bound receptors results in down regulation of surface receptors, which may account for decreased insulin sensitivity in some pathological states associated with chronic hyperinsulinemia.

Regulation of Insulin Secretion

As might be expected of a hormone whose physiological role is promotion of fuel storage, insulin secretion is greatest immediately after eating and decreases during between-meal periods (Fig. 17). Coordination of insulin secretion with the nutritional state as well as with fluctuating demands for energy production is achieved through stimulation of beta cells by metabolites, hormones, and neural signals. Because insulin plays the primary role in regulating storage and mobilization of metabolic fuels, the beta cells must be constantly apprised of bodily needs, not only with regard to feeding and fasting, but also to the changing demands of the environment. Energy needs differ widely when individuals are at peace with their

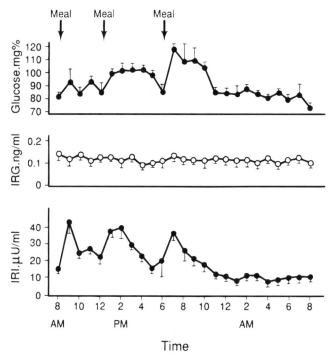

FIG. 17. Changes in the concentrations of plasma glucose, immunoreactive glucagon (*IRG*), and immunoreactive insulin (*IRI*) throughout the day. Values are the mean ± the standard error of the mean (n = 4). From Tasaka, Y., Sekine, M., Wakatsuki, M., et al. (1975): Levels of pancreatic glucagon, insulin, and glucose during twenty-four hours of the day in normal subjects. *Horm. Metab. Res.*, 7:205.

surroundings and when they are fighting for survival. Maintaining constancy of the internal environment is achieved through direct monitoring of circulating metabolites by the beta cells themselves. This input can be overridden or enhanced by hormonal or neural signals that prepare the individual for rapid storage of an influx of food or for massive mobilization of fuel reserves to permit a suitable response to environmental demands.

Glucose

Glucose is the most important regulator of insulin secretion. In the normal individual, its concentration in blood is maintained within the narrow range of 70 to 80 mg/dl after an overnight fast to perhaps about 150 mg/dl immediately after a glucose-rich meal. When the blood glucose level increases above a threshold value of about 100 mg/dl, insulin secretion increases proportionately. At lower concentrations, adjustments in insulin secretion are largely governed by other stimuli (see subsequent discussion) that act as amplifiers or inhibitors of the effects of glucose. The effectiveness of these agents therefore decreases as glucose concentration decreases.

Other Circulating Metabolites

Amino acids are important stimuli for insulin secretion. The transient increase in plasma amino acids after a protein-rich meal is accompanied by increased secretion of insulin. Arginine, lysine, and leucine are the most potent amino acid stimulators of insulin secretion. Insulin secreted at this time may facilitate storage of dietary amino acids as protein and prevents their diversion to gluconeogenesis. Amino acids are effective signals for insulin release only when blood glucose concentrations are adequate. Failure to increase insulin secretion when glucose is in short supply prevents hypoglycemia that might otherwise occur after a protein meal that contains little carbohydrate. Fatty acids and ketone bodies may also increase insulin secretion, but only when they are present at rather high concentrations. Because fatty acid mobilization and ketogenesis are inhibited by insulin, their ability to stimulate insulin secretion provides a feedback mechanism to protect against excessive mobilization of fatty acids and ketosis.

Hormonal and Neural Control

In response to carbohydrate in the lumen, the duodenal mucosa secretes a factor that stimulates the pancreas to release insulin even though blood glucose levels have not yet risen. This anticipatory secretion of insulin prepares tissues to cope with the coming influx of glucose and dampens what might otherwise be a large increase in blood sugar. Various gastrointestinal hormones, including gastrin, secretin, entero-glucagon, and gastric inhibitory peptide (GIP), can evoke insulin secretion when tested experimentally, but of these hormones, only GIP appears to be secreted in sufficient quantity in response to a meal.

The secretion of insulin in response to food in the intestine may also be mediated by a neural pathway. Sometimes the taste or smell of food or the expectation of eating increases insulin secretion. Parasympathetic fibers in the vagus nerve stimulate the beta cells by releasing acetylcholine or peptide neurotransmitters, such as vasoactive intestinal peptide (VIP). Activation of this pathway may be initiated within the brain and involves input from sensory endings in the mouth, stomach, or small intestine.

Insulin secretion by the human pancreas is virtually shut off by epinephrine or norepinephrine delivered to beta cells by either the circulation or sympathetic neurons. This inhibitory effect is seen even when the blood glucose level is high, and it is mediated through α_2 receptors on the surface of the beta cells. Physiological circumstances that activate the sympathetic nervous system thus can shut down insulin secretion and, thereby, remove the major restraint on mobilization of metabolic fuels needed to cope with an emergency.

The secretory activity of beta cells is also enhanced by growth hormone and cortisol by mechanisms that are not yet understood. Although they do not directly evoke a secretory response, basal insulin secretion is increased when these hormones are present in excess, and beta cells become hyperresponsive to signals for insulin secretion. Conversely, insulin secretion is reduced when either is deficient. Excessive growth hormone or cortisol decreases tissue sensitivity to insulin and can produce diabetes (see Chapter 9). The factors that regulate insulin secretion are shown in Fig. 18.

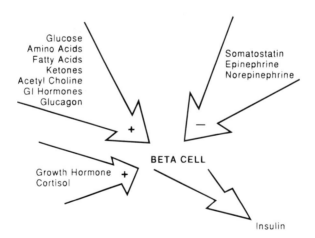

FIG. 18. Metabolic, hormonal, and neural influences on insulin secretion.

Cellular Events

Beta cells increase their rate of insulin secretion within 30 seconds of exposure to increased concentrations of glucose and can shut down secretion as rapidly. The question of how the concentration of glucose is monitored and translated into a rate of insulin secretion has not been answered completely, but some of the important steps are known. The beta cell has specific receptors for glucagon, acetylcholine, and other compounds that increase insulin secretion by promoting the formation of cyclic AMP or IP_3 and DAG (see Chapter 1), but it does not appear to have specific receptors for glucose. To affect insulin secretion, glucose must be metabolized by the beta cell, indicating that some consequence of glucose oxidation, rather than glucose itself is the critical determinant. Glucose is transported across beta cell membranes by GLUT 2, which has a high capacity, but relatively low affinity, for glucose. Consequently, as glucose concentrations increase above about 100 mg/dl, glucose enters the beta cell at a rate that is limited by its concentration and not by availability of transporters. It is likely that glucokinase behaves as a glucose sensor. It is specific for glucose, has the requisite kinetic characteristics, and catalyzes the rate-determining reaction for glucose metabolism in beta cells. Mutations that affect the function of this enzyme result in decreased insulin secretion in response to glucose that may be severe enough to cause a form of diabetes.

The secretion of insulin, like other peptide hormones, requires increased cytosolic calcium. Perhaps through the agency of a calmodulin-activated protein kinase, calcium promotes the movement of secretory granules to the periphery of the beta cell, the fusion of the granular membrane with the plasma membrane, and the consequent extrusion of the granular contents into the extracellular space. To increase insulin secretion, increased metabolism of glucose must somehow bring about an increase in intracellular calcium level. The linkage between glucose metabolism and intracellular calcium concentration appears to be achieved by their mutual relationship to cellular concentrations of adenosine triphosphate (ATP) and diphosphate (ADP).

In resting pancreatic beta cells, efflux of potassium through open potassium channels maintains the membrane potential at about -70 mV. Some potassium channels in these cells are sensitive to ATP, which inhibits (closes) them, and to ADP, which activates (opens) them. When blood glucose concentrations are low, the effects of ADP predominate, even though its concentration in beta cell cytoplasm is about 1,000 times lower than that of ATP. Because glucose transport is not rate limiting in beta cells, increased concentrations in the blood accelerate glucose oxidation and promote ATP formation at the expense of ADP. As a result, ADP levels become insufficient to counter the inhibitory effects of ATP, and potassium channels close. The consequent buildup of positive charge within the beta cell causes the membrane to depolarize, which activates voltage-sensitive calcium channels. Calcium rushing in through newly opened channels reverses the membrane potential and produces an electrical discharge that resembles an action potential. Recordings made in mouse beta cells indicate that the frequency and duration of electrical discharges increase as

glucose concentrations increase. In addition to triggering insulin secretion, elevated
intracellular calcium inhibits voltage-sensitive calcium channels and activates calcium-sensitive potassium channels, allowing potassium to exit and the cell to repolarize (Fig. 19).

Some evidence suggests that voltage-sensitive calcium channels may be substrates

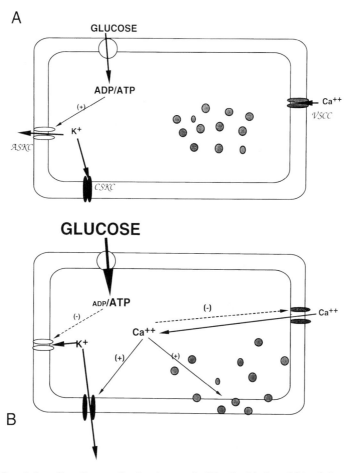

FIG. 19. Regulation of insulin secretion by glucose. **A:** "Resting" beta cell (blood glucose, <100
mg/dl). The ADP/ATP ratio is high enough so that ATP-sensitive potassium channels (*ASKC*)
are open, and the membrane potential is about −70 mV. The voltage-sensitive calcium channels
(*VSCC*) and calcium-sensitive potassium channels (*CSKC*) are closed. **B:** The beta cell response
to increased blood glucose. In response to the increased glucose entry and metabolism, the
ratio of ADP/ATP decreases, and the ATP-sensitive potassium channels close. The VSCC are
activated; calcium enters and stimulates insulin secretion. Increased cytosolic calcium inhibits
the VSCC and activates the CSKC, thereby allowing the cell membrane to repolarize and the
calcium channels to close. The persistence of high glucose levels results in repeated spiking of
electrical discharges and oscillation of intracellular calcium concentrations.

for protein kinase A and that phosphorylation may lower their threshold for activation. This might explain how glucagon and other hormones that activate adenylyl cyclase increase insulin secretion. Agents like acetylcholine increase IP_3 and may thus stimulate the release of calcium from intracellular storage sites. Norepinephrine blocks insulin secretion by way of the inhibitory guanine nucleotide binding protein, Gi (see Chapter 1), which may directly inhibit voltage-sensitive calcium channels as well as adenylyl cyclase.

SOMATOSTATIN

Biosynthesis, Secretion, and Metabolism

Somatostatin was originally isolated from hypothalamic extracts that inhibited the secretion of growth hormone. Somatostatin is widely distributed in many neural tissues where it presumably functions as a neurotransmitter. It is found in many secretory cells (delta cells) outside of the pancreatic islets, particularly in the lining of the gastrointestinal tract. Somatostatin is stored in membrane-bound vesicles and secreted by exocytosis. Measurable increases in the somatostatin concentration can be found in peripheral blood after ingestion of a meal rich in fat or protein. It is cleared rapidly from the blood and has a half-life of only about 3 minutes.

Physiological Actions

Aside from its role in the regulation of growth hormone secretion (see Chapter 10), the physiological importance of somatostatin is not understood. It inhibits secretion of both insulin and glucagon, perhaps by acting in a paracrine fashion, and inhibits secretion of various gastrointestinal hormones. In addition, somatostatin decreases intestinal motility and may slow the rate of absorption of nutrients from the digestive tract. Increased fecal excretion of fat is a prominent feature in patients suffering from somatostatin-secreting tumors. At the cellular level, the inhibitory effects of somatostatin are mediated by surface receptors that act through the inhibitory guanine nucleotide binding protein, Gi to inhibit adenylyl cyclase (see Chapter 1).

Regulation of Secretion

Increased concentrations of glucose or amino acids in blood stimulate somatostatin secretion. In addition, glucose or fat in the gastrointestinal tract elicits a secretory response by delta cells, mediated perhaps by glucagon or gastrointestinal hormones. Somatostatin secretion is also increased by norepinephrine and inhibited by acetyl-choline.

SUGGESTED READING

Becker, A. B., and Roth, R. A. (1990): Insulin receptor structure and function in normal and pathological conditions. *Annu. Rev. Med.*, 41:99–116.

Burant, C. F., Sivitz, W. I., Fukumoto, H., Kayano, T., Nagamatsu, S., Seino, S., Pessin, J. E., and Bell, G. I. (1991): Mammalian glucose transporters: structure and molecular regulation. *Recent Prog. Horm. Res.*, 47:349–387.

Goldfine, I. G. (1987): The insulin receptor: molecular biology and transmembrane signaling. *Endocr. Rev.*, 8:235–255.

Lawrence, J. C., Jr. (1992): Signal transduction and protein phosphorylation in the regulation of cellular metabolism by insulin. *Annu. Rev. Physiol.*, 54:177–193.

Miller, R. E. (1981): Pancreatic neuroendocrinology: peripheral neural mechanisms in the regulation of the islets of Langerhans. *Endocr. Rev.*, 2:471–494.

Pilkis, S. J., and Granner, D. K. (1992): Molecular physiology of the regulation of hepatic gluconeogenesis and glycolysis. *Annu. Rev. Physiol.*, 54:885–909.

Prentki, M., and Matschinski, F. M. (1987): Ca^{+2}, cAMP, and phospholipid-derived messengers in coupling mechanisms of insulin secretion. *Physiol. Rev.*, 67:1185–1248.

Rajan, A. S., Aguilar-Bryan, L., Nelson, D. A., Yaney, G. C., Hsu, W. H., Kunze, D. L., and Boyd, A. E., III (1990): Ion channels and insulin secretion. *Diabetes Care.*, 13:340–363.

Taylor, S. I., Cama, A., Accili, D., Barbetti, F., Quon, M. J., de la Luz Sierra, M., Suzuki, Y., Koller, E., Levy-Toledano, R., Wertheimer, E., Moncada, V. Y., Kadowaki, H., and Kadowaki, T. (1992): Mutations in the insulin receptor gene. *Endocr. Rev.*, 13:566–595.

Simpson, I. A., and Cushman, S. W. (1986): Hormonal regulation of mammalian glucose transport. *Annu. Rev. Biochem.*, 55:1059–1089.

Unger, R. H., and Orci, L. (1976): Physiology and pathophysiology of glucagon. *Physiol. Rev.*, 56:778–838.

6

Principles of Hormonal Integration

Until now, we have considered individual endocrine glands, and some basic information about their physiological functions. While it is helpful for the student first to understand one hormone at a time or one gland at a time, it must be recognized that life is considerably more complex and that endocrinological solutions to physiological problems require integration of a large variety of simultaneous events. In this section, we will consider some of the general principles of endocrine integration. In the ensuing chapters, we will see the application of these principles to the solution of physiological problems.

REDUNDANCY

Survival in a hostile environment has been made possible by the evolution of failsafe mechanisms to govern crucial functions. Just as each organ system has a built-in excess capacity, giving it the potential to function at levels beyond the usual day-to-day demands, so too, is there an excess regulatory capacity provided in the form of seemingly duplicative or overlapping controls. Simply put, the body has more than one way to achieve a given end. For example, as we have seen, the conversion of liver glycogen to blood glucose can be signaled by at least two hormones, glucagon from the alpha cells of the pancreas and epinephrine from the adrenal medulla (Fig. 1). Both of these hormones increase cyclic adenosine monophosphate (AMP) production in the liver and, thereby, activate the enzyme, phosphorylase, which catalyzes glycogenolysis. Two hormones secreted from two different tissues, sometimes in response to different conditions, thus produce the same end result.

Further redundancy can also be seen at the molecular level. Using the same example of conversion of liver glycogen to blood glucose, there are even two ways that epinephrine can activate phosphorylase. By stimulating β-adrenergic receptors, epinephrine increases cyclic AMP formation as already mentioned. By stimulating α-adrenergic receptors, epinephrine also activates phosphorylase, but these receptors

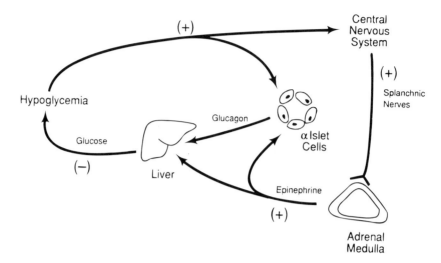

FIG. 1. Redundant mechanisms to stimulate hepatic glucose production.

operate through the agency of increased intracellular calcium concentrations produced by the release of inositol 1,4,5 trisphosphate (Fig. 2).

Redundant mechanisms not only ensure that a critical process will take place, but they also offer the opportunities for flexibility and subtle fine tuning of a process. Though redundant in the respect that two different hormones may have some overlapping effects, the actions of the two hormones are usually not identical in all respects. Within the physiological range of its concentrations in blood, glucagon's action is restricted to the liver; epinephrine produces a variety of other responses in many extrahepatic tissues while increasing glycogenolysis in the liver. Variations in the

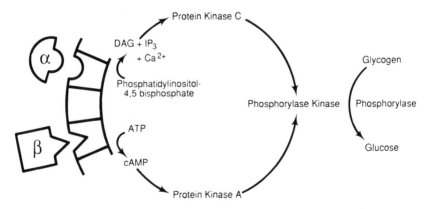

FIG. 2. Redundant mechanisms to activate glycogen phosphorylase by a single hormone, epinephrine, acting through both α and β receptors.

relative input from both hormones allows for a wide spectrum of changes in blood glucose concentrations relative to such other effects of epinephrine as increased heart rate.

Two hormones which produce common effects may differ, not only in their range of actions, but also in their time constants (Fig. 3). One may have a more rapid onset and shorter duration of action, while another may have a longer duration of action, but a slower onset. For example, epinephrine increases blood concentrations of free fatty acids (FFA) within seconds or minutes, and this effect dissipates as rapidly when epinephrine secretion is stopped. Growth hormone similarly increases blood concentrations of FFA, but its effects are seen only after a lag period of two or three hours and persist for many hours. A hormone like epinephrine may therefore be used to meet short-term needs, and another, like growth hormone, may answer sustained needs.

Redundancy also pertains to processes in which the same end may be achieved by more than one physiological means. For example, blood concentrations of calcium may be increased by an action of the parathyroid hormone to mobilize calcium stored in bone crystals (Chapter 7), or by an action of vitamin D to promote calcium absorption from the gut. These processes, as might be expected, have different time constants as well.

Finally, redundancy may also lead to the phenomenon of *synergism* or *potentiation*. Two or more hormones are said to act synergistically when the response to their simultaneous administration is greater than the sum of the responses to each when given alone. For example, both growth hormone and cortisol modestly increase lipolysis in adipocytes. When given simultaneously, however, glycerol production was nearly twice as great as the sum of the effects of each (Fig. 4).

One of the implications of redundancy for our understanding both of normal physiology and endocrine disease, is that partial, or perhaps even complete, failure

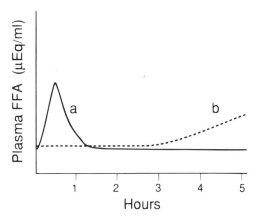

FIG. 3. Idealized representation of the effects of epinephrine and growth hormone on plasma concentrations of FFA.

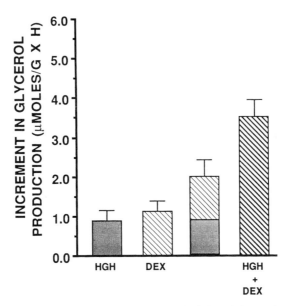

FIG. 4. Synergistic effects of human growth hormone (*HGH*) and the synthetic glucocorticoid dexamethasone (*DEX*) on glycerol production in rat adipocytes. The unlabeled column shows the algebraic sum of the individual effects of HGH and DEX which is only about half as large as that produced by these hormones in combination (HGH and DEX). From Gorin, E., Tai, L.-R., Honeyman, T.W., et al. (1990): Evidence for a role of protein kinase C in the stimulation of lipolysis by growth hormone and isoproterenol. *Endocrinology.* 126:2973.

of one mechanism can be compensated by increased reliance on another mechanism. Thus, functional deficiencies may only be evident in subtle ways and may not show up readily as overt disease. Some deficiencies may only become apparent after appropriate provocation or perturbation of the system. Conversely, strategies for therapeutic interventions designed to increase or decrease the rate of a process must take into account the redundant inputs that regulate that process. Merely accelerating or blocking one regulatory input may not produce the desired effect since independent adjustments in redundant pathways may completely compensate for the intervention.

REINFORCEMENT

It is an oversimplification to think of any hormone as simply having a single unique effect. In accomplishing any end, most hormones act at several locales either within a single cell, or in different tissues or organs to produce separate but mutually reinforcing responses. In some cases, a hormone may produce radically different responses at different locales, which, nevertheless, reinforce each other from the perspective of the whole organism. Let us consider, for example, just some of the ways insulin acts on the fat cell to promote storage of triglycerides.

1. It increases the uptake of glucose which serves as substrate for fatty acid synthesis and for the α-glycerol phosphate needed to trap any free fatty acids formed by spontaneous lipolysis of triglyceride stores.
2. It activates several enzymes critical for fatty acid synthesis, e.g., pyruvate dehydrogenase, pyruvate carboxylase, and acetyl coenzyme A carboxylase.
3. It inhibits the breakdown of already formed triglycerides.
4. It induces the synthesis of the extracellular enzyme, lipoprotein lipase, needed to take up lipids from the circulation.

Any one of these effects might accomplish the end of increasing fat storage, but collectively, these different effects make possible an enormously broader range of response in a shorter time frame. These effects of insulin will be considered further in Chapter 9.

Reinforcement can also take the form of a single hormone acting in different ways in different tissues to produce complementary effects. A good example of this is the action of glucocorticoid hormones to promote gluconeogenesis. As we have seen (Chapter 4, Fig. 13), glucocorticoids promote protein breakdown in the muscle and lymphoid tissues and the consequent release of amino acids into the blood. In the liver, glucocorticoids induce the formation of the enzymes necessary to convert amino acids and other substrates into glucose. Either the extrahepatic action to provide the substrate or the hepatic action to increase the capacity to utilize that substrate would increase gluconeogenesis. Together, these complementary actions increase the overall magnitude and speed of the response.

PUSH–PULL MECHANISMS

As discussed in Chapter 1, many critical processes are under dual control by agents that act antagonistically either to stimulate or to inhibit them. Such dual control allows for more precise regulation through negative feedback. The example cited was hepatic production of glucose, which is increased by glucagon and inhibited by insulin. In emergency situations or during exercise, epinephrine and norepinephrine released from the adrenal medulla and sympathetic nerve endings override both negative feedback systems by inhibiting insulin secretion and stimulating glucagon secretion (Fig. 5). The effect of adding a stimulatory influence and simultaneously removing an inhibitory influence is a rapid and large response, more rapid and larger than could be achieved by simply affecting either hormone alone, or than could be accomplished by the direct glycogenolytic effect of epinephrine or norepinephrine.

Another type of push–pull mechanism can be seen at the molecular level. The net synthesis of glycogen from glucose depends upon the activity of two enzymes, glycogen synthase, which catalyzes the formation of glycogen from glucose, and glycogen phosphorylase, which catalyzes glycogen breakdown (Fig. 6). Net reaction rate is determined by the balance of the activity of these two enzymes. The activity of both enzymes is subject to regulation by phosphorylation, but in opposite directions, i.e., addition of a phosphate group activates phosphorylase but inactivates

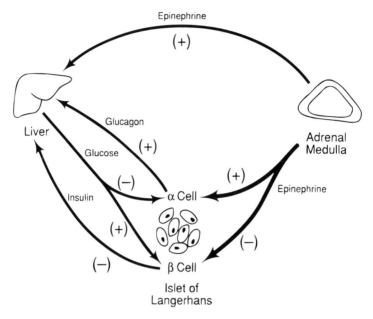

FIG. 5. Push–pull mechanism. Epinephrine inhibits insulin secretion while promoting glucagon secretion.

synthase. In this case, a single agent, cyclic AMP, which activates protein kinase A, increases the activity of phosphorylase and simultaneously inhibits synthase.

MODULATION OF RESPONDING SYSTEMS

In discussing the responses of tissues to stimulation by hormones, we have spoken as though a given amount of hormone always produces the same amount of response, i.e., that both the sensitivity of target tissues to hormonal stimulation and their capacity to respond are constant. This is often not the case. The sensitivity to stimulation and the capacity to respond are two separate though related aspects of hormonal response. *Sensitivity* describes the acuity of a cell's ability to recognize a signal and to respond in proportion to the intensity of that signal. We can define sensitivity in terms of the concentration of hormone that will bring about 50% of the maximum response. The *capacity to respond,* or the maximum response that a tissue is capable of giving, depends upon the amount of competent or differentiated cells in that tissue as well as the level of development of the enzymatic machinery within those cells (Figs. 7 A and B). Hormones regulate both the sensitivity and the capacity of target tissues to respond either to themselves or to other hormones.

One mechanism by which hormones determine the sensitivity of target tissues is by regulation of hormone receptors. It should be recalled that the initial event in

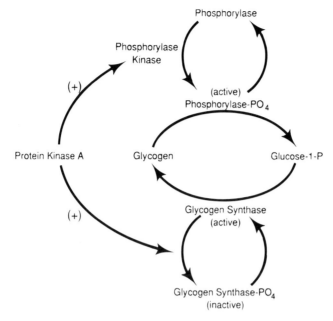

FIG. 6. Push–pull mechanism to activate glycogen phosphorylase while simultaneously inhibiting glycogen synthase.

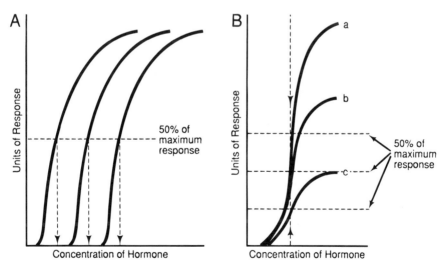

FIG. 7. A: Dose–response curves showing different levels of sensitivity. The *arrows* indicate the concentrations of hormone needed to produce a half-maximal response. **B:** Dose response curves showing different capacities to respond. Note that the concentration needed for the half maximal response shown by the arrows is identical for all these curves.

producing a hormonal response is the interaction of the hormone with its receptor. The higher the concentration of hormone, the more likely it is that there will be an interaction with receptors. If there are no hormone receptors, however, there can be no response, and the more receptors that are available to interact with a given amount of hormone, the more likely is there to be a response. In other words, the likelihood that hormone–receptor interaction will occur is related to the abundance of both the hormone and the receptor. Although the affinity of the receptor for its hormone may also be modulated, in general, it appears to be the number of receptors, rather than their affinity for hormone, that is usually modulated.

Some hormones decrease the number of their own receptors in target tissues. This so-called *down regulation* was originally recognized as a real phenomenon in modern endocrinology when it was shown that the decreased sensitivity of some cells to insulin in hyperinsulin states resulted from a decrease in the number of receptors on the cell surface. However, a similar phenomenon was observed many years earlier by Cannon and Rosenblueth who described the ''supersensitivity of denervated tissues.'' Cannon's original discovery of this phenomenon concerned the hypersensitivity of the denervated heart to circulating epinephrine and norepinephrine. The generality of this phenomenon for both endocrine and neural control systems is further indicated by the increase in acetylcholine receptors that occurs after a muscle is denervated and the restoration to normal after reinnervation. The phenomenon of *tachyphylaxis*, or loss of responsiveness to a pharmacological agent upon repeated or constant exposure, may be another example of down regulation of receptors. Down regulation may result from the inactivation of the receptors at the cell surface, an increased rate of destruction of internalized hormone receptor complexes, or decreased receptor synthesis.

Down regulation is not limited to the effects of a hormone on its own receptor or to the surface receptors for the water-soluble hormones. One hormone can down regulate the receptors for another hormone. This appears to be the mechanism by which triiodothyronine decreases the sensitivity of the thyrotropes of the pituitary to thyrotropin-releasing hormone (see Chapter 3). Similarly, progesterone may down regulate both its own receptor and that of estrogen as well.

Up regulation, or the increase in available receptors, also occurs and can be seen both for receptors on the cell surface and for the internal receptors of the lipid-soluble hormones. Prolactin, and possibly growth hormone, may up regulate their receptors in responsive cells. Estrogen up regulates both its own receptors and those of luteinizing and follicle-stimulating hormones in ovarian cells during the menstrual cycle (see Chapter 12). The molecular mechanisms for up regulation are not understood at this time and are the subject of intensive research. It appears that up regulation, such as that produced by estrogen, is initiated by a change in gene expression.

The sensitivity to hormonal stimulation can also be modulated in ways that may not involve receptors. Postreceptor modulation may affect any of the steps in the biological pathway through which hormonal effects are produced. For example, the activity of cyclic AMP phosphodiesterase increases in adipose tissue in the absence of pituitary hormones. It may be recalled (see Chapter 1) that this enzyme catalyzes the degradation of cyclic AMP, and when its activity is increased, less cyclic AMP can accumulate after the stimulation of adenylyl cyclase by a hormone such as epinephrine. Therefore, if all other things were equal, a higher concentration of epinephrine would be needed to produce a given amount of lipolysis than might be necessary in the presence of normal amounts of pituitary hormones, and hence, the sensitivity to epinephrine appears to be reduced.

Increased activity of phosphodiesterase is only one of several factors contributing to decreased sensitivity to epinephrine in adipose tissue of hypopituitary animals. These tissues also have a defect in their capacity to respond to cyclic AMP because of deficiencies in hormone-sensitive lipase. Therefore, even when all of the receptors are occupied, the maximum response that these tissues can make is below normal. Hormones can also increase the capacity of target cells or tissues to respond to other stimuli. For example, estradiol increases the synthesis of prolactin in pituitary lactotropes (see Chapter 13) and, hence, increases prolactin secretion in response to physiological stimuli. An even more obvious way that a hormone can increase the capacity of a tissue to respond to physiological stimuli is to increase or decrease the number of cells in the target tissues. For example, the gradual increase in estradiol secretion seen in the early part of the menstrual cycle reflects the activity of an increasing number of granulosa cells rather than a change in gonadotropin secretion.

Another aspect of hormone modulation that is related to these examples has been called *permissive action*. This was already discussed in Chapter 4 for the adrenal cortical hormones. A hormone acts permissively when its presence is necessary for, or permits, a biological response to occur, even though the hormone does not initiate the response. Permissive effects were originally described for the adrenal cortical hormones, but they appear to occur for other hormones as well. Permissive actions are not limited to responses to hormones but pertain to any cellular response to any signal.

7

Regulation of Sodium and Water Balance

H. Maurice Goodman and John C. S. Fray

OVERVIEW

Sodium and water balance are precisely regulated by the endocrine system. Osmolality of the extracellular fluid is monitored and adjusted by regulating water excretion by the kidney in response to antidiuretic hormone (ADH) which is secreted by the posterior lobe of the pituitary gland. Constancy of blood osmolality ensures constancy of cellular volume, but if it were attained only by adjusting water retention, the vascular volume would fluctuate widely. Therefore, blood volume must also be precisely regulated so that it is sufficient to ensure perfusion of body tissues but not so expanded that blood pressure is increased. Maintenance of vascular volume depends on maintenance of sodium balance. Renal mechanisms that govern retention or loss of sodium are regulated by the renin–angiotensin–aldosterone system and the atrial natriuretic hormone. Also ADH contributes directly to volume regulation, and when demands for constancy of osmolality are in conflict with demands for constancy of volume, the latter prevails. These hormonal mechanisms operate largely by regulating renal function, but they also regulate salt and water intake.

GENERAL CONSIDERATIONS

All cells of the body have an uninterrupted requirement for nutrients and oxygen and produce waste materials. In addition, many cells must receive signals from other parts of the body to perform their specialized tasks, which in some cases, includes the production of some product that must be transported to other specialized cells. The cardiovascular system accommodates these nutritive, excretory, and communicative needs. Blood readily equilibrates with the fluid that bathes each cell and, thereby, preserves the integrity of the extracellular environment, delivers chemical messages, and transports excretory and secretory products. The integrity of the blood

152

is restored as it flows through such organs as the kidneys, lungs, and liver, whose specialized functions renew the blood's composition and maintain its constancy.

Perfusion of tissues is ensured by maintaining both a sufficient volume of arterial blood and an adequate pressure to drive it through the capillaries. Blood flow to a region is matched to changing requirements of cells by locally initiated adjustments in arteriolar tone. Circularly oriented smooth muscle cells in arterioles relax in response to products of cellular metabolism and thus decrease resistance to flow. Increased flow washes away accumulated products, and with removal of the signal for vasodilation, arterioles regain their former tone. The circulatory system can thus be viewed as a central reservoir of pressurized fluid that can be tapped on demand at any locale to provide needed renewal of the cellular environment.

Several factors go into maintenance of the central reservoir of pressure: (a) the beating of the heart that provides energy, (b) a high degree of arteriolar tone that slows dissipation of the energy imparted by each beat of the heart, (c) low compliance of the arterial tree that allows pressure to build up, and (d) a sufficient volume of blood to fill the system. Central control exerted through the autonomic nervous system provides the minute-to-minute adjustments to cardiac function and arteriolar constriction that maintain the blood pressure relatively constant. Volume is regulated largely by the endocrine system, but volume and pressure are closely interrelated. Changes in volume can offset changes in arteriolar tone and vice versa to maintain constancy or at least adequacy of the central pressure reservoir. It is not surprising, therefore, that hormones that play decisive roles in regulating blood volume also constrict or dilate arterioles.

Permeability of capillaries to small molecules allows blood in the vascular compartment to equilibrate quickly with interstitial fluid. Blood and interstitial fluid together comprise the extracellular compartment, which contains about one third of total body water. Water distributes freely between the vascular compartment and the interstitial compartment, usually in a ratio of 1:3. In some pathological states, however, the interstitial compartment becomes disproportionately enlarged, and edema may be considerable. Major determinants of this distribution are the protein content of plasma, principally albumin, and blood pressure within the capillaries. It appears that the volume of the interstitial compartment is not directly monitored or regulated. Rather, control of interstitial volume is achieved indirectly by controlling pressure, composition, and volume of the vascular compartment.

The volumes of fluid in the intracellular and extracellular compartments are also determined by their solute contents. With a few important exceptions in the kidney, biological membranes are freely permeable to water. Net movement of water into or out of cells is determined by the osmotic gradient. Osmotic flow of water is independent of the identity of solutes and responds simply to the discrepancy in number of solute particles (osmolytes) on either side of the cell membrane. Addition or depletion of water in one compartment therefore is followed by compensatory changes in the other. Concentrations of particular solutes on the extracellular or intracellular sides of the plasma membrane are different, however, and are determined by the properties of the membrane.

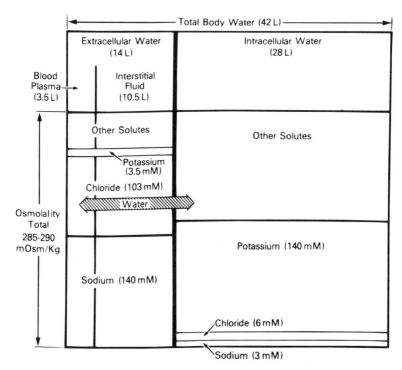

FIG. 1. The distribution of body water and the principal electrolytes. Note that water and electrolytes equilibrate freely between plasma and interstitial fluid, but only water equilibrates between the intracellular and extracellular compartments.

The major intracellular cation is potassium, whose concentration in cellular water is nearly 35 times higher than that in extracellular water. The major extracellular cation is sodium (Fig. 1), which is nearly absent in intracellular water. Blood plasma is in osmotic equilibrium with interstitial and intracellular fluids; therefore, regulation of plasma osmolality regulates total body osmolality. Because sodium is the major contributor to osmolality of blood and because it is largely excluded from the intracellular compartment, changes in sodium balance can change both the distribution of body water and its total volume. Thus, homeostatic regulation of blood volume depends on regulation of intake and excretion of sodium as well as water.

SALT AND WATER BALANCE

Salt and water balance are maintained remarkably constant despite wide variations in intake and loss of both sodium and water. Intake of sodium may vary from almost none in salt-poor environments to several grams during a binge of potato chips and pretzels. Output is primarily in urine, but smaller losses are also incurred in sweat and feces. Large losses can result from excessive sweating, vomiting, diarrhea, burns, or hemorrhage. The kidney is a powerful regulator of sodium output and can preserve sodium balance even when daily intake varies over the 4,000-fold range between 50 mg and 200 g.

Under basal conditions, the typical adult turns over about 1.75 liters of water each day. Most of it originates in the diet in the form of solid and liquid foods, and the remainder is formed metabolically from the oxidation of carbohydrate and fat. Unavoidable losses occur by evaporation from the lungs and skin, as well as by elimination of wastes in the urine and feces. Environment, climate, daily activities, and personal habits impose additional needs for either intake or excretion that must be perfectly offset to maintain physiological balance. So long as intake exceeds obligatory losses, balance can be achieved by controlling excretion. Intake, however, is a voluntary act and varies widely. Thirst and salt appetite are increased when intake falls below the amount needed to maintain balance.

Blood volume is monitored indirectly, primarily as a function of pressure. The concentration of sodium, which is the principal osmolyte of plasma and the primary determinant of blood volume, is monitored only indirectly as a function of osmolality. The kidney is the primary effector of regulation, and at least four hormones—ADH, aldosterone, angiotensin II, and atrial natriuretic hormone (also called atrial natriuretic peptide, ANP, or atriopeptin)—are used to signal regulatory adjustments.

Antidiuretic Hormone

Antidiuretic hormone (ADH) which is also called arginine vasopressin, is primarily responsible for signaling changes in water balance; it is also a potent arteriolar constrictor. As indicated in Chapter 2, it is synthesized in hypothalamic neurons whose cell bodies are located in the supraoptic and paraventricular nuclei. Axons of these cells pass down the pituitary stalk and terminate in the posterior lobe of the pituitary gland from whence the hormone is secreted. Antidiuretic hormone acts on cells of the collecting ducts in the kidney to regulate water balance and on arterioles in skeletal muscle and skin to produce its vasoconstrictor effects.

Antidiuretic Effect

To understand how ADH promotes net absorption of water, we must first consider some basic aspects of renal function. Urine is generated as an ultrafiltrate of blood plasma, and hence, its solute content initially is nearly identical to that of plasma. The final composition of urine is determined by selective reabsorption and secretion of solutes as the tubular fluid passes down the length of the nephron (Fig. 2). Water is reabsorbed passively and follows reabsorption of solute. About two thirds of the fluid is reabsorbed isosmotically in the initial segment of the nephron, the proximal convoluted tubule. The volume is further reduced in the next segment, but more importantly, the activity of cells that form this portion of the tubule generate an

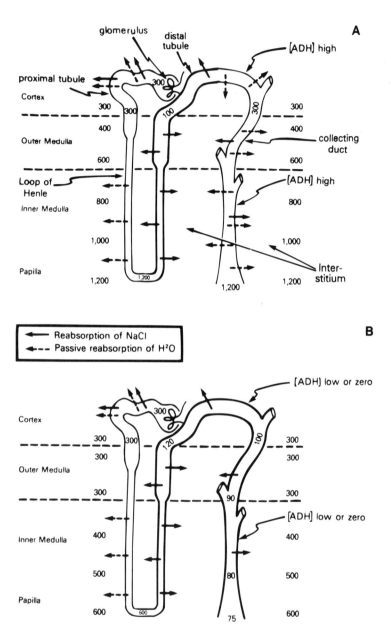

FIG. 2. A typical nephron, showing the principal sites of salt and water reabsorption in the presence (**A**) and absence (**B**) of ADH. *Heavy lines* outline the portions of the nephron that are impermeable to water. The numbers indicate (in milliosmoles per kilogram of water) the osmolality of interstitial and tubular fluid at various levels within the kidney. ADH produces the cellular changes that make the collecting ducts permeable to water and, thus, permits tubular fluid to equilibrate osmotically with interstitial fluid. Modified from Valtin, H. (1983): *Renal Function*, 2nd ed., p. 162, Little, Brown, Boston.

osmotic gradient. This part of the nephron, called the loop of Henle, is shaped like a hairpin, and doubles back on itself in the renal medulla. The combination of this unusual geometry, selective ion movements, and flow of urine within the tubule concentrates solutes in the tubular and interstitial fluid. In the deepest portions of the medulla, the osmolality may be four to five times that of plasma, and it diminishes progressively in more superficial regions of the medulla. After passage through the loop of Henle, tubular fluid is hypoosmolar with respect to blood. Selective reabsorption of ions in the the initial segment of the distal convoluted tubule makes the fluid even more dilute by the time it enters the cortical portion of the collecting ducts.

The collecting ducts extend from the cortex through the medulla and terminate in the renal pelvis. Therefore, fluid that is hypoosmolar when it enters the collecting ducts must pass through regions of increasing osmolality before entering the ureter. The amount of water excreted or reabsorbed is determined by the permeability of the collecting ducts. When they are freely permeable to water, osmotic equilibrium can occur, water (and urea) can flow from the lumen into the interstitium, and a maximally concentrated urine is produced. That is, there is disproportionately more excretion of solutes than of water, and hence, ''free water'' is retained. If, on the other hand, the collecting ducts remain impermeable to water, a dilute urine is produced, and free water is excreted.

Antidiuretic hormone promotes water conservation by stimulating cellular changes that make the collecting ducts permeable to water. In addition, ADH contributes to development of the osmotic gradient by increasing sodium chloride transport by cells of the thick portion of the ascending limb of Henle's loop. In the absence of ADH, the kidney can produce only a dilute urine. The disease state associated with a deficiency of ADH is called *diabetes insipidus* and is characterized by copious production of dilute urine. With this condition, more than 20 liters of water may be excreted per day. The term insipidus, meaning tasteless, was adopted to distinguish the consequences of ADH deficiency from those of insulin deficiency (diabetes mellitus) in which there is copious production of glucose-laden urine (see Chapter 5). *Nephrogenic diabetes insipidus* is the disease that results from failure of the kidney to respond to ADH. In the *syndrome of inappropriate secretion of ADH*, death may result from profound dilution of plasma electrolytes because of an inability to excrete a dilute urine and, hence, free water.

The mechanisms that regulate permeability of cells in the collecting ducts are not fully understood. Upon binding to specific receptors on the basolateral surface of target cells, ADH activates adenylyl cyclase. The consequent generation of cyclic AMP and activation of protein kinase A mediates molecular changes that lead to increased permeability to water (Fig. 3). According to the current view, ADH mobilizes certain proteins in intracellular storage vesicles and promotes their insertion into the luminal membrane of the duct cells. These proteins are thought to serve as channels that allow passage of water across cell membranes. This mechanism is analogous to the mobilization of glucose carriers and their insertion into fat cell

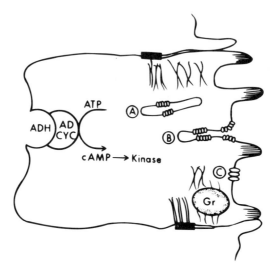

FIG. 3. An ADH-sensitive cell. *A,* cytoplasmic tubule containing water-conducting channels; *B,* fusion and delivery of channels to the luminal membrane; *C,* channels inserted in the membrane; *Gr,* large granule of unknown function; *AD CYC,* adenylyl cyclase. From Hays, R.M. (1983): Alteration of luminal membrane structure by antidiuretic hormone. *Am. J. Physiol.,* 245:289.

membranes described in Chapter 5 to account for increased glucose transport in response to insulin.

Effects on Blood Pressure

Antidiuretic hormone owes its other name, vasopressin, to its ability to constrict vascular smooth muscle and, therefore, increase blood pressure. Vasopressor and antidiuretic effects are mediated by two different receptors called V_1 and V_2. The V_1 receptor is found in smooth muscle while the V_2 receptor is found in renal tubules. The V_1 receptors have a lower affinity for ADH than V_2 receptors (i.e., they require a higher concentration of hormone to be stimulated), and they signal cellular changes with the diacylglycerol–inositol trisphosphate messenger system instead of the cyclic adenosine monophosphate (AMP) system utilized by the V_2 receptors.

Vasopressin may be the most potent naturally occurring constrictor of vascular smooth muscle. On a molar basis, it is at least ten times more active than norepinephrine or angiotensin II in stimulating contraction of isolated strips of artery. Increases in total peripheral resistance are observed at concentrations of ADH that fall within the upper part of the range that promotes water reabsorption. Small increases in peripheral resistance produced by ADH are not accompanied by increased systemic blood pressure, however, because the baroreceptor reflexes mediate compensatory decreases in heart rate and cardiac output and because ADH may decrease cardiac contractility secondary to coronary arteriolar constriction. Because not all arterioles are equally sensitive to it, ADH does not increase resistance uniformly in all vascular beds. Consequently, there is a redistribution of blood flow, which decreases most profoundly in the skin and skeletal muscle. Redistribution can compensate for decreased blood volume by making a disproportionate share of the cardiac output available to essential tissues, such as the brain. Arteriolar constriction also changes the distribution of fluid between the vascular and interstitial compartments. By constricting arterioles, ADH lowers capillary and venular blood pressure and, thereby, promotes net reabsorption of interstitial fluid in the skin and skeletal muscle. The intravascular volume increases, therefore, at the expense of the interstitial compartment.

Regulation of ADH Secretion

Plasma Osmolality

The most important stimulus for ADH secretion is an increase in blood osmolality. Little or no ADH is secreted so long as the osmolality of the plasma remains at or below a threshold value of about 280 mOsm/liter. The osmoreceptors are exquisitely sensitive and elicit increased secretion of ADH when the osmolality increases by as little as 1% to 2%. Above the osmolar threshold, the concentration of ADH in plasma changes in direct proportion to the increase in plasma osmolality (Fig. 4) and decreases urine volume significantly.

The osmoreceptors behave as though they are surrounded by a selectively permeable membrane that allows water to pass freely but restricts movement of most solutes. Sodium chloride, which is largely excluded from cells, is perhaps the most potent osmolyte, as judged by its ability to increase ADH secretion; a more permeant molecule, such as urea, has only a small effect. The osmoreceptors are thought to reside in the *organum vasculosum* in the anteroventral region of the third ventricle. This region lies outside the blood–brain barrier and derives its blood supply from the internal carotid artery. The osmoreceptors communicate with ADH-producing cells in the supraoptic and paraventricular nuclei to form a typical neuroendocrine reflex. In rats, intracarotid injection of concentrated saline increased the electrical activity of nerve cells in the supraoptic and paraventricular nuclei.

Blood Volume

Changes in blood volume are sensed by receptors in both the arterial (high pressure) and venous (low pressure) sides of the circulation. Volume is monitored indirectly as the tension exerted on stretch receptors located (a) on the arterial side, in the carotid sinuses and aortic arch, and (b) on the venous side, in the atria and perhaps the thoracic veins. Low-pressure receptors monitor central venous pressure, which can vary widely with a redistribution of blood, as might occur with changes in posture, physical activity, and ambient temperature. Central venous pressure can

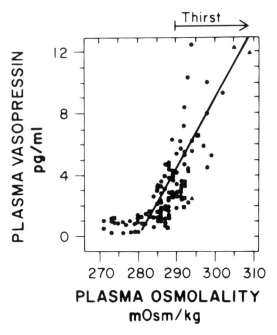

FIG. 4. The relationship between vasopressin (ADH) and osmolality in plasma of unanesthetized rats. Note the appearance of thirst (increased drinking behavior) when plasma osmolality exceeds 290 mOsm/kg. From Robertson, G.L. and Berl, T. (1986): Water Metabolism. In: *The Kidney*, 3rd ed., edited by Brenner, B.M. and Rector, F.C., Jr. p. 392, Saunders, Philadelphia.

fall by as much as 10% to 15% when an individual simply rises from a recumbent to an upright posture. Thus, there is a wide range over which deviations in venous pressure are not reliable indicators of true variations in volume. Because of the extensive buffering capacity of the baroreceptor reflexes, changes in arterial pressure are seen only after large decreases in blood volume. Thus, changes in volume on the order a few percent are difficult to detect and do not elicit compensatory adjustments in fluid balance.

At normal osmolality, ADH secretion is minimal so long as the blood volume remains at or above its physiological threshold or set point. Because the volume receptors are not equipped to detect small changes, stimulation of ADH secretion is not initiated until a relatively large depletion has occurred. The minimal change needed for low-pressure receptors to signal ADH secretion is a 10% to 15% reduction in volume. Similarly, a loss of 10% to 15% of the blood volume can occur before the threshold for the high-pressure volume receptors is reached. Secretion of ADH in response to a decrease in volume is thus an emergency response and not a fine tuner of blood volume. Retention of free water alone is not an effective means of defending the plasma volume. Because it distributes in all compartments, only about

1 ml of every 12 ml of free water retained remains in the vascular compartment. However, when volume falls below a critical threshold value, a potentially life-threatening event is perceived and vigorous secretion of ADH increases blood levels exponentially (Fig. 5).

Because the ADH-secreting cells of the supraoptic and paraventricular nuclei are stimulated by two inputs—increased osmolality and decreased volume—they must be able to integrate these signals and respond appropriately. Decreases in volume or pressure heighten the sensitivity of the osmoreceptors and lower the threshold for ADH secretion in response to increased osmolality (Fig. 6). Volume depletion and increased osmolality, as might result from dehydration, for example, stimulate ADH secretion and reinforce each other. Situations can arise, however, when inputs from osmotic and volume receptors conflict. As a general rule, osmolality is preferentially guarded when the depletion of volume is small. When volume loss is large, however, osmolality is sacrificed in order to maintain the integrity of the circulation.

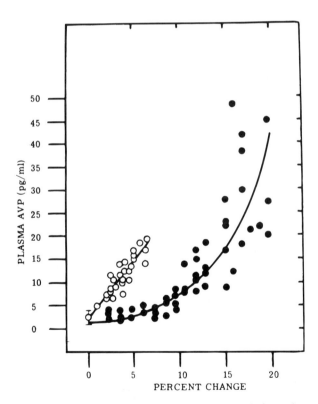

FIG. 5. The relationship between changes in osmolality (*open circles*) or volume (*solid circles*) and ADH (AVP) in plasma of unanesthetized rats. From Dunn, F.L., Brennan, T.J., Nelson, A.E., et al. (1973): The role of blood osmolality and volume in regulating vasopressin secretion in the rat. *J. Clin. Invest.*, 52:3212.

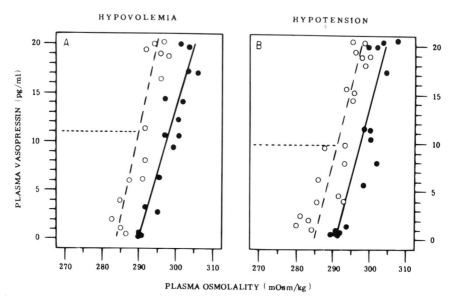

FIG. 6. The relationship between vasopressin (ADH) concentrations and osmolality in plasma of unanesthetized rats made hypovolemic or hypotensive. In normal animals (*solid circles*), the plasma concentrations of ADH increased sharply as the plasma osmolality increased above 290 mOsm/kg. A similar increase occurred in hypovolemic or hypotensive animals (*open circles*), but these animals were more sensitive to changes in osmolality, as indicated in the leftward shift in the curves. The threshold for increased ADH secretion shifted from about 290 mOsm/kg in the normal animals to less than 285 mOsm/kg in the hypovolemic or hypotensive animals. From Robertson, G.L. (1977): The regulation of vasopressin function in health and disease. *Recent Prog. Horm. Res.*, 33:333.

ALDOSTERONE

As already detailed in Chapter 4, aldosterone is an adrenal steroid that plays a pivotal role in maintaining salt and water balance. Angiotensin II is the primary stimulus for aldosterone secretion, although corticotropin (ACTH) and high concentrations of potassium are also potent stimuli. Aldosterone secretion may also be stimulated by a profound decrease in the plasma sodium concentration, but the required concentration of sodium is well below that found under normal physiological circumstances.

Aldosterone is secreted by cells of the zona glomerulosa and acts principally on the cortical portion of the renal collecting ducts to promote absorption of sodium and excretion of potassium and hydrogen ions. It may be recalled that aldosterone does not stimulate a simple one-for-one exchange of sodium for potassium in the nephron. More sodium is retained than potassium is excreted. Selective retention of sodium obligates simultaneous reabsorption of water by the nephron and expands the vascular volume accordingly. The renal effects of aldosterone are augmented by similar effects on sweat and salivary glands and by a poorly understood effect on

TABLE 1. *Comparison of aldosterone and ADH*

Parameter	Aldosterone	ADH
Actions	↑Na retention, ↓K excretion	↑H$_2$O retention
Site of action	Cortical collecting duct and distal tubule	Collecting duct, ascending thick limb of Henle loop (NaCl transport)
Source	Zona glomerulosa of adrenal cortex	Neurons in supraoptic and paraventricular nuclei of hypothalamus
Stimulus for secretion		
Direct	Angiotensin II	↑Osmolality of blood, ↓blood volume, Angiotensin II
Indirect	↓Blood volume as detected by ↓pressure in afferent arteriole, ↓NaCl in distal tubule, ↑sympathetic input, to JG cells from volume, receptors	
Rapidity of response	At least 30-min lag	Instantaneous
Duration of action	Hours	Minutes
Mode of action	RNA and protein synthesis	Cyclic AMP
Chemistry	Steroid	Peptide

ADH, antidiuretic hormone; JG, juxtaglomerular; RNA, ribonucleic acid; AMP, adenosine monophosphate.

the brain that increases the appetite for sodium chloride. Table 1 compares some properties of aldosterone and ADH.

ANGIOTENSIN II

Angiotensin II, a peptide whose properties and production were introduced in Chapter 4, is the primary stimulus for aldosterone secretion. Its formation in blood is limited by the availability of the enzyme renin, which is secreted by the kidney. Renin cleaves circulating angiotensinogen to the decapeptide angiotensin I, which is then converted to the active octapeptide by the ubiquitous converting enzyme. Normally, angiotensinogen is present in blood in abundance, but under some circumstances, e.g., liver disease, availability of this substrate for renin may limit angiotensin II production. Angiotensin II production is controlled primarily by regulating the release of renin from the juxtaglomerular cells. The principal stimuli for renin secretion are (a) decreased pressure in the afferent glomerular arterioles, (b) decreased sodium and chloride flux through the macula densa area of the distal convoluted tubule, and (c) norepinephrine released from sympathetic neurons innervating the juxtaglomerular apparatus.

Although the kidney is the primary regulator of the angiotensin II concentration in blood, angiotensin II is also produced locally in a variety of other tissues, including the walls of blood vessels and the brain, where it may function as a neurotransmitter.

These extrarenal tissues synthesize angiotensinogen as well as renin and may form angiotensin II intracellularly.

Stimulation of aldosterone secretion is only one of the ways in which angiotensin II contributes to maintenance of salt and water balance. Like ADH, it is a powerful constrictor of vascular smooth muscle, but unlike ADH, angiotensin II also constricts venules and, hence, may actually increase capillary pressure. Therefore, under the influence of angiotensin II, net filtration may be increased. Angiotensin II also acts centrally on hypothalamic neurons, and by exciting sympathetic vasomotor outflow, it may reinforce its direct vasoconstrictor action. It also acts directly on cardiac myocytes to increase calcium influx, and thereby increase cardiac contractility. The combination of these effects markedly increases blood pressure and makes angiotensin II the most potent pressor agent known. Vasoconstrictor effects are not uniformly expressed in all vascular beds. Therefore, angiotensin II redistributes blood flow in favor of the brain, heart, and skeletal muscle at the expense of the skin and visceral organs.

Angiotensin II formed within the renal vasculature also acts on the kidney to influence the composition of urine. It promotes sodium chloride and water reabsorption by a direct action on the proximal tubule. In addition, although it stimulates constriction of both the afferent and efferent glomerular arterioles, the efferent arterioles are constricted to a greater degree. As a result, the physical forces that govern fluid uptake in the proximal convoluted tubule are intensified, and sodium and water reabsorption are increased. These effects are seen at low concentrations of angiotensin II.

Angiotensin II, acting both as a hormone and as a neurotransmitter, stimulates thirst, appetite for sodium, and the secretion of ADH through actions exerted on the hypothalamus and perhaps other regions of the brain. Blood-borne angiotensin II can interact with receptors present on hypothalamic cells in the *subfornical organ* and the *organum vasculosum of the stria terminalis,* which lie outside the blood–brain barrier and project to the supraoptic and paraventricular nuclei and other hypothalamic sites. In addition, ADH-producing cells in the paraventricular nuclei also have receptors for angiotensin II and release ADH when angiotensin II is presented to them by intraventricular injection or added to them *in vitro* and, presumably, when released from impinging axons. Finally, at concentrations well below those needed to stimulate aldosterone secretion or aortic constriction, angiotensin II stimulates water absorption from the colon. These mutually reinforcing actions are consistent with volume conservation, i.e., increased drinking behavior is rendered more effective by increased water absorption from the gut and decreased water loss from the kidney, regardless of blood osmolality. These multiple effects of angiotensin II are illustrated in Fig. 7.

Atrial Natriuretic Peptide (Atriopeptin)

Atriopeptin is the most recently discovered hormonal regulator of sodium and water balance. It is synthesized, stored, and secreted by cardiac myocytes located

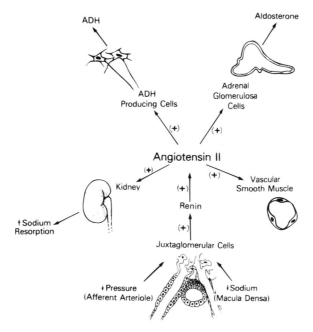

FIG. 7. Major actions of angiotensin II.

primarily in the right atrium, but a substantial amount may also be present in the left atrium. Secretion of ANP, accompanied by a loss of storage granules, is stimulated by volume expansion or excess sodium chloride intake. The major immunoreactive form present in human blood is a 28-amino acid peptide, representing the carboxy terminal region of a 126-amino acid precursor, which is the principal storage form. Enzymatic processing to remove amino acids at both the amino and carboxy terminal ends yields a 20-amino acid peptide, atriopeptin II, which may be the most potent form. Atrio peptin is destroyed rapidly and disappears from plasma with a half-life of about 3 minutes. Its biological effects disappear equally rapidly. Atriopeptin is removed from blood and extracellular fluid by a receptor-mediated process. Membranes of renal and vascular cells contain large numbers of the so-called type II ANP receptor which, instead of signaling a hormonal effect, serves to internalize atriopeptin molecules and deliver them to lysosomes.

Physiological Actions

The kidney is the principal target for atriopeptin, which increases the urine volume and, as its name implies, sodium loss. Atriopeptin increases the glomerular filtration rate, usually without increasing renal blood flow. Simultaneous dilation of afferent and constriction of efferent glomerular arterioles increases pressure in glomerular capillaries and the driving force for filtration of sodium and water. In addition, atriopeptin relaxes glomerular mesangial cells, thereby increasing glomerular permeability. Atriopeptin also decreases reabsorption of sodium and water in the proximal tubule by mechanisms that are not yet understood but which probably involve hemodynamic effects. As a consequence of these actions, increased amounts of salt and water reach the loop of Henle and "wash out" the osmotic gradient. In addition, atriopeptin acts directly on the collecting ducts to decrease salt and water reabsorption. The net result is increased sodium excretion in a large volume of dilute urine, which reduces blood volume and total body sodium. It is noteworthy that the vasodilator effects of atriopeptin are not limited to the renal vasculature but include systemic arterioles as well. Therefore, atriopeptin lowers arterial pressure by decreasing both peripheral resistance and vascular volume.

Not surprisingly, atriopeptin interacts with other hormones that regulate salt and water balance (Fig. 8). It directly and indirectly inhibits secretion of renin and, therefore, secondarily decreases aldosterone secretion. At the same time, atriopeptin acts directly on adrenal glomerulosa cells to antagonize the actions of angiotensin II on steroidogenesis. Atriopeptin also antagonizes the actions of angiotensin II on vascular smooth muscle and on thirst and ADH secretion as well.

There are two classes of atriopeptin receptors, based upon molecular structure, kinetic characteristics, and function. The most abundant by far are the C type, which as already mentioned, function only to clear atriopeptin from the blood. Biologically active B-type receptors are also widely distributed and are found in the kidney cortex, principally in cells associated with the glomerulus and the medullary collecting ducts. In addition, atriopeptin receptors are widespread in vascular smooth muscle cells as well as juxtaglomerular, adrenal glomerulosa, and ADH-secreting cells, which are probably direct targets for atriopeptin. The B-type receptors bind atriopep-

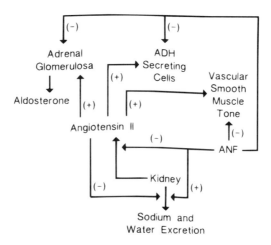

FIG. 8. Actions of atriopeptin (*ANF*).

tin in their extracellular domain and have guanylyl cyclase activity in their cytosolic domain. Increased production of cyclic guanosine monophosphate (GMP) probably accounts for all of the actions of atriopeptin. Although all of its exact cellular mechanisms are poorly understood, cyclic GMP may lower the concentrations of cellular calcium by stimulating calcium adenosine triphosphatase (ATPase) and lower cyclic AMP by stimulating cyclic AMP phosphodiesterase.

Regulation of Secretion

Atriopeptin is secreted in response to increased blood volume or central venous pressure, which apparently is sensed directly by myocytes as increased tension in the atrial wall. Experimental manipulations that increase central venous volume increase atriopeptin secretion. One such manipulation, immersion in water, redistributes blood from peripheral venous plexes to the thoracic vessels. Immersion in water increases the concentration of atriopeptin in blood and simultaneously decreases plasma renin and aldosterone concentrations (Fig. 9). Although increased osmolality also stimulates atriopeptin secretion, increased right atrial pressure is a more potent signal than increased plasma sodium concentration.

INTEGRATED COMPENSATORY RESPONSES TO CHANGES IN SALT AND WATER BALANCE

Hormones contribute in multiple ways to the regulation of salt and water balance. To gain some understanding of how the various endocrine pathways interact, we next consider several examples of perturbations in salt and water balance and the hormonal mechanisms that restore homeostasis. Volume changes can take several forms and may or may not be accompanied by changes in osmolality (sodium balance), as shown in Table 2.

Hemorrhage

With hemorrhage, the vascular volume is decreased without a change in osmolality. To cope with blood loss, especially if it is large, a three-part strategy is usually followed: (a) prevention of further fluid loss, (b) redistribution of remaining fluid to maximize its usefulness, and (c) replacement of the water and sodium losses. The sympathetic nervous system is indispensable for survival during the initial moments after hemorrhage. Hormonal contributions may augment the initial sympathetic reactions and are largely responsible for mediating the later aspects of recovery.

The immediate response to hemorrhage is massive vasoconstriction driven by the sympathetic nervous system. This response sustains arterial pressure and redistributes the cardiac output to ensure adequate blood flow to essential tissues. Renal blood flow and glomerular filtration are markedly reduced. Although slower in onset,

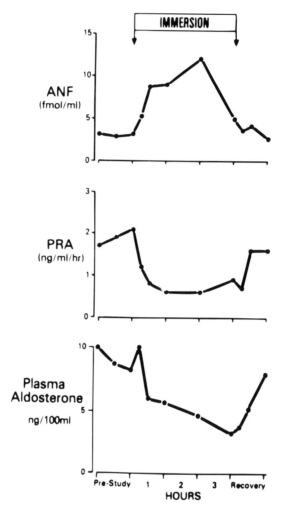

FIG. 9. The effect of water immersion to the neck on the plasma immunoreactive atrial natriuretic peptide (*ANF*), plasma renin activity (*PRA*), and plasma aldosterone in a normal male subject. From Atlas, S.A. (1986): Atrial natriuretic factor: A new hormone of cardiac origin. *Recent Prog. Horm. Res.*, 42:207.

hormonal responses nevertheless may contribute to maintenance of arterial blood pressure through the vasoconstrictor actions of angiotensin II, ADH, and adrenomed-ullary hormones. The sum of these responses transfers extracellular water to the vascular compartment by promoting net fluid absorption by the capillaries and ven-ules. Figure 10 shows the pathways that eventually lead to restoration of blood volume. Initially, hemorrhage, especially if it is severe (30% of blood volume), decreases venous return and thereby reduces right atrial pressure. Cardiac output is

TABLE 2. *Examples of changes in fluid volume*

	Expansion	Contraction
Isosmolar ingestion, hemorrhage	Hyperaldosteronism, heart failure	↑Salt and water, hypoalbuminemia
Hypoosmolar	Excessive water intake, syndrome of inappropriate ADH secretion	Excessive sweating followed by water intake
Hyperosmolar	Excessive salt intake	Dehydration

ADH, antidiuretic hormone.

thus decreased, which at least transiently decreases arterial blood pressure and triggers the sympathetic response.

Response of the Renin–Angiotensin System

Decreased arterial pressure is one of the signals for renin secretion and is directly sensed by the juxtaglomerular cells in the afferent arterioles. This input is nullified if arterial pressure is fully restored by the increase in total peripheral resistance, but direct sympathetic stimulation of the juxtaglomerular cells also increases renin secretion. In addition, decreased renal blood flow and glomerular filtration decrease

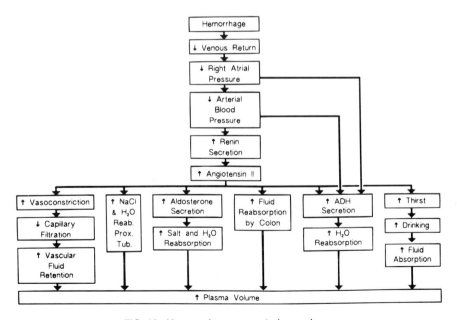

FIG. 10. Hormonal responses to hemorrhage.

sodium and chloride flux through the distal tubule, which acts as yet another stimulus for renin secretion. Redundant pathways for evoking renin secretion, and therefore angiotensin production, ensure that this crucial system is activated by hemorrhage.

Angiotensin II has a wide variety of temporally and spatially separate actions that summate to restore plasma volume and compensate for hemorrhage. This situation is a good example of how different actions of a hormone expressed in different target cells reinforce each other to produce a cumulative response. They were discussed previously and, therefore, are summarized here only in terms of the temporal sequence. Constriction of arteries and arterioles occurs within seconds, but the consequent mobilization of extravascular fluid requires several minutes. Also on the order of minutes may be direct stimulation of salt and water reabsorption in the proximal tubule by angiotensin II. The concentration of angiotensin II required to activate this mechanism is considerably below that required for vasoconstriction, but obviously, this action is of little consequence when the hemorrhage is so severe that renal blood flow is nearly completely shut down.

Other results of angiotensin action are considerably slower to appear. The consequences of stimulating adrenal glomerulosa cells to secrete aldosterone are not seen for almost an hour. Because aldosterone is not stored, it must be synthesized *de novo,* and as long as 10 to 15 minutes may be required to achieve peak production rates. Furthermore, aldosterone, like other steroid hormones, requires a lag period of at least 30 minutes before its effects are evident. The final contribution of angiotensin II is stimulation of salt appetite, thirst, and fluid absorption by the colon. Depending on the severity of the blood loss and the availability of water and salt, many hours or even days may pass before the renin–angiotensin system can restore the plasma volume to its prehemorrhage levels.

Response of the ADH System

Even though osmolality is unchanged, decreased pressure sensed by receptors in the atria, aorta, and carotid sinuses stimulates ADH secretion. Here we have another case of redundancy because ADH and angiotensin II have overlapping actions on arteriolar smooth muscle. These hormones also reinforce each other's actions at the level of the renal tubule because they increase water reabsorption at different sites and by different mechanisms. Although ADH is secreted almost instantaneously in response to hemorrhage, its physiological importance for the early responses is questionable because vascular smooth muscle may already be maximally constricted by sympathetic stimulation, which is even faster. In addition, when renal shutdown is severe, little urine reaches the collecting ducts, and hence, even maximal antidiuresis can conserve little water. However, ADH is an indispensable component of the recovery phase. Thirst and salt-conserving mechanisms would be of little benefit without ADH to promote renal retention of water.

Response of Aldosterone

Like ADH, aldosterone is of little consequence for the immediate reactions to hemorrhage. It acts too slowly. Furthermore, decreased glomerular filtration is far more important quantitatively in conserving sodium. Increased secretion of aldosterone, which is initiated promptly by the renin–angiotensin system and reinforced by increased ACTH secretion, can be regarded as an anticipatory response to ensure sodium conservation when renal blood flow is restored. Aldosterone is indispensable for replenishing blood volume by conserving the sodium ingested during recovery and probably by stimulating sodium intake.

Response of Atriopeptin

It almost goes without saying that the same sensors of depleted vascular volume transmit inhibitory signals for the secretion of atriopeptin; this situation is the converse of that depicted in Fig. 9. We thus have a push–pull mechanism wherein secretion of an inhibitory influence on salt and water retention as well as on the actions of angiotensin II is shut off by the same events that increase secretion of angiotensin II and ADH.

Dehydration

Dehydration (water deficit) is a commonly encountered derangement of homeostasis and may result from severe sweating, diarrhea, vomiting, fever, excessive alcohol ingestion, or simply insufficient fluid intake. Because dehydration usually involves a greater deficit of water than of solute, the osmolality of both the intracellular and extracellular compartments increases. Consequently, the ADH pathway is the principal means for correcting this derangement in water homeostasis. As osmolality increases above its threshold value, ADH secretion promptly increases, and water is reabsorbed in excess of solute until resting osmolality is restored. This action prevents further loss of water in urine, but cannot restore the volume deficit that usually accompanies dehydration. Decreased volume stimulates the renin–angiotensin—-aldosterone system to facilitate vascular adjustments, stimulate thirst, and prepare for replenishment from increased intake of salt and water. Decreased volume also reinforces the osmotic stimulation of ADH secretion. The atriopeptin system is probably not activated because it responds to increased pressure and volume more readily than to increased sodium concentration. Figure 11 illustrates the endocrine responses to dehydration and the series of events that restore osmolality and volume to normal.

Salt Loading and Depletion

Although sodium chloride is scarce in many regions of the world, it is in oversupply in most Western diets. The endocrine system plays a pivotal role in maintaining

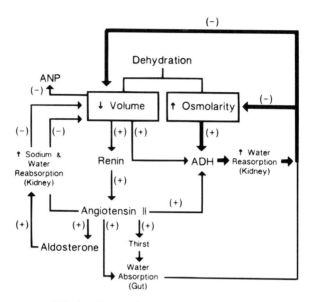

FIG. 11. Hormonal responses to dehydration.

homeostasis and normal blood pressure in the face of salt loading or depletion. Figure 12 shows the responses of normal human subjects who volunteered to consume diets that contained high, low, or standard amounts of sodium. Salt-loaded subjects excreted more than ten times as much sodium in their urine as salt-deprived subjects, but the concentration of sodium in plasma and systolic blood pressure were virtually identical in all three groups. Although extracellular fluid volume was expanded on the high-salt diet and contracted on the low-salt diet, the osmolality and sodium concentration of body fluids remained remarkably constant.

Changes in blood concentrations of angiotensin II (as reflected in renin levels), aldosterone, ADH, and atriopeptin elicited by different amounts of sodium intake are shown in Fig. 12. Plasma renin activity and aldosterone secretion decreased as sodium intake increased. The high rate of sodium loss by subjects on the high-sodium diet may be explained by decreased reabsorption of sodium in the proximal tubule, as a result of decreased angiotensin II and increased atriopeptin, and in the cortical collecting ducts, as a result of decreased aldosterone. As might be expected, the atriopeptin concentration was increased when sodium intake was increased and decreased when sodium intake was low. The reciprocal relationship between atrio-peptin and angiotensin II acts as a push–pull mechanism to promote sodium loss in the sodium-loaded individual and sodium conservation in the salt-deprived subject.

Angiotensin II is important for maintenance of blood pressure when sodium intake is low. Pharmacological blockade of angiotensin formation or action in persons ingesting low amounts of sodium produces marked hypotension. Secretion of ADH was also increased in subjects on a high-salt intake, probably in response to the

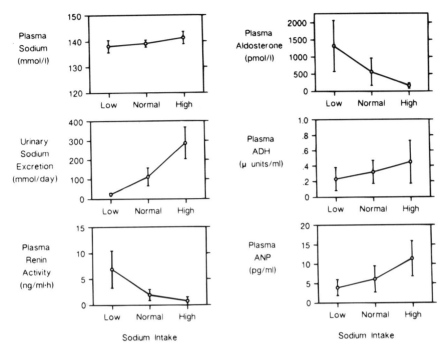

FIG. 12. Responses to sodium loading and sodium depletion. Drawn from the data of Sagnella, G.A., Markandu, N.D., Shore, A.C., et al. (1987): Plasma atrial natriuretic peptide: Its relationship to changes in sodium intake, plasma renin activity and aldosterone in man. *Clin. Sci.*, 72:25.

small increase in plasma osmolality. Plasma sodium concentrations in these subjects was 2% higher than in subjects on the low-sodium diet and 1.4% higher than in subjects on the normal diet. The ADH secreted in response to the osmotic stimulus prevented the loss of water that might otherwise have accompanied the increased amounts of sodium in the urine.

SUGGESTED READING

Brenner, B. M., Ballermann, B. J., Gunning, M. E., and Zeidel, M. L. (1990): Diverse biological actions of atrial natriuretic peptide. *Physiol. Rev.*, 70:665–699.

Campbell, D. J. (1987): Circulating and tissue angiotensin systems. *J. Clin. Invest.*, 79:1–6.

de Bold, A. J. (1985): Atrial natriuretic factor: a hormone produced by the heart. *Science.*, 230:767–769.

Ganong, W. F, and Barbieri, C. (1982): Neuroendocrine components in the regulation of renin secretion. *Front. Neuroendocrinol.*, 7:231–262.

Gibbons, G. H., Dzau, V. J., Farhi, E. R., and Barger, A. C. (1984): Interaction of signals influencing renin release. *Annu. Rev. Physiol.*, 46:291–308.

Laragh, J. H. (1985): Atrial natriuretic hormone, the renin-aldosterone axis, and blood pressure–electrolyte homeostasis. *N. Engl. J. Med.*, 313:1330–1340.

Reid, I. A, and Schwartz, J. (1984): Role of vasopressin in the control of blood pressure. *Front. Neuroendocrinol.*, 8:177–197.

Rosensweig, A., and Seidman, C. E. (1991): Atrial natriuretic factor and related peptide hormones. *Annu. Rev. Biochem.*, 60:229–252.

Sklar, A. H., and Schrier, R. W. (1983): Central nervous system mediators of vasopressin release. *Physiol. Rev.*, 63:1243–1280.

Wade, J. B. (1986): Role of membrane fusion in hormonal regulation of epithelial transport. *Annu. Rev. Physiol.*, 48:213–224.

8

Hormonal Regulation of Calcium Metabolism

OVERVIEW

Adequate amounts of calcium in its ionized form, Ca^{+2}, are needed for normal function of all cells. Calcium ion[1] regulates a wide range of biological processes and is one of the principal constituents of bone. In terrestrial vertebrates, including humans, maintenance of adequate concentrations in the extracellular fluid requires the activity of two hormones, parathyroid hormone (PTH) and a derivative of vitamin D called $1\alpha,25$-dihydroxycholecalciferol ($1,25(OH)_2D_3$) or calcitriol. In more primitive vertebrates living in a marine environment, guarding against excessively high concentrations of calcium requires another hormone, calcitonin, which appears to have only vestigial activity in humans.

Body calcium ultimately is derived from the diet, and daily intake is usually offset by urinary loss. The skeleton acts as a major reservoir of calcium and can buffer the concentration of calcium in extracellular fluid by taking up or releasing calcium phosphate. Parathyroid hormone promotes the transfer of calcium from bone, the glomerular filtrate, and intestinal contents into the extracellular fluid. It acts directly on bone cells to promote calcium mobilization and on renal tubules to reabsorb calcium and excrete phosphate. It promotes intestinal transport of calcium and phosphate indirectly by increasing the formation of $1,25(OH)_2D_3$ required for calcium uptake by intestinal cells. This vitamin D metabolite also promotes calcium mobilization from bone and reinforces the actions of PTH on this process. In addition, $1,25(OH)_2D_3$ promotes reabsorption of calcium and phosphate by renal tubules. The rate of PTH secretion is inversely related to the concentration of blood calcium, which directly inhibits secretion by the chief cells of the parathyroid glands. Calcitonin inhibits the activity of bone-resorbing cells and, thus, blocks inflow of calcium to the extracellular fluid compartment. Its secretion is stimulated by high concentrations of blood calcium.

---

[1] Calcium is present in several forms within the body, but only the ionized form, Ca^{+2}, is monitored and regulated. In this discussion, calcium refers to the ionized form, except when otherwise specified.

GENERAL FEATURES OF CALCIUM BALANCE

Calcium enters into a wide range of cellular and molecular processes. Changes in its concentration within cells regulate enzymatic activities and such fundamental cellular events as muscular contraction, secretion, and cell division. As already discussed (see Chapter 1), calcium and calmodulin also act as intracellular mediators of hormone action. In the extracellular compartment, calcium is vital for blood clotting and maintenance of normal membrane function. Calcium is the basic mineral of bones and teeth and thus plays a structural as well as a regulatory role. Not surprisingly, its concentration in extracellular fluid must be maintained within narrow limits. Deviations in either direction are not readily tolerated and, if severe, may be life threatening.

The electrical excitability of cell membranes increases when the extracellular concentration of calcium is low, and the threshold for triggering action potentials may be lowered almost to the resting potential. This results in spontaneous, asynchronous, and involuntary contractions of skeletal muscle called *tetany*. A typical attack of tetany involves muscular spasms in the face and characteristic contortions of the arms and hands. Laryngeal spasm and contraction of the respiratory muscles may compromise breathing. Pronounced *hypocalcemia* (low blood calcium) may produce more generalized muscular contractions and convulsions.

Increased concentrations of calcium in blood (*hypercalcemia*) may cause calcium salts to precipitate out of solution because of their low solubility at physiological pH. ''Stones'' form, especially in the kidney, where they may produce severe painful damage (renal colic), which may lead to renal failure and hypertension.

Distribution of Calcium in the Body

The adult human body contains approximately 1,000 g of calcium, about 99% of which is sequestered in bone, primarily in the form of hydroxyapatite crystals $(Ca_{10}(PO_4)_6(OH)_2)$. In addition to providing structural support, bone serves as an enormous reservoir for calcium salts. Each day about 600 mg of calcium is exchanged between bone mineral and the extracellular fluid. Much of this exchange reflects resorption and reformation of bone as the skeleton undergoes constant remodeling, but some also occurs by exchange with a labile calcium pool in the bone.

Most of the calcium that is not in bone crystals is found in cells of soft tissues bound to proteins within the sarcoplasmic reticulum, mitochondria, and other organelles. Energy-dependent transport of calcium by these organelles and the cell membrane maintains the resting concentration of free calcium in the cytosol at low levels, i.e., 0.1 to 1 μM. Cytosolic calcium can increase 1,000-fold or more, however, with just a brief change in the membrane permeability or affinity of intracellular binding proteins. The rapidity and magnitude of changes in cytosolic calcium are consistent with its role as a biological signal.

The concentration of calcium in interstitial fluid is about 1.5 mM. Interstitial calcium consists mainly of free, ionized calcium, but some is complexed with such anions as citrate, lactate, or phosphate. Both ionized and complexed calcium pass freely through capillary membranes and equilibrate with calcium in blood plasma. The total calcium concentration in blood is nearly twice that of interstitial fluid because calcium is avidly bound by albumin and other proteins. Total calcium in blood plasma is normally about 10 mg/dl (5 mEq/liter or 2.5 mM), but only the ionized component appears to be monitored and regulated. Because so large a fraction of blood calcium is protein bound, diseases that produce substantial changes in albumin concentrations may produce striking abnormalities in total plasma calcium content, even though the concentration of ionized calcium may be normal.

Calcium Balance

Normally, adults are in calcium balance, i.e., on average, daily intake equals daily loss in urine and feces. Except for lactation and pregnancy, deviations from balance reflect changes in the metabolism of bone. Immobilization of a limb, bed rest, weightlessness, and malignant disease are examples of circumstances that produce negative calcium balance. Dietary intake of calcium in the United States typically varies between 500 and 1,500 mg per day, primarily from dairy products. For example, an 8-oz glass of milk contains about 290 mg of calcium. Calcium absorbed from the gut exchanges with the various body pools and ultimately is lost in the urine. These relationships are illustrated in Fig. 1.

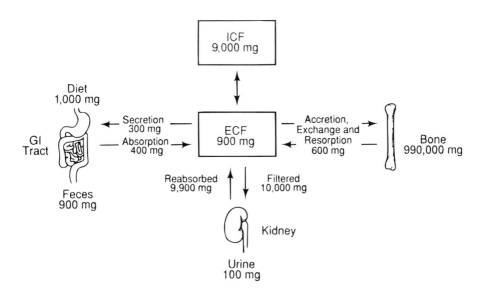

FIG. 1. Daily calcium balance in a typical adult.

Intestinal Absorption

Calcium is taken up along the entire length of the small intestine, but uptake is greatest in the ileum and jejunum. Secretions of the gastrointestinal tract are rich in calcium and add to the minimum load that must be absorbed to maintain balance. Net uptake is usually in the range of 100 to 200 mg per day. Absorption of calcium requires metabolic energy and the activity of specific carrier molecules in the luminal membrane (brush border) of intestinal cells. Although detailed understanding is not yet at hand, it appears that carrier-mediated transport across the brush border determines the overall rate. Calcium is carried down its concentration gradient into the cytosol of intestinal epithelial cells and is extruded from the basolateral surfaces in exchange for sodium, which must then be pumped out at metabolic expense. The overall transfer of calcium from the intestinal lumen to the interstitial fluid proceeds against a concentration gradient and is largely dependent on $1,25(OH)_2D_3$ (see subsequent discussion). Although some calcium is taken up passively, simple diffusion is not adequate to meet the body's needs even when the concentration of calcium in the intestinal lumen is high.

Bone

Understanding the regulation of calcium balance requires at least a rudimentary understanding of the physiology of bone. Metabolic activity in bone must satisfy two needs. The skeleton must attend to its own structural integrity through continuous remodeling and renewal, and it must respond to systemic needs for adequate amounts of calcium in the extracellular fluid. By and large, maintenance of adequate concentrations of calcium in blood takes precedence over maintenance of structural integrity of bone. However, the student must recognize that these two homeostatic functions, though driven by different forces, are not completely independent. Diseases of bone that disrupt skeletal homeostasis may have consequences in regard to overall calcium balance, and conversely, inadequacies of calcium balance lead to inadequate mineralization of bone.

The *extracellular matrix* is the predominant component of bone. One third of the bony matrix consists of collagen and other proteins, and two thirds is comprised of highly ordered mineral crystals. The organic component, called osteoid, provides the framework on which bone mineral is deposited. Collagen molecules in osteoid aggregate and cross-link to form fibrils of precise structure. Spaces between the ends of collagen molecules within fibrils provide initiation sites for crystal formation. Most calcium phosphate crystals are found within collagen fibrils and have their long axes oriented in parallel with the fibrils.

Cortical (compact) bone is the most prevalent form and is found in the shafts of long bones and on the surfaces of the pelvis, skull, and other flat bones. The basic unit of cortical bone is called an *osteon* and consists of concentric layers, or lamellae, of bone arranged around a central channel (haversian canal), which contains the

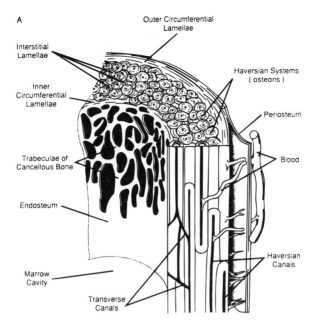

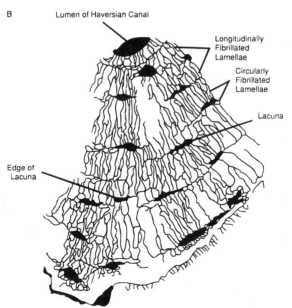

FIG. 2. Sector of a cross section of a haversian system from human bone. Note the concentric lamellae. Each lacuna is normally filled with an osteocyte whose processes fill the extensive network of canaliculi. From Fawcett, D.W. (1986): *A Textbook of Histology*, 11th ed., p. 204, Saunders, Philadelphia.

capillary blood supply. Osteons are usually 200 to 300 mm in diameter and several hundred millimeters long. They are arranged with their long axes oriented in parallel with the shaft of bone. Other canals, which run roughly perpendicularly, penetrate the osteons and form an anastomosing array of channels through which blood vessels in haversian canals connect with vessels in the *periosteum*. Tightly packed osteons are surrounded on both inner and outer aspects by several lamellae that extend circumferentially around the shaft. The entire bone is surrounded on its outer surface by the periosteum and is separated from the marrow by the *endosteum* (Fig. 2).

Cancellous (trabecular) bone is found at the ends of the long bones; in the vertebrae; and in the internal portions of the pelvis, skull, and other flat bones. It is also called spongy bone, a term which well describes its appearance in section (Fig. 3). Although only about 20% of the skeleton is comprised of trabecular bone, its spongelike organization provides at least five times as much surface area for metabolic exchange as does compact bone. The trabeculae of spongy bone are not penetrated by blood vessels, but the spaces between them are filled with blood sinusoids or highly vascular marrow. The trabeculae are completely surrounded by endosteum.

Distributed throughout the lamellae of both forms of bone are tiny chambers, or lacunae, each of which houses an *osteocyte*. The lacunae are interconnected by a network of canaliculi, which extend to the endosteal and periosteal surfaces. Osteo-

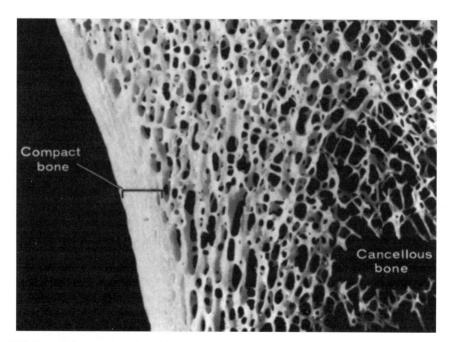

FIG. 3. A thick ground section of the tibia illustrating the cortical compact bone and the lattice of trabeculae of the cancellous bone. From Fawcett, D.W. (1986): *A Textbook of Histology*, 11th ed., p. 201, Saunders, Philadelphia.

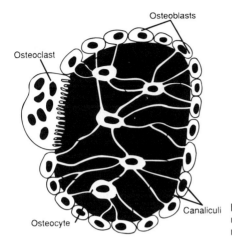

FIG. 4. Cross section through a bony trabecula. The *shaded area* indicates mineralized matrix.

cytes receive nourishment and biological signals by way of cytoplasmic processes that extend through the canaliculi to form gap junctions with each other and cells of the endosteum or periosteum (Fig. 4).

It is important to recognize that the mineralized matrix in both forms of bone is separated from the extracellular compartment of the rest of the body by a continuous layer of cells sometimes called the *bone membrane*. This layer of cells is comprised of the endosteum, periosteum, osteocytes, and cells that line the haversian canals. Crystallization or solubilization of bone mineral is determined by physicochemical equilibria which are related to the concentrations of calcium, phosphate, hydrogen, and other constituents in bone water. Net flux of calcium and phosphate into or out of the small pools of fluid that equilibrate with bone crystals involves active participation of the cells of the bone membrane. Hormones regulate the calcium concentration in the extracellular fluid compartment and the mineralization of bone by regulating the activities of these cells.

Osteoblasts are the cells responsible for the formation of bone. They arise from progenitors in connective tissue and form a continuous sheet on the surface of newly forming bone. When actively laying down bone, osteoblasts are cuboidal or low columnar in shape. They have a dense rough endoplasmic reticulum consistent with their role in synthesis and secretion of collagen and other proteins of bone matrix. Osteoblasts probably also promote mineralization, but their role in this regard and details of the mineralization process are somewhat controversial. Under physiological conditions, calcium and phosphate are in metastable solution. That is, their concentrations in extracellular fluid would be sufficiently high for them to precipitate out of solution were it not for other constituents, particularly pyrophosphate, which stabilize the solution. During mineralization, osteoblasts secrete alkaline phosphatase, which cleaves pyrophosphate and thus removes a stabilizing influence, and at the same time increases local concentrations of phosphate, which promotes crystallization. In addition, during bone growth and probably during remodeling of mature bone, osteoblasts secrete calcium-rich vesicles into the calcifying osteoid.

During growth or remodeling of bone, some osteoblasts become entrapped in matrix and differentiate into osteocytes. Upon completion of growth or remodeling, surface osteoblasts dedifferentiate to become the flattened, spindle-shaped cells of the endosteum that lines most of the surface of bone. These cells may be reactivated in response to stimuli for bone formation. Thus, osteoblasts, osteocytes, and quiescent lining cells represent three stages of the same cellular lineage and together comprise most, or perhaps all, of the bone membrane.

Osteoclasts are responsible for bone resorption (Fig. 4). They are large cells that arise by fusion of mononuclear cells; they may have as many as 50 nuclei. Precursors of osteoclasts are thought to originate in bone marrow and migrate through the circulation from the thymus and other reticuloendothelial tissues to sites of bone destined for resorption. Mononuclear precursors of osteoclasts are probably attracted to sites of bone resorption by partially degraded products of osteoid. In histological sections, osteoclasts are usually found on the surface of bone in pits created by their erosive action. The part of the osteoclast that comes in contact with bone is thrown into many folds called the ruffled border. The ruffled border sweeps over the surface of bone, continuously changing its configuration as it releases acids and hydrolytic enzymes that dissolve the protein matrix and mineral crystals. Small bone crystals are often seen in phagocytic vesicles deep in its folds. Upon completion of resorption, osteoclasts are inactivated and lose some of their nuclei. Inactivation involves fission of the giant, polynucleate cell back into mononuclear cells. Some multinuclear cells remain quiescent on the bone surface interspersed among the lining cells.

Resorption of bone is precisely coupled with bone formation, suggesting that osteoblasts and osteoclasts somehow communicate with each other. The nature of their cross talk is not known but apparently involves a variety of paracrine factors, including prostaglandins, growth factors, and partially digested components of osteoid. The pattern of events in bone remodeling typically begins with activation of osteoclasts followed sequentially by bone resorption, osteoblast activation, and finally, bone formation.

Kidney

Both ionized and complexed calcium pass freely through the glomerular membranes. Normally, 98% to 99% of the 10,000 mg of calcium filtered by the glomeruli each day is reabsorbed by the renal tubules. About two thirds of calcium reabsorption occurs in the proximal tubule, tightly coupled to sodium reabsorption; for the most part, calcium is dragged passively along with water. Much of the remaining calcium is reabsorbed in the loop of Henle and is also tightly coupled to sodium reabsorption. Normally, only about 10% of the filtered calcium reaches the distal nephron. The reabsorption of calcium in the vicinity of the junction of the distal convoluted tubules and the collecting ducts is governed by an active, saturable process that is independent of sodium reabsorption. Active transport of calcium in this region is hormonally regulated (see subsequent discussion).

Phosphorus Balance

Because of their intimate relationship, the fate of calcium cannot be discussed without also considering phosphorus. Calcium is usually absorbed in the intestines accompanied by phosphorus, and deposition and mobilization of calcium in bones always occurs in conjunction with phosphorus. Phosphorus is as ubiquitous in its distribution and physiological role as is calcium. The high-energy phosphate bond of adenosine triphosphate (ATP) and other metabolites is the coinage of biological energetics. Phosphorus is indispensable for biological information transfer. It is a component of nucleic acids and second messengers, such as cyclic adenosine monophosphate (AMP) and inositol 1,4,5 trisphosphate (IP_3), and as the addend that increases or decreases enzymatic activities.

About 90% of the 500 to 800 g of phosphorus in the adult human is deposited in the skeleton. Much of the remainder is incorporated into organic phosphates distributed throughout soft tissues in the form of phospholipids, nucleic acids, and soluble metabolites. Daily intake of phosphorus is in the range of 1,000 to 1,500 mg, mainly in dairy products. Organic phosphorus is digested to inorganic phosphate before it is absorbed in the small intestine by both active and passive processes. Net absorption is linearly related to intake and appears not to saturate. The concentration of inorganic phosphate in blood is about 3.5 mg/dl. About 55% is present as free ions, about 35% is complexed with calcium or other cations, and 10% is protein bound. Phosphate concentrations are not tightly controlled and may vary widely under such influences as diet, age, and sex. Ionized and complexed phosphate pass freely across glomerular and other capillary membranes. Phosphate in the glomerular filtrate is actively reabsorbed by a sodium-linked cotransport process in the proximal tubule. These relationships in daily phosphorus balance are shown in Fig. 5.

PARATHYROID GLANDS AND PTH

The parathyroid glands arose relatively recently in vertebrate evolution, coincident with the emergence of ancestral forms onto dry land. They are not found in fish and are seen in amphibians such as the salamander only after metamorphosis to the land-dwelling form. The importance of the parathyroids in normal calcium economy was established during the latter part of the 19th century when it was found that parathyroidectomy resulted in lethal tetany. Diseases resulting from overproduction or underproduction of PTH are relatively uncommon.

Human beings typically have four parathyroid glands, but as few as two and as many as eight have been observed. Each gland is a flattened ellipsoid measuring

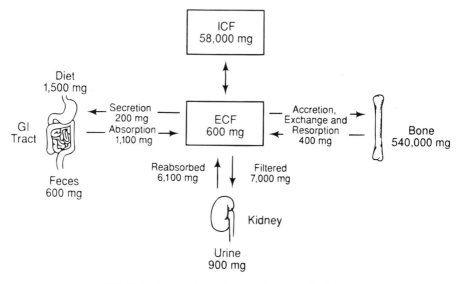

FIG. 5. Daily phosphorus balance in a typical adult.

about 6 mm in its longest diameter. The aggregate mass of the adult parathyroid glands is less than 150 mg. These glands adhere to the posterior surface of the thyroid gland or occasionally are embedded within the thyroid tissue. They are well vascularized and derive their blood supply mainly from the inferior thyroid arteries. Parathyroid glands comprise two cell types (Fig. 6). The *chief cells* predominate and are arranged in clusters or cords. They are the source of PTH and have all of the cytological characteristics of cells that produce protein hormones: rough endoplasmic reticulum, prominent Golgi apparatus, and some membrane-bound storage granules. The *oxyphil cells*, which appear singly or in small groups, are larger than the chief cells and contain a remarkable number of mitochondria. Oxyphil cells have no known function and are thought by some to be degenerated chief cells. Their cytological properties are not characteristic of secretory cells. Few oxyphil cells are seen before puberty, but their number increases thereafter with age.

Biosynthesis, Storage, and Secretion of PTH

The secreted form of PTH is a simple straight-chain peptide of 84 amino acids. There are no disulfide bridges. As many as 50 amino acids can be removed from the carboxyl terminus without compromising its biological potency, but removal of just the serine at the amino terminus virtually inactivates the hormone. Like other peptide hormones, PTH is synthesized as a larger "preprohormone." Sequential cleavage forms first a 90-amino acid prohormone and then the mature hormone. The larger, transient forms have little or no biological activity and are not released

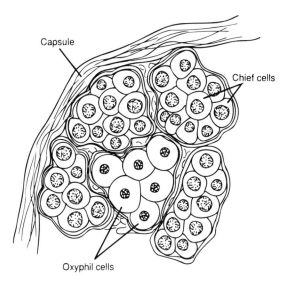

FIG. 6. Section through a human parathyroid gland showing small chief cells and larger oxyphil cells. The cells are arranged in cords surrounded by loose connective tissue. From Borysenko and Beringer (1984): *Functional Histology,* 2nd ed., p. 316, Little, Brown, Boston.

into the circulation even at times of intense secretory activity. Although PTH is synthesized continuously at a high rate, the glands store little hormone.

Parathyroid cells are unusual in the respect that hormone degradation as well as synthesis is adjusted according to physiological demand for secretion. As much as 90% of the hormone synthesized may be destroyed within the chief cells, which break down PTH at an accelerated rate when plasma calcium concentrations are high. The breakdown products are biologically inert and are released into the circulation. Similar fragments are produced by degradation of PTH in the liver and also enter the blood stream. Fragments of PTH remain in the blood hours longer than the intact hormone, which has a half-life of only a few minutes, and are cleared from the blood by filtration at the glomeruli. The intact 84-amino acid peptide is the only biologically active form of PTH in blood.

Standard radioimmunoassays overestimate active PTH in blood because most antisera cannot distinguish the fragments from the intact hormone. The use of two site immunometric or ''sandwich'' assays has overcome this difficulty. These assays use two antibodies that recognize different segments of PTH. One antibody is covalently labeled with a fluorescent or radioactive molecule, and the second is coupled to an insoluble support. The intact hormone serves as a bridge between the labeled antibody and the insoluble antibody, so that the label can be precipitated only when both antibodies are bound to the same molecule. The amount of label recovered in the precipitate form is proportional to the amount of intact hormone present in the plasma sample.

A substance closely related to PTH, *parathyroid hormone-related peptide (PTHrP),* is found in the plasma of patients suffering from certain malignancies. The gene for PTHrP was isolated from some tumors and found to encode a peptide whose first 13 amino acid residues are remarkably similar to the first 13 amino acids of PTH; thereafter, the structures of the two molecules diverge. The PTHrP binds to the PTH receptor and, therefore, produces the same biological effects as PTH. The PTHrP may play an important role in fetal calcium metabolism or as an autocrine or paracrine factor in postnatal life, but little or none is found in blood plasma of normal individuals. Although PTH and PTHrP are both recognized by the PTH receptor, they are immunologically distinct and do not cross react in immunoassays.

Mechanisms of PTH Actions

Interaction of PTH with receptors on the surfaces of target cells increases the formation of cyclic AMP and of IP_3 and diacylglycerol (DAG, see Chapter 1). The PTH receptor is coupled to adenylyl cyclase through a stimulatory G protein (G_s) and to phospholipase C through another G protein. Consequently, protein kinases A and C are also activated, and intracellular calcium is increased. Rapid responses almost certainly result from protein phosphorylation, while delayed responses result from altered gene expression mediated presumably by transcription factors that are substrates for cyclic AMP-dependent protein kinase. It is likely that the two second messenger pathways activated by PTH are redundant and reinforce each other. The importance of cyclic AMP for the action of PTH is underscored by the occurrence of a rare disease called *pseudohypoparathyroidism* in which patients are unresponsive to PTH. About one half of the reported cases of unresponsiveness to PTH are attributable to a genetic defect in G_s. These patients also have decreased responses to other cyclic AMP-dependent signals.

Physiological Actions of PTH

Parathyroid hormone is the principal regulator of the calcium concentration in extracellular fluid. It increases the calcium concentration and decreases the phosphate concentration in blood by various direct and indirect actions on bone, kidney, and intestine. In its absence, the concentration of calcium in blood, and hence interstitial fluid, decreases dramatically over a period of several hours while the concentration of phosphate increases. Hypoparathyroidism may result from insufficient production of active hormone or defects in the responses of target tissues; acutely, it produces all the symptoms of hypocalcemia, including tetany and convulsions. Chronically, neurological, ocular, and cardiac deficiencies may also be seen. Hyperparathyroidism results in kidney stones and excessive demineralization leading to weakening of bone.

Actions on Bone

Bone responds quickly to small changes in PTH concentration. The initial response, observable within 2 to 3 hours, is limited to resorption of calcium with little or no accompanying degradation of osteoid. This early response is thought to result mainly from activity of osteocytes and cells in the bone membrane and has been called *osteocytic osteolysis*. Although preformed osteoclasts are also activated, on the whole, their involvement in the early phase of the response is slight. PTH increases the permeability of osteocytes and other cells of the bone membrane to calcium in the surrounding bone fluid compartment. Calcium enters the cytosol (driven by a steep concentration gradient) and is then extruded vectorially into the extracellular fluid compartment on the other side of the bone membrane. Uptake of calcium by osteocytes lowers its concentration in the bone fluid compartment that is in rapid equilibrium with bone crystals and shifts the equilibrium toward solubilization. The few osteoclasts present throughout the bone membrane secrete lactic and other acids, and the resulting lower pH contributes further to solubilization of bone crystals. These events are shown in Fig. 7. Initially, PTH inhibits the bone-forming activity of osteoblasts, and production of osteoid is sharply reduced.

A second phase of the response to PTH becomes evident after about 12 hours and is characterized by widespread resorption of both mineral and organic components of the matrix, particularly in trabecular bone. Osteoclastic activity predominates, as

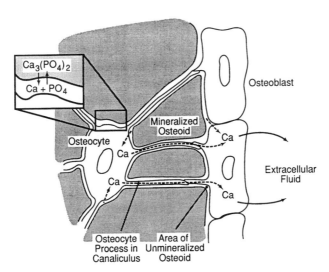

FIG. 7. Osteolytic osteolysis. The hormone PTH increases the permeability of osteocytes and osteoblasts to calcium in the bone fluid compartment, which lies between the mineralized osteoid and bone cells. Lowering the concentration of ionic calcium favors the solubilization of calcium in amorphous calcium phosphate crystals. Calcium that enters osteocytes is transferred to osteoblasts through long cytoplasmic processes, which form gap junctions with osteoblasts in the endosteum. Calcium is then pumped into extracellular fluid.

evidenced by increased urinary excretion of hydroxyproline and other products of collagen breakdown. Although the activity of all bone cell types is increased by PTH, it appears that only osteocytes and osteoblasts have receptors for PTH. Activation and recruitment of osteoclasts must then be accomplished indirectly by some endocrine or paracrine signal produced by osteocytes or osteoblasts. Monocytic precursors of osteoclasts are recruited from reticuloendothelial tissues and migrate to bone, where they fuse to form active polynuclear giant cells. Even later, osteoblasts, which were inhibited in the early phases of PTH action, become active as a result of the biological coupling discussed previously, and new bone is laid down. However, with prolonged exposure to high concentrations of PTH, as occurs with hyperparathyroidism, osteoclastic activity is greater than osteoblastic activity, and bone resorption predominates.

Actions on Kidney

In the kidney, PTH produces three distinct effects, each of which contributes to the maintenance of calcium homeostasis. In the distal nephron, it promotes the reabsorption of calcium, and in the proximal tubule, it inhibits reabsorption of phosphate and promotes hydroxylation, and hence, activation of vitamin D (see subsequent discussion).

Calcium Reabsorption

The kidney reacts quickly to changes in PTH concentration in blood and is primarily responsible for minute-to-minute adjustments in blood calcium. PTH acts directly on the distal portion of the nephron to decrease urinary excretion of calcium well before significant amounts of calcium can be mobilized from bone. About 90% of the filtered calcium is reabsorbed in the proximal tubule and the loop of Henle, independently of PTH. Therefore, because its actions are limited to the distal reabsorptive mechanism, PTH can provide only fine tuning of calcium excretion. Even small changes in the fraction of calcium reabsorbed from the glomerular filtrate, however, can be of great significance. Hypoparathyroid patients whose blood calcium is maintained in the normal range excrete about three times as much urinary calcium as do normal subjects.

Even when maximally stimulated, the PTH-sensitive mechanism has a low capacity that saturates when the filtered load of calcium is high. The filtered load of calcium is determined in part by the plasma calcium concentration and, hence, may be increased by PTH. Because reabsorption of calcium in the proximal portions of the nephron is proportional to sodium and water reabsorption, a nearly constant fraction of the filtered load reaches the distal nephron. Consequently, when the filtered load is high, more calcium may reach the distal nephron than the reabsorbing mechanism can handle. This circumstance accounts for the paradoxical increase in urinary calcium seen in later phases of PTH action. Regardless of the amount excreted, however, PTH decreases the fraction of filtered calcium that escapes in the urine.

Phosphate Excretion

Parathyroid hormone powerfully inhibits tubular reabsorption of phosphate and, thus, increases the amount excreted in urine. This effect is seen within minutes after injection of PTH and is exerted mainly in the proximal tubules, where the bulk of phosphate reabsorption occurs. In producing this so-called *phosphaturic effect*, PTH activates adenylyl cyclase in the basolateral membranes of tubular cells. Cyclic AMP then diffuses across these cells and activates protein kinase A at the luminal pole. Phosphorylation of the sodium–phosphate cotransporter in the brush border may be responsible for decreased uptake of phosphate. Some cyclic AMP escapes from renal tubular cells and appears in the urine. About one half of the cyclic AMP found in the urine arises in the kidney and is attributable to the actions of PTH. Only trivial quantities of phosphate are excreted as cyclic AMP.

Effects on Intestinal Absorption

Calcium balance ultimately depends on intestinal absorption of dietary calcium. Calcium uptake is severely reduced in hypoparathyroid patients and dramatically increased in those with hyperparathyroidism. Within 1 to 2 days after treatment of hypoparathyroid subjects with PTH, calcium uptake increases. Intestinal uptake of calcium is stimulated by an active metabolite of vitamin D. PTH stimulates the renal enzyme that converts vitamin D to its active form (see subsequent discussion), but has no direct effects on intestinal transport of either calcium or phosphate.

Regulation of PTH Secretion

The chief cells of the parathyroid glands are exquisitely sensitive to changes in extracellular calcium and secrete PTH at a rate that is inversely related to the concentration of ionized calcium in blood. The resulting increases or decreases in blood levels of PTH produce either positive or negative changes in the plasma calcium concentration and, thereby, provide negative feedback signals for regulation of PTH secretion. The activated form of vitamin D, whose synthesis depends on PTH, is also a negative feedback inhibitor of PTH secretion (see following discussion). Although blood levels of phosphate are also affected by PTH, phosphate has no effect on the secretion of PTH. A decrease in ionized calcium in blood appears to be the only physiologically relevant signal for PTH secretion.

The cellular mechanisms by which extracellular calcium regulates PTH secretion are poorly understood. It appears that chief cells synthesize and secrete PTH unless inhibited by calcium. Cyclic AMP concentrations rise and fall in parallel with PTH secretion, suggesting that cyclic AMP-mediated events may govern PTH secretion.

Extracellular calcium concentrations apparently are monitored by membrane calcium receptors that are coupled through the inhibiting guanine nucleotide binding protein, Gi, and perhaps other G proteins to membrane calcium channels and to the phosphatidylinositol phosphate second-messenger pathway (see Chapter 1). When extracellular calcium increases, calcium channels open and allow extracellular calcium to enter. At the same time, IP$_3$ triggers the release of calcium from intracellular stores. Although increased cytosolic calcium is associated with increased secretion in other secretory cells, the resulting increase in intracellular calcium inhibits PTH secretion by chief cells. This effect of increased calcium apparently results in a decrease in cyclic AMP within the chief cells. While it is still not certain that decreases in cyclic AMP alone can explain the inhibitory effects of calcium on PTH secretion, it is likely that calcium activates cyclic AMP phosphodiesterase and, hence, accelerates cyclic AMP degradation. The membrane calcium receptors may inhibit adenylyl cyclase by activating Gi. In addition, protein kinase C that is activated by DAG and calcium may phosphorylate and, thereby, inhibit adenylyl cyclase. These events are summarized in Fig. 8.

CALCITONIN

Cells of Origin

Calcitonin is sometimes also called *thyrocalcitonin* to describe its origin in the parafollicular cells of the thyroid gland. These cells, which are also called C cells, occur singly or in clusters in or between thyroid follicles. They are larger and stain less densely than do the follicular cells in routine preparations (Fig. 9). Like other peptide hormone-secreting cells, they contain membrane-bound storage granules. Parafollicular cells arise embryologically from neuroectodermal cells that migrate to the last branchial pouch and, in submammalian vertebrates, give rise to the ultimobranchial glands. In addition to producing calcitonin, parafollicular cells can take up and decarboxylate amine precursors and, thus, have some similarity to pancreatic alpha cells and cells of the adrenal medulla. This relationship may account for the frequent association of malignancies in more than one of these organs in a hereditary syndrome of multiple endocrine neoplasias. Parafollicular cells give rise to a unique neoplasm, *medullary carcinoma of the thyroid*, which may secrete large amounts of calcitonin.

Biosynthesis, Secretion, and Metabolism

Calcitonin consists of 32 amino acids and has a molecular weight of about 3,400 Daltons. Like other peptide hormones, it is initially formed as a larger precursor. Except for a seven-member disulfide ring at the amino terminus, calcitonin has no remarkable structural features. Immunoreactive circulating forms are heterogeneous in size, reflecting the presence of precursors, partially degraded hormone, and disulfide-linked dimers and polymers. The active hormone has a half-life in plasma of about 5–10 minutes and is cleared from blood primarily by the kidney.

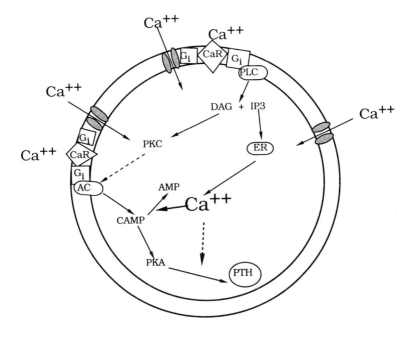

CHIEF CELL

FIG. 8. Proposed mechanism for regulation of PTH secretion by calcium. Extracellular calcium (*CA⁺⁺*) binds to membrane calcium receptors (*CaR*) which communicate with membrane calcium channels, phospholipase C (*PLC*), and adenylyl cyclase (*AC*) by way of G proteins (*G$_i$*). Increased intracellular Ca⁺⁺ released from the endoplasmic reticulum (*ER*) or entering through Ca⁺⁺ channels inhibits PTH secretion by accelerating cyclic AMP (*CAMP*) degradation to *AMP* and perhaps interfering with subsequent actions of protein kinase A (*PKA*). These actions are reinforced by the inhibitory effects of protein kinase C (*PKC*) on AC.

The gene that encodes calcitonin also encodes a neuropeptide called *calcitonin gene-related peptide* (CGRP). This gene contains six exons, but only the first four are represented in the messenger ribonucleic acid (mRNA) transcript that codes for the precursor of calcitonin. In the mRNA that codes for CGRP, the portion corresponding to exon 4 is deleted and replaced by exons 5 and 6. Since the first exon codes for a nontranslated region, and the peptide corresponding to exons 2 and 3 is removed in posttranslational processing, the mature products have no common amino acid sequences. This is an interesting example of how a single gene can give rise to completely different products when expressed in different cells with different enzymatic machinery.

Physiological Actions of Calcitonin

Calcitonin escaped discovery for many years mainly because no obvious derangement in calcium balance or other homeostatic function results from its deficient or

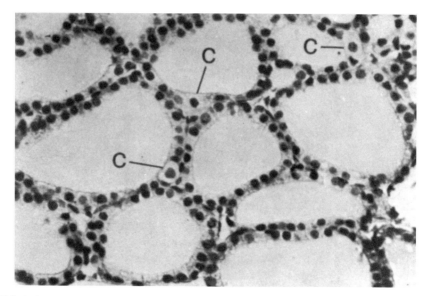

FIG. 9. Low-power photomicrograph of a portion of the thyroid gland of a normal dog. Parafollicular (*C*) cells are indicated in the walls of the follicles. From Ham, A.W. and Cormack, D.H. (1979): *Histology*, 8th ed., p. 802, Lippincott, Philadelphia.

excessive production. Thyroidectomy does not produce a tendency toward hypercalcemia, and thyroid tumors that secrete massive amounts of calcitonin do not cause hypocalcemia. Attention was drawn to the possibility of a calcium-lowering hormone by the experimental finding that direct injection of calcium into the thyroid artery caused a more rapid fall in blood calcium than did parathyroidectomy. Indeed, calcitonin promptly and dramatically lowers the blood calcium concentration in many experimental animals. Calcitonin is not a major factor in calcium homeostasis in humans, however, and does not participate in minute-to-minute regulation of blood calcium concentrations. Rather, the importance of calcitonin may be limited to protection against excessive bone resorption.

Actions on Bone

Calcitonin lowers blood calcium and phosphate primarily by inhibiting osteoclastic activity. The decrease in blood calcium produced by calcitonin is greatest when osteoclastic bone resorption is most intense and is least evident when osteoclastic activity is minimal. Interaction of calcitonin with receptors on the osteoclast surface promptly increases cyclic AMP formation, and within minutes, the expanse and activity of the ruffled border diminishes. Osteoclasts pull away from the bone surface and begin to dedifferentiate. Synthesis and secretion of lysosomal enzymes is inhibited. In less than an hour, fewer osteoclasts are present, and those that remain have decreased bone-resorbing activity.

Osteoclasts are the principal, and probably only, target cells for calcitonin in bone. Osteoblasts do not have receptors for calcitonin and are not directly affected by it. Curiously, although they are uniquely expressed in either osteoblasts or osteoclasts, PTH and calcitonin receptors are closely related and have about one third of their amino acid sequences in common, suggesting that they evolved from a common ancestral molecule. Because of the coupling phenomenon in the cycle of bone resorption and bone formation discussed earlier, inhibition of osteoclastic activity by calcitonin eventually decreases osteoblastic activity as well. All cell types appear quiescent in histological sections of bone that was chronically exposed to high concentrations of calcitonin.

Actions on Kidney

At high concentrations, calcitonin may increase urinary excretion of calcium and phosphorus, probably by acting on the proximal tubules. In humans, these effects are small, last only a short while, and are unlikely to be physiologically important for lowering blood calcium levels. The renal effects of calcitonin are not important in patients with thyroid tumors that secrete large amounts of calcitonin. Kidney cells "escape" from prolonged stimulation with calcitonin and become refractory to it, possibly as a result of down regulation of receptors.

Regulation of Secretion

Parafollicular cells respond directly to ionized calcium in the blood. Circulating concentrations of calcitonin are low when the blood calcium level is in the normal range or below, but they increase proportionately when the calcium concentration rises above about 9 mg/dl (Fig. 10). The concentration of calcitonin in blood may also increase after eating. Gastrin, a hormone produced by gastric mucosal cells, stimulates the parafollicular cells to secrete calcitonin. Other gastrointestinal hormones that have the same four amino acids at their carboxyl terminus, including cholecystokinin-pancreozymin, glucagon, and secretin, have similar effects, but gastrin is the most potent. Secretion of calcitonin in anticipation of an influx of calcium from the intestine may guard against excessive concentrations of plasma calcium. This phenomenon is analogous to the anticipatory secretion of insulin after a carbohydrate-rich meal (see Chapter 5). Although the importance of this response in humans is not established, the sensitivity of parafollicular cells to gastrin has been exploited clinically as a provocative test for diagnosing medullary carcinoma of the thyroid.

THE VITAMIN D–ENDOCRINE SYSTEM

A derivative of vitamin D_3, $1,25(OH)_2D_3$, is indispensable for maintaining adequate concentrations of calcium in the extracellular fluid and adequate mineralization of bone matrix. Vitamin D deficiency leads to inadequate calcification of bone matrix and severe softening of the skeleton, called *osteomalacia*, which may lead

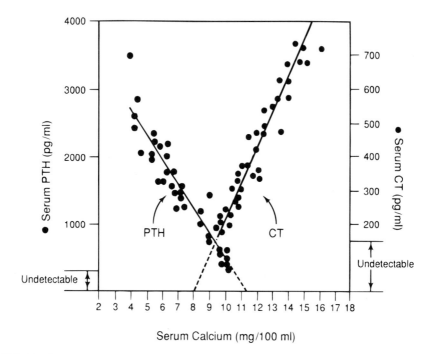

FIG. 10. Concentrations of immunoreactive PTH and calcitonin (*CT*) in pig plasma as a function of the plasma calcium level. From Arnaud, C.D., Littledike, T., and Tsao, H.S. (1969): Simultaneous measurement of calcitonin and parathyroid hormone in the pig. In: *Proceedings of the Symposium on Calcitonin and C Cells,* edited by Taylor, S. and Foster, G.V. Heinemann, London.

to deformities and fractures. Osteomalacia in children is called *rickets* and may result in permanent deformities of the weight-bearing bones (bowed legs). Although vitamin D is now often called the vitamin D–endocrine system, when it was discovered as the factor in fish oil that prevents rickets, its hormone-like nature was not suspected. One important distinction between hormones and vitamins is that hormones are synthesized within the body from simple precursors, but vitamins must be provided in the diet. Actually, vitamin D_3, can be synthesized endogenously in humans, but the rate is limited by a nonenzymatic reaction that requires radiant energy in the form of light in the near-ultraviolet range—hence, the name *sunshine vitamin.* The immediate precursor for vitamin D_3, 7-dehydrocholesterol, is synthesized from acetyl coenzyme A and is stored in the skin. Conversion of 7-dehydrocholesterol to vitamin D_3 proceeds spontaneously in the presence of sunlight that penetrates the epidermis to the outer layers of the dermis. Vitamin D deficiency became a significant public health problem as a byproduct of industrialization. Urban living, smog, and increased indoor activity limit exposure of the populace to sunshine and, hence, endogenous production of vitamin D_3. This problem is readily addressed by adding vitamin D to foods, particularly milk.

    1,25(OH)$_2$D$_3$ also fits the description of a hormone in the respect that it travels through the blood in small amounts from its site of production to affect cells at distant sites. Another major difference between a vitamin and a hormone is that vitamins usually are cofactors in metabolic reactions, whereas hormones behave as regulators and interact with specific receptors. $1,25(OH)_2D_3$ produces many of its biological effects in a manner characteristic of steroid hormones (see Chapter 1). It binds to a specific intracellular receptor, which in turn binds to chromatin and induces RNA and protein synthesis. In fact, the $1,25(OH)_2D_3$ receptor belongs to the same family as other steroid hormone receptors.

Synthesis and Metabolism

The form of vitamin D produced in mammals is called cholecalciferol, or vitamin D_3; it differs from vitamin D_2 (ergosterol), which is produced in plants, only in the length of the side chain. Irradiation of the skin results in photolysis of the bond that links carbons 9 and 10 in 7-dehydrocholesterol and, thus, opens the B ring of the steroid nucleus (Fig. 11). The resultant cholecalciferol is biologically inert but, unlike its precursor, has a high affinity for a vitamin D-binding protein in plasma. Vitamin D_3 is transported by the blood to the liver, where it is oxidized at carbon 25 to form 25-hydroxycholecalciferol ($25OH-D_3$), and is again released into the blood. Although $25OH-D_3$ is the major circulating form of vitamin D, it has little biological activity. In the proximal tubules of the kidney, a second hydroxyl group is added at carbon 1 to yield the compound, $1,25(OH)_2D_3$, which is about 1,000 times as active as $25OH-D_3$. This compound probably accounts for all the biological activity of vitamin D. It is considerably less abundant in blood and binds less tightly to vitamin D-binding globulin than its precursor $25OH-D_3$. Consequently, $1,25(OH)_2D_3$ has a half-life in blood of 15 hours compared to 15 days for $25OH-D_3$.

The kidney also has the requisite enzymes to hydroxylate either $25OH-D_3$ or $1,25(OH)_2D_3$ at carbon 24 to produce $24,25(OH)_2D_3$ or $1,24,25(OH)_3D_3$. Of these, $24,25(OH)_2D_3$ is by far the most important quantitatively and is the major product of vitamin D metabolism. It is about 100 times more abundant in blood than $1,25(OH)_2D_3$ but has an even lower affinity for the vitamin D receptor in intestinal mucosal cells than does $25OH-D_3$. Although some investigators have suggested special biological functions for the 24-hydroxylated metabolites, it appears that oxidation at carbon 24 is the initial reaction of a degradative or inactivating pathway. Subsequent reactions include oxidation of the side chain and biliary excretion.

Physiological Actions of $1,25(OH)_2D_3$

Overall, the principal physiological actions of $1,25(OH)_2D_3$ increase calcium and phosphate concentrations in extracellular fluid. These effects are exerted primarily on intestine and bone and, to a lesser extent, on kidney. Vitamin D receptors are widely distributed, however, and a variety of other actions have been described, including regulation of intracellular calcium concentrations, enzyme induction, and cell growth and differentiation. Because these latter effects are neither well under-

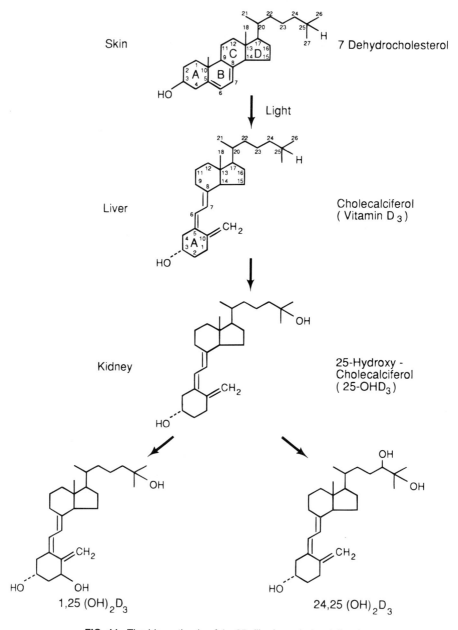

FIG. 11. The biosynthesis of 1α,25-dihydroxycholecalciferol.

stood nor germane to regulation of calcium balance, they will not be discussed further.

Actions on Intestine

Uptake of dietary calcium and phosphate depends on active transport by epithelial cells lining the small intestine. A deficiency of vitamin D severely impairs intestinal transport of both calcium and phosphorus. Although calcium uptake is usually accompanied by phosphate uptake, the two ions are transported by independent mechanisms, both of which are stimulated by $1,25(OH)_2D_3$. Increased uptake of calcium is seen about 2 hours after $1,25(OH)_2D_3$ is given to deficient subjects and is maximal within 4 hours. A much longer time is required when vitamin D is given, presumably because of the time needed for sequential hydroxylations in liver and kidney.

Details of how $1,25(OH)_2D_3$ increases ion transport are still not known. As with other steroid hormones, $1,25(OH)_2D_3$ produces its biological effects by inducing the production of new proteins. At least three vitamin D-dependent proteins are known, but just how they relate to increased transport of calcium and phosphate is not yet understood. Increased uptake of calcium is accompanied by increased production of a specific cytosolic high-affinity calcium binding protein called *calbindin*, alkaline phosphatase, and calcium-dependent ATPase (Fig. 12). We can speculate that $1,25(OH)_2D_3$ may increase calcium permeability of the brush border membrane. The binding protein may keep the cytosolic calcium concentration low and, thus, maintain a gradient favorable for calcium influx. It may also act as a shuttle to deliver calcium to the sodium–calcium exchange pump in the basolateral membranes. The mechanism by which $1,25(OH)_2D_3$ increases phosphate transport is even less well understood.

Some evidence obtained in experimental animals and in cultured cells suggests

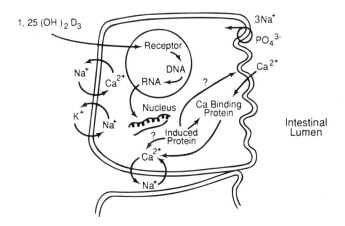

FIG. 12. The actions of $1,25(OH)_2D_3$ on intestinal transport of calcium.

that $1,25(OH)_2D_3$ may also produce some rapid actions that are not mediated by altered genomic expression. Among these are rapid transport of calcium across the intestinal epithelium by a process that may involve both the IP_3–DAG and the cyclic AMP messenger systems (see Chapter 1) and the activation of membrane calcium channels. The physiological importance of these rapid actions of $1,25(OH)_2D_3$ and the nature of the receptor that signals them are not known.

Actions on Bone

Although the most obvious consequence of vitamin D deficiency is decreased mineralization of bone, $1,25(OH)_2D_3$ apparently does not directly increase bone formation or calcium phosphate deposition in osteoid. Rather, mineralization of osteoid occurs spontaneously when adequate amounts of these ions are available. Ultimately, increased bone mineralization is made possible by increased intestinal absorption of calcium and phosphate. Paradoxically, perhaps, $1,25(OH)_2D_3$ acts directly on bone to promote resorption in a manner that resembles the late effects of PTH. Like PTH, $1,25(OH)_2D_3$ increases both the number and activity of osteoclasts. As is seen for PTH, osteoblasts rather than osteoclasts have receptors for $1,25(OH)_2D_3$, suggesting again that osteoblasts communicate with osteoclasts and their precursor cells. Although they act by different mechanisms, some overlap is likely in the actions of $1,25(OH)_2D_3$ and PTH on bone. Both agents probably express their actions through some final common pathway. The sensitivity of bone to PTH decreases with vitamin D deficiency; conversely, in the absence of PTH, 30 to 100 times as much $1,25(OH)_2D_3$ is needed to mobilize calcium and phosphate.

Actions on Kidney

When given to vitamin D-deficient subjects, $1,25(OH)_2D_3$ increases reabsorption of both calcium and phosphate. The effects on phosphate reabsorption are probably indirect. Secretion of PTH tends to be increased in vitamin D deficiency (*secondary hyperparathyroidism*) because of the low concentration of ionized calcium in blood and because $1,25(OH)_2D_3$ directly inhibits PTH secretion. As $1,25(OH)_2D_3$ normalizes the plasma calcium concentration, decreased secretion of PTH allows proximal tubular reabsorption of phosphate to increase. The effects of $1,25(OH)_2D_3$ on calcium reabsorption are probably direct. Specific receptors for $1,25(OH)_2D_3$ are found in the distal nephron where selective uptake of calcium occurs. These cells also contain the same vitamin D-dependent calcium-binding protein as found in intestinal cells. It is unlikely that $1,25(OH)_2D_3$ regulates calcium balance on a minute-to-minute basis. Instead, it may act in a permissive way to support the actions of PTH, which is the primary regulator.

Regulation of $1,25(OH)_2D_3$ Production

As is true of any hormone, the concentration of $1,25(OH)_2D_3$ in blood must be appropriate for prevailing physiological circumstances if it is to exercise its proper

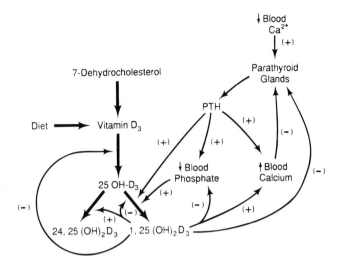

FIG. 13. The regulation of 1α,25-dihydroxycholecalciferol synthesis.

role in maintaining homeostasis. Production of $1,25(OH)_2D_3$ is subject to feedback regulation in a fashion quite similar to that of other hormones. The most important regulatory step is the hydroxylation of carbon 1 by cells in the proximal tubules of the kidney. This reaction, which converts a nearly inactive precursor to a highly active hormone, is stimulated primarily by PTH, which thus acts as a tropic hormone, and by low concentrations of phosphate. Although 1α-hydroxylase activity may be increased by cyclic AMP, the principal effect of PTH is to increase synthesis of this enzyme, which has a half-life of only a few hours. In the absence of PTH, the concentration of 1α-hydroxylase in renal cells quickly falls.

Like other steroid hormones, $1,25(OH)_2D_3$ is a negative feedback inhibitor of its own production. It inhibits hydroxylation of carbon 1 in the kidney and of carbon 25 in the liver. In addition, $1,25(OH)_2D_3$ stimulates hydroxylation of carbon 24, which diverts precursor to a degradative pathway. Finally, the results of its actions, increased calcium and phosphate concentrations in blood, directly or indirectly silence the two activators of its production, PTH and low phosphate. The regulation of $1,25(OH)_2D_3$ production is summarized in Fig. 13.

INTEGRATED ACTIONS OF CALCITROPIC HORMONES

Response to a Hypocalcemic Challenge

Because some calcium is always lost in urine, even a short period of total fasting can produce a mild hypocalcemic challenge. More severe challenges are produced by a diet deficient in calcium or anything that might interfere with intestinal or renal

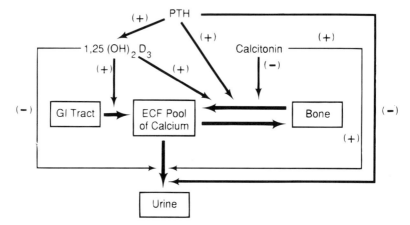

FIG. 14. The overall regulation of calcium balance by PTH, calcitonin and 1,25(OH)$_2$D$_3$.

absorption of calcium. The parathyroid glands are exquisitely sensitive to even a small decrease in ionized calcium and promptly increase PTH secretion (Fig. 14). The effects of PTH on osteocytic osteolysis and reabsorption of calcium from the glomerular filtrate are evident after about 1 hour, providing the first line of defense against a hypocalcemic challenge. These actions are adequate only to compensate for a mild or brief challenge. Osteocytic osteolysis is limited to a rather small pool of labile bone mineral, and even if renal tubular reabsorption of calcium were 100% efficient, it is simply a mechanism to reduce further calcium loss, and cannot replenish blood calcium.

When the hypocalcemic challenge is large and sustained, additional, delayed responses to PTH are needed. After about 24 hours, increased formation of 1,25(OH)$_2$D$_3$ increases the efficiency of calcium absorption from the gut. Osteoclastic bone resorption in response to both PTH and 1,25(OH)$_2$D$_3$ taps the almost inexhaustible reserves of calcium in the skeleton. If calcium intake remains inadequate, skeletal integrity may be sacrificed in favor of maintaining adequate blood calcium concentrations.

Response to a Hypercalcemic Challenge

Hypercalcemia is rarely seen under normal physiological circumstances, but it may be a complication of a variety of pathological conditions. Hypercalcemia might result, for example, when a subject who has been living for some time on a calcium-deficient diet ingests calcium-rich food. Under the influence of high concentrations of PTH and 1,25(OH)$_2$D$_3$, osteoclastic bone resorption and osteocytic osteolysis actively transfer bone mineral to the extracellular fluid. In addition, calcium absorptive mechanisms in the intestine and renal tubules are stimulated to their maximal efficiency. Consequently, the calcium that enters the gut is absorbed efficiently, and the blood calcium is increased by a few tenths of a milligram per deciliter. Although PTH secretion promptly decreases and its effects on osteocytic osteolysis and calcium and phosphate transport in renal tubules quickly diminish, several hours pass before hydroxylation of 25OH-D_3 and osteoclastic bone resorption diminish. Even after its production is shut down, many hours are required for responses to $1,25(OH)_2D_3$ to decrease. Although some calcium phosphate may precipitate in demineralized osteoid, renal loss of calcium is the principal means of lowering blood calcium. The rate of renal loss, however, is limited to only 10% of the calcium present in the glomerular filtrate, or about 40 mg per hour, even after complete shutdown of PTH-sensitive transport. Under these circumstances, we might expect calcitonin secretion to increase and to cause the flux of calcium from bone to blood to decrease as the osteoclasts are inhibited.

OTHER HORMONES AFFECTING CALCIUM BALANCE

In addition to the primary endocrine regulators of calcium balance discussed previously, it is apparent that many endocrine and paracrine factors influence calcium balance. Bone growth and remodeling appear to involve a poorly understood interplay of local and circulating factors, including insulin-like growth factor (IGF-I, see Chapter 10) and such osteoclast activating factors as the cytokines, interleukin-1 (see Chapter 4) and tumor necrosis factor. Some of these factors such as transforming growth factor-β may be responsible for coupling of bone resorption and bone formation as discussed earlier in this chapter. The prostaglandins (see Chapter 4) also have calcium mobilizing activity and stimulate bone lysis. Pathological changes in calcium metabolism can thus result from interference with the production or action of the various growth factors as well as with the production, metabolism, or actions of PTH, calcitonin, and $1,25(OH)_2D_3$.

Many of the systemic hormones directly or indirectly have an impact on calcium balance. Obviously, special demands are imposed on overall calcium balance during growth, pregnancy, and lactation. All of the hormones that govern growth, principally growth hormone, the IGFs, and thyroid and gonadal hormones (see Chapter 10) directly or indirectly influence the activity of bone cells and calcium uptake and excretion. The gonadal hormones play a role in maintaining bone mass, which decreases in their absence, leading to *osteoporosis*. This condition is characterized by an imbalance between bone resorption and bone formation and is common in postmenopausal women.

Defects in calcium metabolism are seen in hyperthyroidism or in conditions of excess or deficiency of adrenal cortical hormones. These hormonal effects are imperfectly understood. Thyroid hormones may act directly on bone cells to increase resorption, and in excess produce a decrease in bone mass. This action may lead to mild hypercalcemia and, secondarily, may suppress PTH secretion, which in turn, may account for increased urinary loss of calcium and decreased intestinal absorption. Excessive glucocorticoid concentrations also decrease skeletal mass. Glucocorticoids antagonize the actions and formation of $1,25(OH)_2D_3$ and directly inhibit calcium uptake in the intestine. In addition, they may interfere with maturation of osteoblasts. Adrenal insufficiency may lead to hypercalcemia due largely to decreased renal excretion of calcium.

CONCLUDING COMMENTS

The regulation of calcium homeostasis provides good examples of some of the principles of hormonal integration discussed in Chapter 6. The principle of cooperativity is illustrated by the multiple actions of PTH on different tissues to produce a variety of effects that contribute to the central theme of increasing calcium in the extracellular compartment. The overlapping effects of PTH and $1,25(OH)_2D_3$ illustrate redundancy. The opposing actions of PTH and calcitonin on osteoclasts are typical of a push–pull system. The thoughtful student will undoubtedly find other examples in this exquisitely coordinated system.

SUGGESTED READING

Bell, N. H. (1985): Vitamin D-endocrine system. *J. Clin. Invest.*, 76:1–6.

Brommage, R., and DeLuca, H. F. (1985): Evidence that 1,25-dihydroxyvitamin D_3 is the physiologically active metabolite of vitamin D_3. *Endocr. Rev.*, 6:491–511.

Brown, E. M. (1991): Extracellular Ca^{2+} sensing, regulation of parathyroid cell function, and the role of Ca^{2+} and other ions as extracellular (first) messengers. *Physiol. Rev.*, 71:371–411.

Chambers, J. T., and Hall, T. J. (1991): Cellular and molecular mechanisms in the regulation and function of osteoclasts. *Vitam. Horm.*, 46:41–86.

Cohn, D. V., Kumarasamy, R., and Ramp, W. K. (1986): Intracellular processing and secretion of parathyroid gland proteins. *Vitam. Horm.*, 43:283–315.

Habener, J. F., Roseblatt, M., and Potts, J. T., Jr. (1984): Parathyroid hormone: biochemical aspects of biosynthesis, secretion, action, and metabolism. *Physiol. Rev.*, 64:985–1054.

Muff, R., and Fischer, J. A. (1992): Parathyroid hormone receptors in control of proximal tubular function. *Annu. Rev. Physiol.*, 54:67–79.

Nijweide, P. J., Burger, E. H., and Feyen, J. H. M. (1986): Cells of bone: proliferation, differentiation, and hormonal regulation. *Physiol. Rev.*, 66:855–886.

Norman, A. W., Roth, J., and Orci, L. (1982): The vitamin D endocrine system: steroid metabolism, hormone receptors, and biological response (calcium binding proteins). *Endocr. Rev.*, 3:331–366.

Pocotte, S. L., Ehrenstein, G., and Fitzpatrick, L. A. (1991): Regulation of parathyroid hormone secretion. *Endocr. Rev.*, 12:291–301.

Walters, M. R. (1992): Newly identified actions of the vitamin D endocrine system. *Endocr. Rev.*, 13: 719–764.

9

Hormonal Regulation of Fuel Metabolism

OVERVIEW

All cells of the body require an uninterrupted supply of metabolic fuel whether they are at rest or carrying out their unique specialized functions. Although metabolic fuels must ultimately originate in the diet, evolution of the capacity for storage of energy-rich substrates in times of plenty and the ability to draw on these stores in times of want has liberated us from the necessity of constant feedings. We now consider the elaborate hormonal mechanisms that regulate storage and mobilization while maintaining just the right amounts of blood nutrients to meet the varied demands of specialized tissues. The strategy of hormonal regulation of metabolism during starvation or exercise is to provide sufficient substrate to working muscles while maintaining an adequate concentration of glucose in blood to satisfy the needs of the brain and other glucose-dependent cells. When dietary carbohydrate is inadequate, availability of glucose is ensured by: (1) gluconeogenesis from alanine, glycerol, and lactate and (2) inhibition of glucose utilization by those tissues that can satisfy their energy needs with other substrates, notably fatty acids and ketone bodies. We have already considered the metabolic effects of insulin, glucagon (see Chapter 5), and epinephrine (see Chapter 4), which are the immediate regulators of blood glucose. In addition, growth hormone and cortisol (see Chapter 4) contribute to long-term maintenance of fuel reserves, and thyroxine, via triiodothyronine (see Chapter 3) governs the overall rate of fuel consumption. Here, we consider how these hormones interact to solve two common metabolic problems: starvation and exercise.

GENERAL FEATURES OF ENERGY METABOLISM

Body Fuels

Glucose

Glucose is readily oxidized by all cells. One gram yields about 4 Calories. The average 70-kg man requires approximately 2,000 Calories per day and, therefore, would require a reserve supply of approximately 500 g of glucose to ensure sufficient substrate to survive 1 day of food deprivation. If glucose were stored as an isosmolar solution, approximately 10 liters of water (10 kg) would be needed to accommodate a single day's energy needs, and the 70-kg man would have to carry around a storage depot equal to his own weight if he were to survive only 1 week of starvation. Actually, he has only about 20 g of free glucose dissolved in his extracellular fluids, or enough to provide energy for about 1 hour.

Glycogen

Polymerizing glucose to glycogen eliminates the osmotic requirement for large volumes of water. To meet a single day's energy needs, only about 1 kg of "wet" glycogen is required; that is, 500 g of glycogen obligates only about 0.5 liters of water. Glycogen stores in the well-fed 70-kg man are only enough to meet part of a day's energy needs—about 100 g in the liver and about 200 g in the muscle.

Protein

Calories can also be stored in somewhat more concentrated form as protein. Storage of protein, however, also obligates storage of some water, and oxidation of protein creates unique byproducts: ammonia, which must be detoxified to form urea at metabolic expense, and sulfur-containing acids. The body of a normal 70-kg man in nitrogen balance contains about 10 to 12 kg of protein, most of which is in skeletal muscle. Little or no protein is stored as an inert fuel depot, so that mobilization of protein for energy necessarily produces some functional deficits. Under conditions of prolonged starvation, as much as one half of the body protein may be consumed for energy before death ensues, usually from failure of the respiratory muscles.

Fat

Triglycerides are by far the most concentrated storage form of high-energy fuel (9 Calories/g). One day's energy needs can be met by less than 250 g of triglyceride, which is stored without water. Thus, a 70-kg man carrying 10 kg of fat maintains an adequate depot of fuel to meet energy needs for more than 40 days. Most fat is stored in adipose tissue, but other tissues, such as muscle, also contain small reserves of triglycerides.

Problems Inherent in the Use of Glucose and Fat as Metabolic Fuels

1. Fat is the most abundant and efficient energy reserve, but efficiency has its price. When converting dietary carbohydrate to fat, about 25% of the energy is dissipated as heat. More importantly, synthesis of fatty acids from glucose is

an irreversible process. Once the carbons of glucose are converted to fatty acids, there can be no net reconversion to glucose. The glycerol portion of triglycerides remains convertible to glucose, but glycerol represents only about 10% of the mass of triglyceride.

2. The limited water solubility of fat complicates its transport between tissues. Triglycerides are "packaged" as high or low density lipoproteins or as chylomicrons for transport in blood to storage sites. Uptake by cells follows breakdown to fatty acids by lipoprotein lipase at the external surface or within capillaries adjacent to muscle or fat cells. Mobilization of stored triglycerides also requires breakdown to fatty acids, which leave adipocytes in the form of free fatty acids (FFA). The FFA are not very soluble in water and are transported in blood firmly bound to albumin. Because they are bound to albumin, FFA have limited access to tissues such as brain; they can be processed to water-soluble forms in the liver, however, which converts them to four-carbon ketoacids (ketone bodies), which can cross the blood–brain barrier.

3. Energy can be derived from glucose without simultaneous consumption of oxygen, but oxygen is required for the degradation of fat. Therefore, glucose must be constantly available in the blood to satisfy the needs of red blood cells, which lack mitochondria, and cells in the renal medullae, which function under low oxygen tension. Under basal conditions, these cells consume about 50 g of glucose each day and release an equivalent amount of lactate into the blood. Because lactate is readily reconverted to glucose in the liver, however, these tissues do not act as a drain on carbohydrate reserves.

4. In a well-nourished person, the brain relies almost exclusively on glucose to meet its energy demands and consumes nearly 150 g of it per day. The brain cannot derive energy from oxidation of FFA or amino acids. Ketone bodies are the only alternative substrates to glucose, but studies in experimental animals indicate that only certain regions of the brain can substitute ketone bodies for glucose. Total fasting for 4 to 5 days is required before the concentrations of ketone bodies in blood are high enough to provide a significant fraction of the brain's energy needs. Even after several weeks of total starvation, the brain continues to satisfy about one third of its energy needs with glucose. The brain stores little glycogen and, hence, must depend on the circulation to meet its minute-to-minute fuel requirements. The rate of glucose delivery depends on its concentration in arterial blood, the rate of blood flow, and the efficiency of extraction. Although an increased flow rate might compensate for decreased glucose concentration, the mechanisms that regulate blood flow in the brain are responsive to oxygen and carbon dioxide, rather than to glucose. Under basal conditions, the concentration of glucose in arterial blood is about 5 mM (90 mg/dl), of which the brain extracts about 10%. The fraction extracted can double, or perhaps even triple, when the concentration of glucose is low, but when the blood glucose falls below about 30 mg/dl, metabolism and function are compromised. Thus, the brain is exceedingly vulnerable to hypoglycemia, which can quickly produce coma or death.

Fuel Consumption

The amount of metabolic fuel consumed in a day varies widely and normally is balanced by variations in food intake, but the adipose tissue reservoir of triglycerides can shrink or expand to accommodate an imbalance in fuel intake and expenditure. Muscle comprises about 50% of body mass and is by far the major consumer of metabolic fuel. Even at rest, muscle metabolism accounts for about 30% of the oxygen consumed. Although the normal 70-kg man consumes about 2,000 Calories in a typical day, he may require only about 1,200 Calories with complete bed rest or as much as 6,000 Calories with prolonged physical activity. For example, marathon running may consume 3,000 Calories in only 3 hours. Under basal conditions, individuals on a typical mixed diet derive about one half of their daily energy needs from the oxidation of glucose, a small fraction from consumption of protein, and the remainder from fat. With starvation or with prolonged exercise, limited carbohydrate reserves are quickly exhausted unless some restriction is placed on carbohydrate consumption by muscle, whose fuel needs far exceed those of any other tissue and can be met by increased utilization of fat. In fact, simply providing muscle with fat restricts its ability to consume carbohydrate. Hormonal regulation of energy balance is largely accomplished through adjusting the flux of energy-rich fatty acids and their derivatives to muscle and the consequent sparing of carbohydrate and protein.

GLUCOSE–FATTY ACID CYCLE

The self-regulating interplay between glucose and fatty acid metabolism (Fig. 1) is called the *glucose–fatty acid cycle* and constitutes an important biochemical

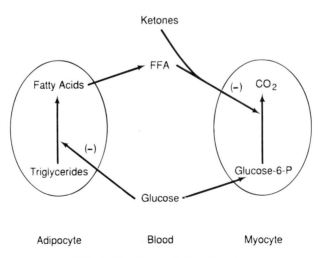

FIG. 1. The glucose–fatty acid cycle.

mechanism for restricting glucose utilization when alternative substrate is available. Fatty acids, produced constantly in adipose tissue in an ongoing cycle of lipolysis and reesterification, may either escape from fat cells to become the FFA, or be retained as triglycerides, depending on the availability of α-glycerol phosphate. The only source of α-glycerol for reesterification is the pool of triose phosphates derived from glucose oxidation because adipose tissue is deficient in the enzyme required to phosphorylate and, hence, reuse the glycerol released from triglycerides. Consequently, when glucose is abundant, α-glycerol phosphate is readily available, and the rate of reesterification is high relative to lipolysis. Conversely, when glucose is scarce, more fatty acids escape and plasma concentrations of FFA increase.

Oxidation of fatty acids inhibits glucose metabolism in muscle by the complex series of events depicted in Fig. 2. The FFA, which are 16 or 18 carbons long, are taken up by muscle in proportion to their concentration in blood and are oxidized within the mitochondria to acetyl coenzyme A (CoA). Ketone bodies are also rapidly converted to acetyl CoA by muscle. Acetyl CoA condenses with oxaloacetate to form citrate and, thereby, enters the tricarboxylic acid cycle for final conversion to carbon dioxide. Formation of acetyl CoA from long-chain fatty acids or ketone

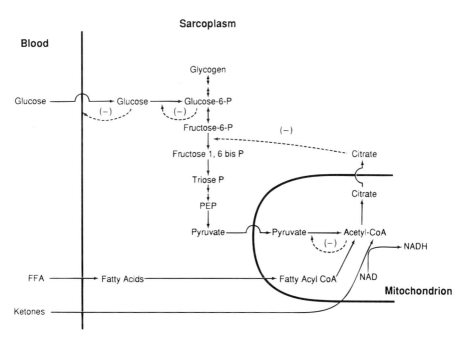

FIG. 2. The inhibition of glucose metabolism in muscle by fatty acids and ketone bodies. Metabolites formed as a consequence of oxidizing fatty acids and ketone bodies inhibit phosphofructokinase and the irreversible conversion of pyruvate to acetyl CoA. Inhibition of phosphofructokinase maintains glycogen and secondarily inhibits glucose uptake. Pyruvate formed from any fructose-6-phosphate that penetrates the barrier at phosphofructokinase may be released as either pyruvate or lactate and be reconverted to glucose in the liver.

bodies is accompanied by conversion of the cofactor nicotinamide adenine dinucleotide (NAD) to its reduced form, NADH. In the nonworking muscle, this process proceeds at a rate that exceeds the oxidative regeneration of this cofactor and, hence, depletes mitochondrial reserves. The resulting scarcity of NAD limits the oxidation of citrate, which accumulates first in the mitochondria and then in the cytosol, where its concentration may increase many fold. Scarcity of NAD also limits decarboxylation of pyruvate and, hence, deters irreversible loss of this basic carbohydrate precursor.

Citrate is a powerful inhibitor of phosphofructokinase. This enzyme, which catalyzes the major rate-determining reaction of glycolysis, acts as the gatekeeper of glucose oxidation. When glycolysis is inhibited at this step, glucose is diverted into glycogen, which therefore accumulates. When the capacity for glycogen storage is saturated, glucose-6-phosphate accumulates and powerfully inhibits phosphorylation of glucose by hexokinase. Glucose enters myocytes by carrier-mediated diffusion driven by the concentration gradient across the cell membrane. When hexokinase is not inhibited by glucose-6-phosphate, glucose is phosphorylated as rapidly as it enters the cell. Its intracellular concentration therefore is exceedingly low, and the concentration gradient for glucose between extracellular and intracellular water is maintained. When hexokinase is inhibited, glucose uptake is also inhibited because free glucose accumulates within the myocytes and reduces the driving force for further uptake (Fig. 2).

In the glucose–fatty acid cycle, glucose indirectly regulates its own rate of oxidation by a negative feedback process that spares glucose for those tissues that cannot make use of alternative substrates. The glucose–fatty acid cycle operates in normal physiology even though the concentration of glucose in blood remains nearly constant. In fact, the contribution of some hormones, notably glucocorticoids and growth hormone, to the maintenance of blood glucose and muscle glycogen depends in part on the glucose–fatty acid cycle. Conversely, in addition to directly stimulating glucose transport in muscle, insulin indirectly increases glucose metabolism by decreasing FFA mobilization from adipose tissue, thereby shutting down the glucose–fatty acid cycle.

OVERALL REGULATION OF BLOOD GLUCOSE CONCENTRATION

Despite vagaries in dietary input and large fluctuations in consumption, the concentration of glucose in blood remains remarkably constant. The concentration of glucose in blood at any time is determined by the rate of input from the liver and the rate of removal by the various body tissues. Under most circumstances, liver glycogen is the immediate source of blood glucose. Gluconeogenesis may contribute to blood glucose directly but is more important for replenishing glycogen stores. The rate of glucose removal from the blood varies over a wide range, depending on physical activity and environmental temperature.

Minute-to-minute regulation of blood glucose depends on (a) insulin, which in promoting fuel storage, drives glucose concentrations down and (b) glucagon and catecholamines, which in mobilizing fuel reserves, drive glucose concentrations up. Effects of these hormones are evident within seconds or minutes and dissipate as quickly. Insulin acts at the level of the liver to inhibit glucose output and on muscle and fat to increase glucose uptake. The liver is more sensitive to insulin than are muscle and fat. Smaller increments in insulin concentration are needed to inhibit glucose production than to promote glucose uptake. Glucagon and catecholamines act on hepatocytes to promote glycogenolysis and gluconeogenesis. They have no direct effects on glucose uptake by peripheral tissues, but epinephrine and norepinephrine may decrease the demand for blood glucose by mobilizing alternative fuels, glycogen and fat, within muscle and adipose tissue. Increased blood glucose is perceived directly by the beta cells, which respond by secreting insulin. Hypoglycemia is perceived, not only by the glucagon-secreting alpha cells of the pancreatic islets, but also by the central nervous system, which activates sympathetic outflow to the islets and the adrenal medullae. Sympathetic stimulation of pancreatic islets increases the secretion of glucagon and inhibits the secretion of insulin. In addition, hypoglycemia evokes the secretion of the hypothalamic releasing hormones that stimulate corticotropin (ACTH) and growth hormone secretion from the pituitary gland (Fig. 3). Cortisol secreted in response to ACTH and growth hormone act only after a substantial delay, and hence, increased amounts are unlikely to contribute to rapid restoration of the blood glucose. However, they are important for withstanding a sustained hypoglycemic challenge.

Long-term regulation, operative on a time scale of hours or perhaps days, depends on direct and indirect actions of many hormones and ultimately ensures (a) that the peripheral drain on glucose reserves is minimized and (b) that the liver contains an adequate reservoir of glycogen to satisfy the minute-to-minute needs of glucose-

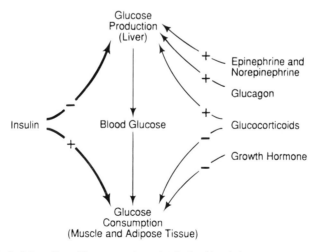

FIG. 3. Interaction of hormones to maintain the blood glucose concentration.

dependent cells. To achieve these ends, peripheral tissues, mainly muscle, must be provided with alternate substrate and limit their consumption of glucose. At the same time, gluconeogenesis must be stimulated and supplied with adequate precursors to provide the 150 to 200 g of glucose needed each day. Long-term regulation includes all of the responses that govern glucose utilization as well as all those reactions that govern storage of fuel as glycogen, protein, or triglycerides.

INTEGRATED ACTIONS OF METABOLIC HORMONES

Metabolic fuels absorbed from the intestine are largely converted to storage forms in liver, adipocytes, and muscle. It is fair to state that storage is virtually the exclusive province of insulin, which stimulates the biochemical reactions that convert simple compounds to more complex storage forms and inhibits fuel mobilization. Hormones that mobilize fuel and defend the glucose concentration of the blood are called *counterregulatory* and include glucagon, epinephrine, norepinephrine, cortisol, and growth hormone (Fig. 4). The secretion of most or all of these hormones is increased whenever there is increased demand for energy. These hormones act synergistically, and together produce effects that are greater than the sum of their individual actions. In the example shown in Fig. 5, glucagon and epinephrine raised the blood glucose level primarily by increasing hepatic production. When cortisol was given simultaneously, these effects were magnified, even though cortisol had little effect when given alone. Triiodothyronine (T_3) must also be considered in this context because its actions increase the rate of fuel consumption and the sensitivity of target cells to insulin and the counterregulatory hormones. Before examining the interactions of these hormones in the whole body, it is useful to summarize their effects on individual tissues.

Adipose Tissue

The central event in adipose tissue metabolism is the cycle of fatty acid esterification and triglyceride lipolysis (Fig. 6). Although reesterification of fatty acids can regulate FFA output from fat cells, regulation of lipolysis and, hence, the rate at which the cycle spins provides a wider range of control. Catecholamines and insulin, through their antagonistic effects on cyclic adenosine monophosphate (AMP) metabolism, increase or decrease the activity of hormone-sensitive lipase. Responses to these hormones are expressed within minutes. Other hormones, especially cortisol and T_3, modulate the sensitivity of adipocytes to insulin and catecholamines. These effects are not due to abrupt changes in hormone concentrations but, rather, seem to reflect long-term tuning of the metabolic machinery. Finally, growth hormone produces a sustained increase in lipolysis after a delay of about 2 hours. Growth hormone and cortisol also decrease fatty acid esterification by inhibiting glucose metabolism. These hormonal effects on adipose tissue are summarized in Table 1.

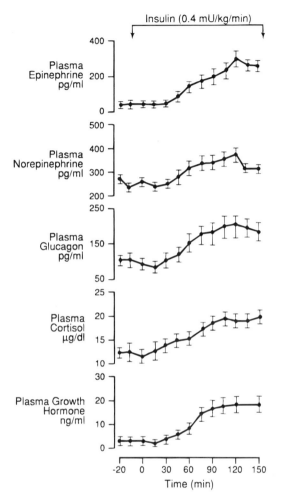

FIG. 4. Counterregulatory hormonal responses to insulin-induced hypoglycemia. The infusion of insulin reduced the plasma glucose concentration to 50 to 55 mg/dl. The *asterisks* indicate the first point at which the rise in plasma hormone concentration was significantly above basal levels. From Sacca, L., Sherwin, R., Hendler, R., et al. (1979): Influence of continuous physiologic hyperinsulinemia on glucose kinetics and counterregulatory hormones in normal and diabetic humans. *J. Clin. Invest.*, 63:849.

Muscle

By inhibiting FFA mobilization, insulin promptly decreases plasma FFA and thus removes a deterrent of glucose utilization in muscle at the same time that it promotes transport of glucose into myocytes. The response to insulin can be divided into two components. Stimulation of glucose transport and glycogen synthesis are direct effects and are seen within minutes. Increased oxidation of glucose that results from

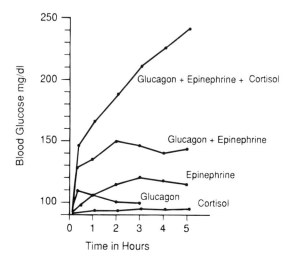

FIG. 5. Synergistic effects of cortisol, glucagon, and epinephrine on increasing the plasma glucose level. Note that the hyperglycemic response to the triple hormone infusion is far greater than the additive response of all three hormones given singly. Redrawn from data of Eigler, N., Sacca, L., and Sherwin, R.S. (1979): Synergistic interactions of physiologic increments of glucagon, epinephrine, and cortisol in the dog. *J. Clin. Invest.,* 63:114.

the release of phosphofructokinase inhibition requires several hours. Epinephrine and norepinephrine promptly increase cyclic AMP production and glycogenolysis. When the rate of glucose production from glycogen exceeds the need for adenosine triphosphate (ATP) production, muscle cells release lactate, which can be reconverted to glucose in liver. Growth hormone and cortisol directly inhibit glucose uptake by muscle and indirectly decrease glucose metabolism in myocytes through the agency of the glucose–fatty acid cycle. By indirectly inhibiting phosphofructokinase, growth hormone and cortisol divert glucose into muscle glycogen and decrease glycogen breakdown. The resulting preservation of muscle glycogen has been called the *glycostatic effect* of growth hormone. Preservation of muscle glycogen is also part of the overall effect of cortisol that gives rise to the term ''glucocorticoid.'' In addition, cortisol inhibits the uptake of amino acids and their incorporation into proteins and simultaneously promotes degradation of muscle protein. As a result, muscle becomes a net exporter of amino acids, which provide substrate for gluconeogenesis in liver. These events are summarized in Table 2.

Liver

The antagonistic effects of insulin and glucagon on gluconeogenesis, ketogenesis, and glycogen metabolism in hepatocytes are described in Chapter 5. Epinephrine and norepinephrine, by virtue of their effects on cyclic AMP metabolism, share all the actions of glucagon. In addition, these medullary hormones activate α_1-adrenergic

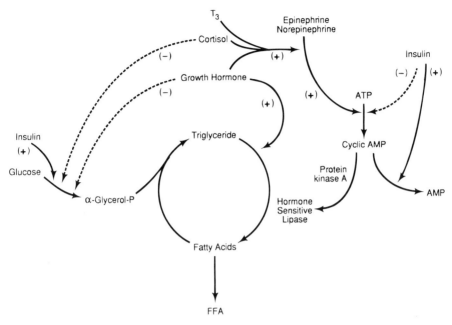

FIG. 6. Hormonal effects on FFA production. Epinephrine and norepinephrine stimulate (+) hormone-sensitive lipase through a cyclic AMP-mediated process. Insulin antagonizes this effect by inhibiting (−) cyclic AMP formation and stimulating its degradation. Cortisol, T_3, and growth hormone increase the response of adipocytes to epinephrine and norepinephrine. Growth hormone also directly stimulates lipolysis. Insulin indirectly antagonizes the production of FFA by increasing reesterification. Growth hormone and cortisol increase FFA release by inhibiting reesterification.

receptors and reinforce these effects through the agency of the diacylglycerol–inositol 1,4,5 trisphosphate–calcium system (see Chapter 1). Cortisol is indispensable as a permissive agent for the actions of glucagon and catecholamines on gluconeogenesis and glycogenolysis. In addition, cortisol induces the synthesis of a variety of enzymes responsible for gluconeogenesis and glycogen storage. By virtue of its actions on muscle, cortisol is also indispensable for providing substrate for gluconeo-

TABLE 1. *Hormonal effects on metabolism in adipocytes*

Hormone	Glucose uptake	Lipolysis	Reesterification	Rate
Insulin	↑	↓	↑	R
Epinephrine and norepinephrine	↑	↑↑	↑	R
Growth hormone	↓	↑	↓	S
Cortisol	↓	↑[a]	↓	S
T_3	↑	↑[a]	↑	S

[a] Permissive effects.
T_3, triiodothyronine; R, rapid; S, slow.

TABLE 2. *Hormonal effects of glucose metabolism in muscle*

	Glucose uptake	Glucose phosphorylation	Glycolysis	Glycogen storage
Insulin	↑ (D)	↑ (I)	↑ (I)	↑ (D)
Epinephrine, norepinephrine	↓[a] (I)	↓[a] (I)	↑	↓ (D)
Growth hormone	↓ (D, I)	↓ (I)	↓ (I)	↑ (I)
Cortisol	↓ (D, I)	↓ (I)	↓ (I)	↑ (I)
T_3	↑	↑	↑	↑ or ↓[b]

[a] Immediate effect is secondary to glycogenolysis; later effect is secondary to the glucose fatty acid cycle.
[b] Dependent on the dose; high rates of oxygen consumption may decrease glycogen.
D, direct; I, indirect via the glucose fatty acid cycle; T_3, triiodothyronine.

genesis. Thyroid hormone promotes glucose utilization in liver by promoting synthesis of enzymes required for glucose metabolism and lipid formation. Growth hormone is thought to increase hepatic glucose production, but the underlying mechanisms are not understood. Growth hormone also increases ketogenesis, largely by increasing the mobilization of FFA. These hormonal influences on hepatic metabolism are summarized in Table 3.

Pancreatic Islets

Alpha and beta cells of pancreatic islets are targets for metabolic hormones as well as producers of glucagon and insulin. Insulin inhibits glucagon secretion, and in its absence, the alpha cells are not shut down by hyperglycemia. Conversely, glucagon can stimulate insulin secretion. Epinephrine and norepinephrine inhibit insulin secretion and stimulate glucagon secretion. Growth hormone, cortisol, and T_3 are required for normal secretory activity of beta cells, whose capacity for insulin secretion is reduced in their absence. The effects of growth hormone and cortisol on insulin secretion are somewhat paradoxical. Although their effects in adipose

TABLE 3. *Hormonal regulation of metabolism in liver*

Hormone	Glucose output	Glycogen synthesis or breakdown	Gluconeogenesis	Ketogenesis	Ureogenesis	Lipogenesis
Insulin	↓ (D)	S	↓ (D)	↓ (I, D)	↓ (I, D)	↑ (D)
Glucagon	↑ (D)	B	↑ (D)	↑ (D)	↑ (D)	↓ (D)
Epinephrine, norepinephrine	↑ (D)	B	↑ (D)	↑ (I, D)	↑ (D)	↓ (D)
Growth hormone	↑ (I)		↑ (I)	↑ (I)	↑[a] (I)	↓ (I)
Cortisol	↑ (I, D)	S	↑ (I, D)	↑ (I)	↑ (I)	↓ (I)
T_3	↑ (I)	B	↑ (I)	↑ (I)	↑ (I)	↑ (D?)

[a] Growth hormone promotes protein synthesis and, hence, decreases the availability of amino acids for ureogenesis.
I, indirect effect; D, direct effect; T_3, triiodothyronine; S, synthesis; B, breakdown

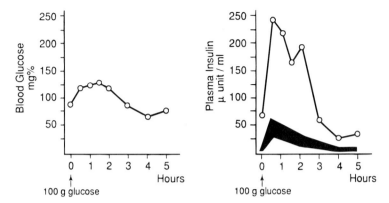

FIG. 7. The plasma insulin response following ingestion of 100 g of glucose in an acromegalic subject with normal glucose tolerance. The *shaded area* represents the plasma insulin response of 43 normal subjects after ingestion of 100 g of glucose. From Daughaday, W.H. and Kipnis, D.M. (1966): The growth-promoting and anti-insulin actions of somatotropin. *Recent Prog. Horm. Res.*, 22:49.

tissue, muscle, and liver are opposite to those of insulin, growth hormone and corti-sol, nevertheless, increase the sensitivity of beta cells to signals for insulin secretion and exaggerate responses to hyperglycemia (Fig. 7). When cortisol or growth hor-mone are present in excess, higher than normal concentrations of insulin are required to maintain blood glucose levels in the normal range. Higher concentrations of insulin itself may contribute to decreased sensitivity by down regulating insulin receptors in fat and muscle. When either growth hormone or glucocorticoids are present in excess for prolonged periods, diabetes mellitus often results. Approxi-mately 30% of patients suffering from excess growth hormone (acromegaly) and a similar percentage of persons suffering from Cushing's disease (excess glucocorti-coids) experience diabetes mellitus as a complication of their disease. In the early stages, diabetes is reversible and disappears when the excess pituitary or adrenal secretion is corrected. Later, however, diabetes may become irreversible, and the islet cells may be destroyed. This so-called *diabetogenic effect* is an important con-sideration with chronic glucocorticoid therapy and argues against the use of growth hormone to build muscle mass in athletes. Hormonal effects on insulin secretion and sensitivity of tissues to insulin are summarized in Table 4.

REGULATION OF METABOLISM DURING FEEDING AND FASTING

Postprandial Period

Immediately after eating, metabolic activity is directed toward the processing and sequestration of energy-rich substrates that are absorbed by the intestines. This phase is dominated by insulin, which is secreted in response to three inputs to the beta

TABLE 4. *Hormonal effects on insulin secretion and sensitivity of target cells to insulin*

	Insulin secretion by beta cells	Sensitivity of target cells to insulin
Insulin		↓[a]
Glucagon	↑	↓[b]
Epinephrine, norepinephrine	↓	↓[b]
Growth hormone	↑ (I)	↓
Cortisol	↑ (I)	↓
T$_3$	↑ (I)	↑

[a] Down regulation of receptors.
[b] Stimulates opposite effect.
I, indirect effect (increases sensitivity to direct stimuli); T$_3$, triiodothyronine

cells. The *cephalic,* or psychological aspect of eating stimulates insulin secretion though acetylcholine and perhaps vasoactive inhibitory peptide (VIP) released from vagal fibers that innervate islet cells. Food in the small intestine stimulates secretion of intestinal hormones, especially gastric inhibitory peptide (GIP), which is a potent secretagogue for insulin. Finally, the beta cells respond directly to increased glucose and amino acid levels in arterial blood (see Chapter 5). During the postprandial period, the concentration of insulin in peripheral blood may rise from a resting value of about 10 μU/ml to perhaps as much as 50 μU/ml. Glucagon secretion may also increase at this time in response to increased amino acid levels in arterial blood. Dietary amino acids may also stimulate growth hormone secretion. Characteristically, the sympathetic nervous system is relatively quiet during the postprandial period, and there is little secretory activity of the adrenal medulla or cortex at this time. Under the dominant influence of insulin, dietary carbohydrate and lipid are transferred to storage depots in liver, adipose tissue, and muscle, and amino acids are converted to proteins in various tissues. Extrahepatic tissues use dietary glucose and fat to meet their needs instead of glucose derived from hepatic glycogen or fatty acids mobilized from adipose tissue. As a result of decreased output of glucose and glycogen formation from dietary sugars, hepatic glycogen increases by an amount equivalent to about one half of the ingested carbohydrate. Fatty acid mobilization is inhibited by the high concentrations of insulin and glucose in blood. Of course, the composition of the diet profoundly affects postprandial responses. Obviously, a diet rich in carbohydrate elicits quantitatively different responses from one that is mainly composed of fat.

Postabsorptive Period

Several hours after eating, when metabolic fuels have largely been absorbed from the intestine, the body begins to draw on fuels that were stored during the postprandial period. During this period, insulin secretion returns to relatively low basal rates and is governed principally by the concentration of glucose in blood, which has returned to about 5 mM. Glucagon, growth hormone, and adrenal hormones are also secreted at relatively low basal rates. In the postabsorptive state, about 75% of the glucose secreted by the liver is derived from glycogen, and the remainder comes from gluco-neogenesis. About 75% of the glucose consumed by extrahepatic tissues during this period is taken up by brain, blood cells, and other tissues whose consumption of fuels is independent of insulin. Muscle and adipose tissue, which are highly dependent on insulin, account for the remaining 25%. Gradually, FFA increase as adipose tissue is relieved of the restraint produced by high levels of insulin during the postprandial period. The blood glucose level remains constant during this period, but glucose metabolism in muscle decreases as the restrictive effects of the glucose–fatty acid cycle become operative. The liver gradually depletes its glycogen stores and begins to rely more heavily on gluconeogenesis from amino acids and glycerol to replace the glucose consumed by extrahepatic tissues.

Fasting

More than 24 hours after the last meal, the individual can be considered to be fasting. At this time, circulating insulin concentrations decrease further, and glucagon and growth hormone increase. Cortisol secretion follows its basal diurnal rhythmic pattern (see Chapter 4) unaffected by fasting at this early stage, but basal concentra-tions of cortisol play their essential permissive role in allowing gluconeogenesis and lipolysis to proceed. Glucocorticoids and growth hormone also exert a restraining influence on glucose metabolism in muscle and adipose tissue. With the further decrease in insulin concentration, any remaining restraint on lipolysis is removed. The lipolytic cycle speeds up, fatty acid esterification decreases, and FFA mobiliza-tion is accelerated. This effect is supported and perhaps accelerated by growth hor-mone and cortisol. Decreased insulin permits a net breakdown of muscle protein, and the amino acids that consequently leave muscle, mainly as alanine, provide the substrate for gluconeogenesis. Fuel consumption after 24 hours of fasting is shown in Fig. 8.

With prolonged fasting of 3 days or more, increased growth hormone and de-creased insulin permit even greater mobilization of FFA, and ketogenesis becomes significant. By about day 3 of starvation, ketone bodies reach concentrations of 2 to 3 mM in blood and begin, not only to provide for an appreciable fraction of the brain's metabolic needs, but also to inhibit protein degradation in muscle. Conse-quently, at the same time that there is decreased demand by the brain for glucose, the production of gluconeogenic substrate decreases as protein reserves are spared. Urinary nitrogen excretion, which increased during the first few days of fasting, decreases to the postabsorptive level or below, reflecting decreased production of glucose from amino acids. During subsequent weeks of total starvation, nitrogen excretion remains low, with just enough degradation of amino acids to account for diminished, but still essential, glucose metabolism in the brain. Virtually all other energy needs are met by oxidation of fat until triglyceride reserves are depleted. In

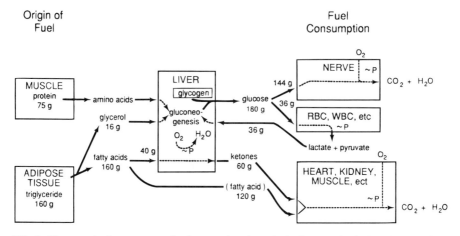

FIG. 8. The quantitative turnover of substrates in a hypothetical person in the basal state after fasting for 24 hours ($-1,800$ Calories). From Cahill, G.F., Jr. (1970): Starvation in man. *N. Engl. J. Med.*, 282:668.

the terminal stages of starvation, proteins are rapidly broken down to amino acids, and gluconeogenesis increases once again.

Table 5 gives some representative values for hormone concentrations in blood in the transition from the fed to the fasting state. The values for cortisol remain unchanged or might even decrease somewhat until late in starvation. The concentrations of cortisol shown in the table represent morning values and change with the time of day in a diurnal rhythmic pattern that is not altered by fasting (see Chapter 4). Even though its concentration does not increase during fasting, cortisol nevertheless is an essential component of the survival mechanism. In its absence, mechanisms for producing and sparing carbohydrates are virtually inoperative, and death from hypoglycemia is inevitable. The role of glucocorticoids in fasting is a good example of permissive action, in which a hormone maintains the instruments of metabolic adjustments so that other agents can manipulate those instruments effectively. Hypo-

TABLE 5. *Representative values for some blood constituents during fasting*

Sampling time	Glucose (mg/dl)	Insulin (mU/ml)	Glucagon (pg/ml)	Cortisol (ng/ml)	GH (ng/ml[a])	T_3 (ng/ml)
Postprandial		150	50		120	<11.2
Postabsorptive		90	15	100	120	21.15
Day 1	80	10 to 12	120	120	2	1.15
Day 3	70	8	150	110	6	0.70
Day 5	70	7	150	110	10	0.60

[a] Mean values for GH concentrations may be misleading. GH secretion is pulsatile (see Chapter 10), and starvation permits the appearance of wide fluctuations in blood concentrations.
GH, growth hormone; T_3, triiodothyronine.

glycemia or perhaps nonspecific stress reactions may account for increased cortisol in the terminal stages of starvation.

The decrease in plasma concentrations of T_3 are not indicative of decreased secretion of thyroid hormone but, rather, reflect decreased conversion of plasma thyroxine to T_3. At least during the first few days of fasting, thyroxine concentrations in plasma remain constant. Recall (see Chapter 3) that T_3, which is formed mostly in extrathyroidal tissue, is the biologically active form of the hormone. Deiodination of thyroxine can lead to the formation of T_3 or the inactive metabolite reverse T_3 (rT_3). With starvation, the concentration of rT_3 in plasma increases, suggesting that the metabolism of thyroxine shifted from the formation of the active to the inactive metabolite. Some of this increase also results from a somewhat slower rate of degradation of rT_3. The mechanism for this effect is unknown. A decrease in the production of T_3 results in an overall decrease in metabolic rate (oxygen consumption) and can be viewed as a mechanism for conservation of metabolic fuels.

The secretion of growth hormone follows a pulsatile pattern that is exaggerated during starvation (see Chapter 10). The values for growth hormone shown in Table 5 represent average daytime concentrations. Because the metabolic changes produced by growth hormone are similar to those produced by the decrease in insulin, the importance of growth hormone in fasting is not clear. Growth hormone decreases glucose utilization and increases glucose production, but these effects are difficult to demonstrate experimentally in normal subjects because they are masked by compensatory changes in insulin secretion. Persons suffering from a genetic deficiency of growth hormone may become hypoglycemic during fasting. Treatment with growth hormone helps to maintain their blood glucose (Fig. 9).

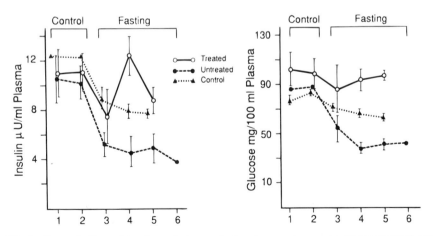

FIG. 9. Concentrations of insulin and glucose in the plasma of normal subjects (control) and patients suffering from an isolated deficiency of growth hormone are shown during control days of normal food intake and while fasting. Some growth hormone-deficient patients were given 5 mg of human growth hormone per day (*treated*). The fast began after the collection of blood on day 2. From Merimee, T.J., Felig, P., Marliss, E., et al. (1971): Glucose and lipid homeostasis in the absence of human growth hormone. *J. Clin. Invest.*, 50:574.

HORMONAL INTERACTIONS DURING EXERCISE

During exercise, overall oxygen consumption may increase 10 to 15 times in a well-trained young athlete. The requirements for fuel are met by mobilization of reserves within muscle cells and from extramuscular fuel depots. The flux of fuel through the blood can potentially deplete, or at least dangerously lower, glucose concentrations and, hence, jeopardize the brain unless some physiological controls are operative. We can consider two forms of exercise: (a) short-term maximal effort, characterized by sprinting for a few seconds, and (b) sustained aerobic work, characterized by marathon running.

Short-Term Maximal Effort

For the few seconds of the 100-yard dash, endogenous ATP reserves in muscle, creatine phosphate and glycogen, are the chief sources of energy. For short-term maximal effort, energy must be released from fuel before circulatory adjustments can provide the required oxygen. The breakdown of glycogen to lactate provides the needed ATP and is activated in part through intrinsic biochemical mechanisms that activate glycogen phosphorylase and phosphofructokinase. For example, calcium released from the sarcoplasmic reticulum in response to neural stimulation not only triggers muscle contraction but also activates glycogen phosphorylase. These intrinsic mechanisms are reinforced by epinephrine and norepinephrine released from the adrenal medullae and sympathetic nerve endings in response to central activation of the sympathetic nervous system.

The endocrine system is important primarily for maintaining or replenishing fuel reserves in muscle. Through the actions of hormones and the glucose–fatty acid cycle already discussed, glycogen reserves in muscle are sustained at or near capacity, so that muscle is always prepared to respond to demands for maximal effort. During the recovery phase, lactate released from working muscles is converted to glucose in the liver and can be exported back to muscle in the classic Cori cycle. Insulin secreted in response to increased dietary intake of glucose or amino acids promotes reformation of glycogen. Alternatively, when sprinting is followed by a period of fasting, muscle glycogen is replaced through the interplay of hormones and the glucose–fatty acid cycle (as discussed previously).

Sustained Aerobic Exercise

The sustained exercise of the marathon runner must be aerobic and relies heavily on utilization of fatty acids, which may provide as much as two thirds of the energy requirements. Table 6 shows the changes in fuel consumption with time in subjects exercising at 30% of their maximal oxygen consumption. With sustained exercise, the glucose consumed is derived in part from blood and in part from muscle glycogen. For reasons that are not fully understood, working muscles, even in the trained

TABLE 6. *Fuels consumed by leg muscles of a man during mild prolonged exercise*

Period of exercise (min)	% Contribution to oxygen uptake		
	Plasma glucose	Plasma free fatty acids	Muscle glycogen
40	27	47	36
90	41	37	22
180	36	50	14
240	30	62	8

From Newsholme, EA. and Leech, AR. (1983): *Biochemistry for the Medical Sciences*, p. 370, Wiley, New York.

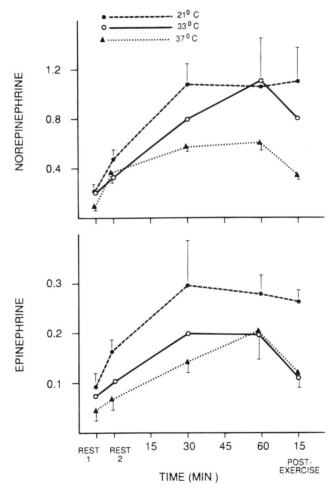

FIG. 10. The mean concentrations of catecholamines in plasma at rest and during swimming (requiring 68% of maximum oxygen consumption (V_{O2} max)) at three water temperatures. From Galbo, H. (1983): *Hormonal and Metabolic Adaptation to Exercise*, Georg Thieme Verlag, Stuttgart, p.12.

athlete, cannot derive more than about 70% of their energy from oxidation of fat. Hypoglycemia and exhaustion occur when muscle glycogen is depleted. With sustained exercise, as with starvation, biochemical mechanisms such as the glucose–fatty acid cycle are critical for preserving carbohydrate, and all of the counter-regulatory hormones participate in supplying fat to the working muscles and maximizing gluconeogenesis (Figs. 10 and 11).

Anticipation of exercise may be sufficient to activate the sympathetic nervous system, which is of critical importance, not only for supplying fuel for the working

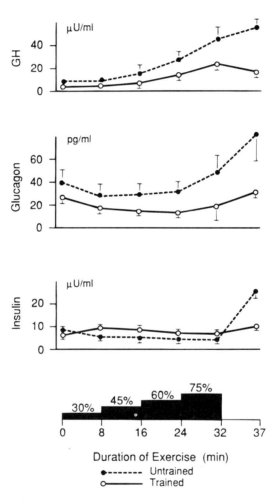

FIG. 11. The effects of graded exercise on hormone concentrations in plasma. Six racing cyclists and six untrained subjects performed upright bicycle exercise. From Galbo, H. (1983): *Hormonal and Metabolic Adaptation to Exercise*, Georg Thieme Verlag, Stuttgart, p. 31.

muscles, but also for making the cardiovascular adjustments that maintain blood flow to carry fuel and oxygen to muscle, gluconeogenic precursors to liver, and heat to sites of dissipation. Insulin secretion is shut down by sympathetic activity. At first glance, this effect seems deleterious for glucose consumption in the muscle. However, the decrease in insulin concentration only decreases the glucose uptake by nonworking muscles. The transport of glucose across the sarcolemma is stimulated by muscle contractions even in the absence of insulin. Glucose metabolism in working muscles is therefore not limited by membrane transport but, rather, by phosphofructokinase, which in turn is responsive to a variety of intracellular metabolites that coordinate its activity with energy demand.

Glycogen reserves of nonworking muscles may provide an important source of carbohydrate for working muscles during sustained exercise and for restoring muscle glycogen after exercise. Epinephrine and norepinephrine stimulate glycogenolysis in nonworking as well as working muscles. The glucose phosphate produced from glycogen is completely broken down to carbon dioxide and water in working muscles, but nonworking muscles convert it to pyruvate and lactate, which escape into the blood. The liver then reconverts these three-carbon acids to glucose, which is returned to the circulation and selectively taken up by the working muscles (Fig. 12).

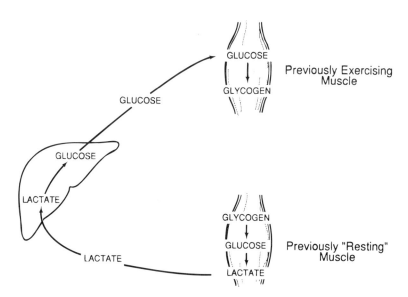

FIG. 12. The postulated interaction between previously exercising muscle and previously resting muscle via the Cori cycle during recovery from prolonged arm exercise. From Ahlborg, G., Wahren, J., and Felig, P. (1986): Splanchnic and peripheral glucose and lactate metabolism during and after prolonged arm exercise. *J. Clin. Invest.*, 77:690.

SUGGESTED READING

Felig, P., Sherwin, R. S., Soman, V., Wahren, J., Hendler, R., Sacca, L., Eigler, N., Goldberg, D., and Walesky, M. (1979): Hormonal interactions in the regulation of blood glucose. *Recent Prog. Horm. Res.*, 35:501–528.

Kraus-Friedmann, N. (1984): Hormonal regulation of hepatic gluconeogenesis. *Physiol. Rev.*, 64:170–259.

Newsholme, E. A., and Leech, A. R. (1983): Chap. 8: Integration of carbohydrate and lipid metabolism. Chap. 9: Metabolism in exercise. Chap. 14: Integration of metabolism during starvation, refeeding and injury. In: *Biochemistry for the Medical Sciences*, Wiley, New York, pp. 336–356.

Randle, P. J., Kerbey, A. L., and Espinal, J. (1988): Mechanisms decreasing glucose oxidation in diabetes and starvation: role of lipid fuels and hormones. *Diabetes Metab. Rev.*, 4:623–638.

Shulman, G. I., and Landau, B.R. (1992): Pathways of glycogen repletion. *Physiol. Rev.*, 72:1019–1035.

Steinberg, D. (1976): Interconvertible enzymes in adipose tissue regulated by cyclic AMP-dependent protein kinase. In: *Advances in Cyclic Nucleotide Research*, edited by Greengard, P., and Robison, G. A. pp. 157–198, Raven, New York.

10

Hormonal Control of Growth

OVERVIEW

The simple word ''growth'' describes a variety of processes, both living and nonliving, that share the common feature of increase in mass. We limit the definition of growth to mean the organized addition of new tissue as occurs normally in development from infancy to adulthood. This process is complex and depends on the interplay of genetic, nutritional, and environmental influences as well as actions of the endocrine system. In this chapter, we examine the hormones that play important roles in growth and their interactions at critical times in development. Although rapid strides are being made, our understanding of the molecular and cellular events that regulate cell division and differentiation is still limited; hence, our understanding of the orchestration of these processes by hormones is even more limited, though not totally deficient.

Growth is most rapid during prenatal life. In only 9 months, body length increases from just a few nanometers to almost 30% of the final adult height. The growth rate decelerates after birth, but during the first year of life, it is rapid enough that the infant increases half again in height to about 45% of its final adult stature. Thereafter, growth decelerates and continues at a slow rate until puberty. Steady growth during this juvenile period contributes the largest fraction, about 40%, to final adult height. With the onset of sexual development, growth accelerates to about twice the juvenile rate and contributes about 15% to 18% of final adult height before stopping altogether.

Our understanding of hormonal influences on growth is limited to the juvenile and adolescent periods. During the juvenile period, the influence of growth hormone (GH) is preeminent, but appropriate secretion of insulin and thyroid hormone is essential for optimal growth. The adolescent growth spurt reflects the added input of androgens and estrogens, which speed up growth and the changes in bone that bring it to a halt (Fig. 1). Throughout the growing period, adrenal glucocorticoids contribute to growth in a positive way in the sense that they are essential for survival and well-being.

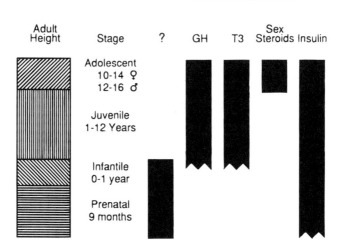

FIG. 1. Hormonal regulation of growth at different stages of life.

GH

The single most important hormone for normal growth is GH, which is also called somatotropin (STH). Attainment of adult size is absolutely dependent on GH; in its absence, growth is severely limited.

Pituitary dwarfism is the failure of growth that results from lack of GH during childhood. Pituitary dwarfs typically are of normal weight and length at birth and grow rapidly and normally during early infancy. By the end of the first year, however, growth is noticeably below the normal rate and continues slowly for many years. Left untreated, they may reach heights of 3 to 4 feet. Typically, the pituitary dwarf retains a juvenile appearance because of the retention of "baby fat" and the disproportionately small size of maxillary and mandibular bones. Pituitary dwarfism is not a single entity and may encompass a range of defects. The deficiency in GH may be accompanied by deficiencies in several or all other anterior pituitary hormones (*panhypopituitarism*) and might result from traumatic injury to the pituitary gland or a tumor that either destroys pituitary cells themselves or their connections to the hypothalamus. These individuals do not mature sexually and suffer from inadequacies of thyroid and adrenal glands as well. The lack of GH may be an isolated inherited defect, with no abnormalities in other pituitary hormones. Aside from their diminutive height, such individuals are normal in all respects and can reproduce normally. Causes of *isolated GH deficiency* are multiple and include derangements in synthesis, secretion, and end-organ responsiveness.

Overproduction of GH may occur either as a result of some derangement in the mechanisms that control secretion by normal pituitary cells or from tumor cells that function autonomously. Overproduction of GH in children results in *gigantism*, in which an adult height in excess of 8 feet has occasionally been reported. Overproduction of GH during adulthood, after the growth plates of long bones have fused (see subsequent discussion), produces growth only by stimulation of responsive osteoblastic progenitor cells in the periosteum. There is thickening of the cranium and mandible and enlargement of some facial bones and bones in the hands and feet. Growth and deformities in these acral parts give rise to the name *acromegaly* to describe this condition. The persistence of responsive cartilage progenitor cells in the costochrondral junction leads to elongation of the ribs to give a typical barrel-chested appearance. In acromegalic patients, there is also thickening of the skin and disproportionate growth of some soft tissues, including the spleen and liver.

When thinking about giants and dwarfs, it is important to keep in mind the limitations of GH action. The pediatric literature makes frequent use of the term "*genetic potential*" in discussions of diagnosis and treatment of disorders of growth. We can think of GH as the facilitator of expression of genetic potential for growth rather than as the primary determinant. The entire range over which GH can influence adult stature in humans is only about 30% of the genetic potential. Persons destined by their genetic makeup to attain a final height of 6 feet will attain a height of about 4 feet even in the absence of GH and are unlikely to exceed 8 feet in height even with massive overproduction of GH from birth. We do not understand what determines the genetic potential for growth, but it is clear that although both arise from a single cell, a hypopituitary elephant is enormously larger than a giant mouse. Within the same species, something other than aberrations in GH secretion accounts for the large differences in size of miniature and standard poodles or Chihuahuas and Great Danes.

Synthesis, Secretion, and Metabolism

Although the anterior pituitary gland produces at least six hormones, more than one third of its cells synthesize and secrete GH. In humans, the 5 to 10 mg of stored GH make it the most abundant hormone in the pituitary, accounting for almost 10% of the dry weight of the gland. More than ten times as much GH is produced and stored as any other pituitary hormone. Ninety percent of the GH produced by somatotropes is comprised of 191 amino acids and has a molecular weight of about 22,000 Daltons. The remaining 10%, called 20K GH, has a molecular weight of 20,000 Daltons and lacks the 15-amino acid sequence corresponding to residues 32 to 46. Both forms are products of the same gene and result from alternate splicing of the ribonucleic acid (RNA) transcript. Both forms of hormone are secreted and have similar growth-promoting activity, although metabolic effects of the 20K form are reduced.

About half of the GH in blood circulates bound to a protein that has the same amino acid sequence as the extracellular domain of the GH receptor (see subsequent discussion). In fact, the plasma GH binding protein is a product of the same gene that encodes the GH receptor and may originate by proteolytic cleavage of the receptor at the outer surface of target cells. We do not understand the physiological importance of the GH binding protein. The monomeric form of free GH can readily cross capillary membranes. Estimates of the half-life of GH in blood vary from 6 to about 20 minutes. The GH that crosses the glomerular membrane is reabsorbed and destroyed in the kidney. Less than 0.01% of the hormone secreted each day reaches the urine in recognizable form. Also, GH is degraded in its various target cells following uptake by receptor-mediated endocytosis.

Like other peptide and protein hormones, GH binds to a receptor on the surface of target cells. The structure of the GH receptor is known, but its manner of initiating a biological response is not. It is a glycoprotein that has a single membrane-spanning region and apparently does not interact with G proteins. It has the curious capacity to bind to either of two sites on the GH molecule so that, in the presence of GH, it forms a dimer that is held together by the hormone. Dimerization of receptors is also seen for other hormones and cytokines and is thought to be important for signal generation. Like the insulin receptor, the GH receptor is phosphorylated on tyrosine residues in the presence of its hormone.

Physiological Effects

Effects on Skeletal Growth

The ultimate height attained by an individual is determined by the length of the skeleton and, in particular, the vertebral column and long bones of the legs. Growth of these bones occurs by a process called *endochondral ossification* in which proliferating cartilage is replaced by bone. The ends of long bones are called epiphyses and arise from separate ossification centers than those responsible for ossification of the diaphysis, or shaft. In the growing individual, the epiphyses are separated from the diaphysis by cartilaginous regions called epiphyseal plates in which continuous production of chondrocytes provides the impetus for diaphyseal elongation. Chondrocytes in epiphyseal growth plates are arranged in orderly columns in parallel with the long axis of the bone (Fig. 2). Frequent division of small, flattened cells in the germinal zone at the distal end of the growth plate provides for continual elongation of columns of chondrocytes. As they grow and mature, chondrocytes produce mucopolysaccharide and collagen, which constitute the cartilage matrix. The cartilage cells hypertrophy, become heavily vacuolated, and degenerate as the surrounding matrix becomes calcified. Ingrowth of blood vessels and migration of osteoblast progenitors from the marrow results in replacement of calcified cartilage with true bone. Proliferation of chondrocytes at the epiphyseal border of the growth plate is balanced by cellular degeneration at the diaphyseal end; so in the normally growing individual, the thickness of the growth plate remains constant as the epiphyses are pushed further and further outward by the elongating shaft of bone. Eventually, progenitors of chondrocytes are either exhausted or lose their capacity to divide.

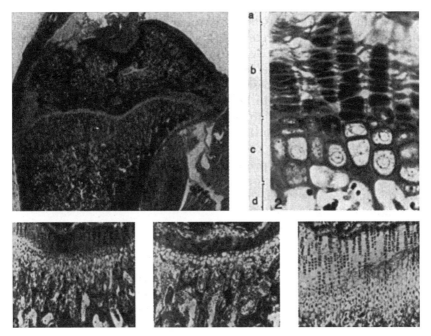

FIG. 2. 1: Transverse section through rat tibia. The *arrow* points to the epiphyseal growth plate. 2: Enlarged area of epiphyseal plate. *a*, germinal zone; *b*, zone of proliferation; *c*, zone of maturation and hypertrophy; and *d*, zone of degeneration. Central area of epiphyseal plate in a 54-day-old female rat. 3: Normal. 4: At 25 days after hypophysectomy. Note the narrowness and atrophic appearance of the growth plate. 5: At 25 days after hypophysectomy but given daily injections of GH for 10 days prior to autopsy. Note the marked widening of the epiphyseal plate and elongated columns of hypertrophied chondrocytes. From Ray, R.D., Evans, H.M., and Becks, H. (1941): Effect of the pituitary growth hormone on the epiphyseal disk of the tibia of the rat. *Am. J. Pathol.*, 17:509.

As remaining chondrocytes go through their cycle of growth and degeneration, the epiphyseal plate becomes progressively narrower and is ultimately obliterated when diaphyseal bone fuses with the bony epiphyses. At this time, the epiphyseal plates are said to be closed, and the capacity for further growth is lost.

In the absence of GH, there is severe atrophy of the epiphyseal plates, which become narrow as proliferation of cartilage progenitor cells slows markedly (Fig. 2, panel 4). Conversely, after GH is given to a hypopituitary subject, resumption of cellular proliferation causes columns of chondrocytes to elongate and epiphyseal plates to widen. This characteristic response has been used as the basis of a biological assay for GH in experimental animals.

Growth of bone requires that diameter as well as length increase. Thickening of long bones is accomplished by proliferation of osteoblastic progenitors from the connective tissue sheath (*periosteum*) that surrounds the diaphysis. As it grows, bone is also subject to continual reabsorption and reorganization, with the incorporation of new cells that originate in both the periosteal and endosteal regions. Remodeling, which is an intrinsic property of skeletal growth, is accompanied by destruction and replacement of calcified matrix, as described in Chapter 8. Treatment with GH often produces a transient increase in urinary excretion of calcium and phosphorus, reflecting bone remodeling. The increased urinary hydroxyproline derives from the breakdown and replacement of collagen in bone matrix.

Somatomedin Hypothesis

Although epiphyseal growth plates are obviously stimulated after GH is given to hypophysectomized animals, little or no stimulation of cell division, protein synthesis, or incorporation of radioactive sulfur into mucopolysaccharides of cartilage matrix was observed when epiphyseal cartilage taken from hypophysectomized rats was incubated with GH. In contrast, when cartilage taken from the same rats was incubated with blood plasma from hypophysectomized rats that had been treated with GH, there was a sharp increase in matrix formation, protein synthesis, and deoxyribonucleic acid (DNA) synthesis. Blood plasma from normal rats produced similar effects, but plasma from hypophysectomized rats that had not been given GH had little effect. These experiments gave rise to the hypothesis that GH may not act directly to promote growth but, instead, may stimulate the liver to produce an intermediate, blood-borne substance that activates chondrogenesis and, perhaps, other GH-dependent processes. This substance was called somatomedin (*somato-tropin mediator*). Subsequently, it was discovered that somatomedin is actually two closely related substances and accounts for the insulin-like activity that persists in plasma even after all the authentic insulin is removed by immunoprecipitation. These substances are now called insulin-like growth factors or IGF-I and IGF-II.

In general, plasma concentrations of IGF-I reflect the availability of GH. They are higher than normal in blood of persons suffering from acromegaly and are very low in GH-deficient individuals (Fig. 3). People who are resistant to the growth-promoting effects of GH, e.g., pygmies of Africa and some families of dwarfs, have normal or even high concentrations of GH in their blood but low concentrations of IGF-I. When GH is injected into GH-deficient patients or experimental animals, IGF-I concentrations increase after a delay of about 6 to 8 hours and remain elevated for more than 1 day. Levels of IGF-I in plasma, however, do not always correlate with those of GH, and are influenced by such other factors as the nutritional state.

While it is clear that IGF-I stimulates cell division in cartilage and many other tissues and can account for much of the growth-promoting action of GH, the somatomedin hypothesis as originally formulated cannot explain some experimental findings. For example, direct injection of small amounts of GH into tibial epiphyseal cartilage in one leg of hypophysectomized rats stimulated growth only in the injected limb. Only a direct action of GH on osteogenesis can explain such localized stimulation of growth because IGF-I in the plasma would be equally available to all tissues. It is now apparent that GH stimulates prechondrocytes and other cells in the epiphyseal plates to synthesize and secrete IGF-I, which acts in an autocrine or paracrine

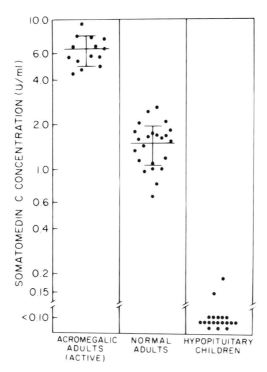

FIG. 3. Serum somatomedin C (*IGF-I*) concentrations in acromegalic adults, normal adults, and untreated hypopituitary children. Bars indicate means ± one standard deviation. From Furnaletto, R.W., Underwood, L.E., Van Wyk, J.J., et al. (1977): Estimation of somatomedin-C levels in normals and patients with pituitary disease by radioimmunoassay. *J. Clin. Invest.*, 60:648.

manner to stimulate cell division (Fig. 4). Evidence to support this model includes the findings of both GH and IGF receptors in the epiphyseal plates along with the messenger RNA for IGF-I. Some IGF-I that is produced in the liver may also reach these cells through the blood and stimulate them to divide. The relative importance of the two sources of IGF-I for regulation of growth is not yet resolved.

Local production of IGF-I has also been implicated in growth processes that are independent of GH, including compensatory hepatic or renal hypertrophy, wound healing, thyroid hyperplasia, and growth and differentiation of granulosa cells of the ovary (see Chapter 12). The involvement of two effector signals, one produced systemically to initiate local production of the other, may be a general mechanism for regulating cellular growth and is reminiscent of the interaction of interleukin-1 (IL-1) and IL-2 in promoting the growth of T lymphocytes (see Chapter 4).

IGF

Both IGF-I and IGF-II are small unbranched peptides and have molecular weights of about 7,500 Daltons. They are encoded in separate genes and are expressed in a

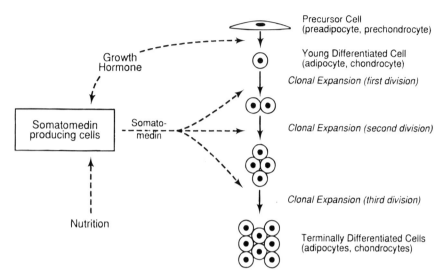

FIG. 4. Dual effectors of GH action. From Green, H., Morikawa, M., and Nixon, T. (1985): A duel effector theory of growth-hormone action. *Differentiation.,* 29:195.

variety of cells. They are very similar in structure to proinsulin (see Chapter 5), both in terms of amino acid sequence and in the arrangement of disulfide bonds. In contrast to insulin, however, the region corresponding to the connecting peptide is not removed from the mature form of the IGFs. The cellular receptors for IGF-I and insulin are also very similar and consist of tetramers of two membrane-spanning β subunits connected by disulfide bonds to two extracellular α subunits (see Chapter 5). Like the insulin receptor, the IGF-I receptor catalyzes phosphorylation of some of its own tyrosine residues as well as those of other proteins when stimulated.

About 90% of the IGF-I in plasma is thought to be produced by the liver and circulates complexed with a specific binding protein. Six different IGF-binding proteins have been found in various biological fluids. The most important IGF-binding protein in blood, called IGFBP-3, is a glycoprotein whose synthesis is also regulated by GH. Virtually all of the IGF-I and IGF-II present in blood is bound to IGFBP-3 which associates with another protein to form a large (approximately 150,000 Dalton) complex. Consequently, IGF does not readily escape from the vascular compartment and has a half-life of about 20 hours. Like IGF-I, the IGF binding proteins are produced locally in target cells for IGF as well as by the liver. Locally produced IGF-binding proteins regulate the access of IGF to its receptor.

Effects of GH on Body Composition

Animals or human subjects that are GH-deficient have a relatively high proportion of fat, compared to water and protein, in their bodies. Treatment with GH changes the proportion of these bodily constituents to resemble the normal juvenile distribution. Body protein stores increase, particularly in muscle, and there is a relative decrease in fat. Even though it diminishes body fat by reducing the amount of intracellular triglycerides, GH seems to be required for differentiation of preadipocytes into fat cells in young children as well as in cultured fibroblasts. Most internal organs grow in proportion to body size, except the liver and spleen, which may be disproportionately enlarged. The heart may also be enlarged in acromegalic subjects, perhaps more from hypertension, which is frequently seen in these individuals, than from direct effects of GH on the heart. The skin and underlying connective tissue also increase in mass, but GH does not appear to influence growth of the thyroid, gonads, or reproductive organs.

Changes in body composition and organ growth can be monitored by studying changes in the biochemical balance of body constituents. When human subjects or experimental animals are given GH repeatedly for several days, there is net retention of nitrogen, in the form of protein, as well as potassium and sodium, reflecting expansion of the intracellular and extracellular compartments (Fig. 5). Urinary nitrogen is decreased, as is the concentration of urea in blood. Decreased hepatic production of urea is thought to result from diversion of amino acids into protein, rather than from direct inhibition of ureogenesis. Immediately after GH is injected, plasma concentrations of amino acids decrease as a result of rapid uptake and conversion to protein.

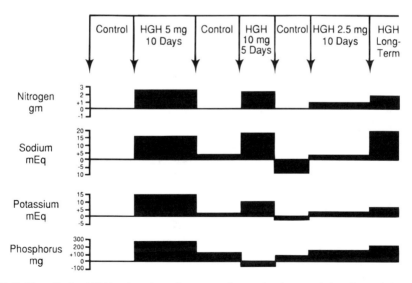

FIG. 5. The effects of GH treatment on nitrogen, sodium, potassium, and phosphorus balances in an 11.5-year-old girl with pituitary dwarfism. Changes above the control baseline represent the retention of the substance; below the line, they represent a loss. From Hutchings, J.J., Escamilla, R.F., Deamer, W.C., et al. (1959): Metabolic changes produced by human growth hormone (Li) in a pituitary dwarf. *J. Clin. Endocrinol. Metab.,* 19:759.

Effects on Energy Metabolism

As already discussed in Chapter 9, GH is also a metabolic hormone. The relationship of its metabolic effects, which are independent of IGF-I, to its growth-promoting effects has not been established. Sometimes, particularly after a period of GH deprivation, GH produces a brief insulin-like response that includes a decrease in blood glucose concentration accompanied by increased uptake and utilization of glucose by muscle and fat. This anomalous effect disappears quickly, and its physiological significance remains a mystery. After about 2 hours, glucose metabolism is inhibited in both muscle and adipose tissue. Not only is there a decrease in the rate of glucose uptake, but glycogen stores in muscle are preserved. In adipose tissue, GH promotes the breakdown of stored triglyceride, which increases the concentration of free fatty acids (FFA) in blood. This effect, coupled with inhibition of glucose metabolism and, hence, synthesis of fatty acids, accounts for the relative loss of body fat described previously. Throughout the course of treatment with GH, there tends to be increased reliance on oxidation of body fat to meet basal energy needs and to fuel accelerated protein synthesis. Increased reliance on fat is said to spare protein by reducing utilization of dietary protein for energy production either directly or after conversion to glucose.

Growth hormone reinforces its direct effects on fat and carbohydrate metabolism by decreasing the sensitivity of muscle and fat to insulin. At the same time, it increases the sensitivity of the beta cells to various stimuli for insulin secretion. It is possible that this effect of GH makes more insulin available to promote net protein synthesis and simultaneously protects against potentially harmful decreases in blood glucose levels that might otherwise ensue. By decreasing insulin sensitivity and glucose metabolism, while promoting mobilization and utilization of body fat, GH is said to have a *diabetogenic* effect. Indeed, prolonged treatment with large doses of GH can induce a state of temporary or even permanent diabetes. Diabetes is a frequent complication of acromegaly.

Regulation of GH Secretion

Growth is a slow, continuous process that takes place over more than a decade. It might be expected, therefore, that concentrations of GH in blood would be fairly static. In contrast to such expectations, however, frequent measurements of GH concentrations in blood plasma throughout the day reveal wide fluctuations, indicative of multiple episodes of secretion. Because the metabolism of GH is thought to be invariant, changes in its plasma concentration imply changes in secretion. In rats, GH is secreted in regular pulses every 3.0 to 3.5 hours in what has been called an ultradian rhythm. In humans, GH secretion is also pulsatile, but the pattern of changes in blood concentrations is less obvious than in rats. Frequent bursts of secretion occur throughout the day, with the largest being associated with the early hours of

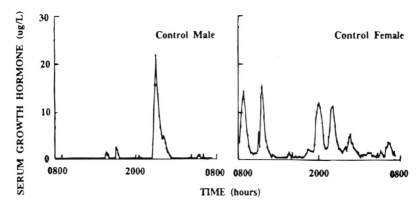

FIG. 6. GH concentrations in blood sampled at 10-minute intervals over a 24-hour period in a normal adult male and a normal adult female subject. The large pulse in the male coincides with the early hours of sleep. Note that the pulses of secretion are more frequent and of greater amplitude in the female. From Asplin, C.M., Faria, H.C.S., Carlsen, E.C., et al. (1989): Alterations in the pulsatile mode of growth hormone release in men and women with insulin-dependent diabetes mellitus. *J. Clin Endocrinol. Metab.,* 69:239.

sleep in men (Fig. 6). In addition, stressful changes in the internal and external environment can produce brief episodes of hormone secretion. Little information or diagnostic insight can therefore be obtained from a single random measurement of the concentration of GH in blood. Because secretory episodes only last a short while, multiple, frequent measurements are needed to evaluate the functional status or to relate GH secretion to physiological events. Alternatively, it is possible to withdraw small amounts of blood continuously over the course of a day, and by measuring GH in the pooled sample, to obtain a 24-hour integrated concentration of GH in blood.

Effects of Age

Using the continuous sampling method, it was found that GH secretion, though most active during the adolescent growth spurt, persists throughout life long after the epiphyses have fused and growth has stopped (Fig. 7). Between age 20 and 40 years, the daily rate of secretion gradually decreases in both men and women, but it is remarkable that, even during middle age, the pituitary continues to secrete over 0.5 mg of GH every day. Low rates of GH secretion in elderly people may be related to the loss of lean body mass in later life. Changes in GH secretion with age reflect changes in both frequency and magnitude of secretory pulses.

Regulators of GH Secretion

In addition to spontaneous pulses, secretory episodes are induced by such metabolic signals as a rapid fall in blood glucose concentration or an increase in certain

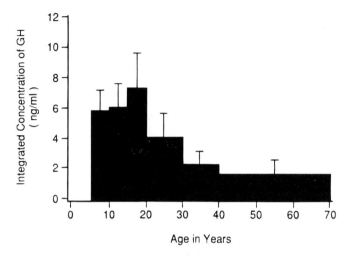

FIG. 7. The relationship between the integrated concentration of GH (*IC-GH*) and age in 173 normal male and female subjects. From Zadik, Z., Chalew, S.A., McCarter, R.J., Jr., et al. (1985): The influence of age on the 24-hour integrated concentration of growth hormone in normal individuals. *J. Clin. Endocrinol. Metab.*, 60:513.

amino acids, particularly arginine and leucine. The physiological significance of these changes in GH secretion is not understood, but provocative tests using these signals are helpful for judging the competence of the GH secretory apparatus (Fig. 8). Traumatic and psychogenic stresses are also powerful inducers of GH secretion in humans and monkeys (Fig. 9), but whether increased secretion of GH is beneficial for coping with stress is not established and is not universally seen in mammals. In rats, for example, GH secretion is inhibited by the same signals that increase it in humans. However, regardless of their significance, these observations indicate that GH secretion is under minute-to-minute control by the nervous system. That control is expressed through the hypothalamohypophyseal portal circulation, which delivers two hypothalamic neuropeptides to the somatotropes: GH-releasing hormone (GHRH) and somatostatin (see Chapter 2). GHRH provides the primary drive for GH secretion. In its absence or when a lesion interrupts hypophyseal portal blood flow, secretion of GH ceases. Somatostatin reduces or blocks the response of the pituitary to GHRH.

Defective hypothalamic production or secretion of GHRH may be a more common cause of GH deficiency than are defects in the pituitary gland. The GH concentrations in plasma are restored to normal in many GH-deficient individuals after treatment with GHRH, suggesting that their somatotropes are competent but not adequately stimulated.

Defects in somatostatin synthesis or secretion are not known to be responsible for disease states, but long-acting analogues of somatostatin can be used to decrease GH secretion.

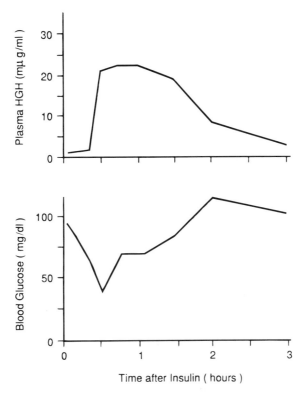

FIG. 8. Acute changes in plasma GH levels in response to insulin-induced hypoglycemia. From Roth, J., Glick, S.M., Yalow, R.S., et al. (1963): Hypoglycemia: A potent stimulus to secretion of growth hormone. *Science.*, 140:987.

In addition to neuroendocrine mechanisms that control secretion in response to changes in the internal or external environment, the secretion of GH is under negative feedback control. As in other negative feedback systems, inhibitory signals are products of GH action, principally IGF-I. Increased concentrations of FFA or glucose, which are also related to GH action, may also exert inhibitory effects and decrease GH secretion in response to a variety of provocative stimuli. IGF-I appears to act both at the hypothalamic level, where it stimulates the secretion of somatostatin, and at the pituitary level, where it decreases the response of somatotropes to GHRH. Increased FFA or glucose similarly increase somatostatin secretion. Some evidence suggests that GH may also have a direct suppressive effect on its own production and may either inhibit the release of GHRH or increase the secretion of somatostatin. These relationships are illustrated in Fig. 10.

Negative feedback control, by itself, sets the overall level of GH secretion but cannot account for secretory pulses that occur spontaneously or in response to such provocative signals as a rapid fall in blood glucose or a rise in blood amino acids.

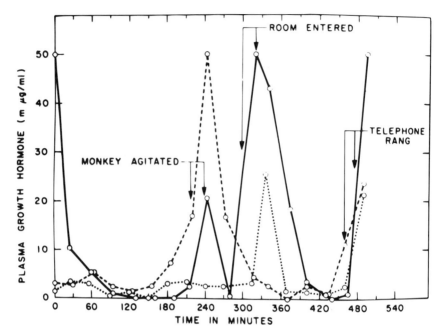

FIG. 9. Plasma GH concentrations in three rhesus monkeys studied simultaneously. From Meyer, V. and Knobil, E. (1967): Growth hormone secretion in the unanesthesized rhesus monkey in response to noxious stimuli. *Endocrinology.*, 80:163.

These pulses of GH secretion are superimposed on negative feedback regulation. Both GHRH and somatostatin contribute to the pulsatile nature of GH secretion, and both appear to be secreted intermittently. Pulsatile secretion of GH is produced by the simultaneous increase in GHRH and decrease in somatostatin secretion. We still do not understand how such reciprocal changes in secretion of these two neurohormones are accomplished, either under basal conditions or in response to environmental perturbations.

Actions of GHRH and Somatostatin on the Somatotrope

Receptors for both GHRH and somatostatin are present on the surface of somatotropes in association with several G proteins, and express their antagonistic effects on GH synthesis and secretion through their opposing influences on cyclic adenosine monophosphate (AMP) production and cytosolic calcium concentrations. GHRH activates adenylyl cyclase through a typical stimulatory G protein-linked mechanism (see Chapter 1). Cyclic AMP promotes the formation of a transcription factor, Pit 1, which in turn increases transcription of the GH gene. In addition, cyclic AMP-dependent phosphorylation of voltage-sensitive calcium channels is thought to lower their threshold and increase their likelihood of opening. Voltage-sensitive calcium

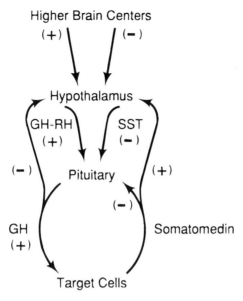

FIG. 10. Regulation of GH secretion. +, stimulation; −, inhibition.

channels are also activated by a G protein-dependent mechanism that depolarizes the somatotrope membrane by direct communication between activated GHRH receptors and sodium channels. The resulting increase in cytosolic calcium causes exocytosis of GH. Increased calcium also limits the secretory event by inhibiting voltage-sensitive calcium channels and promotes membrane repolarization by activating potassium channels. Somatostatin acts through the inhibitory guanine nucleotide binding protein, Gi, to prevent activation of adenylyl cyclase. Somatostatin receptors are also linked to potassium channels through G proteins. Activation of potassium channels hyperpolarizes or blocks depolarization of the plasma membrane, and thereby prevents GHRH from increasing intracellular calcium (Fig. 11).

THYROID HORMONES

As already mentioned in Chapter 3, growth is stunted in children suffering from an unremediated deficiency of thyroid hormones. Thyroidectomy of juvenile experimental animals produces nearly as drastic an inhibition of growth as hypophysectomy, and restoration of normal amounts of triiodothyronine (T_3) or thyroxine (T_4) promptly reinitiates growth. Conversely, excessive secretion of thyroid hormones may somewhat accelerate growth, but the effects of hyperthyroidism are not dramatic and may be somewhat masked by the accelerated catabolism of protein that accompanies the hypermetabolic state. Young mice grow somewhat faster than normal after treatment with thyroxine, but although attained earlier, adult size is no greater than

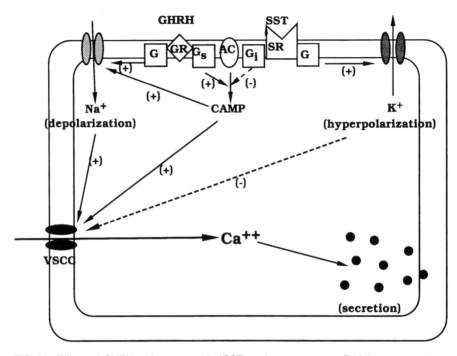

FIG. 11. Effects of *GHRH* and somatostatin (*SST*) on the somatotrope. Both hormones act on adenylyl cyclase through their respective stimulatory or inhibitory guanine nucleotide binding proteins, G_s or G_i. GHRH increases cellular calcium (Ca^{++}) by activating sodium (Na^+) channels, thereby depolarizing the somatotrope and activating voltage-sensitive calcium channels (*VSCC*). Cyclic AMP-dependent phosphorylation of VSCC lowers their threshold. Also SST antagonizes the effects of GHRH by activating potassium (K^+) channels, thereby preventing the activation of VSCC. *AC*, adenylyl cyclase; *GR*, GHRH receptor; *SR*, SST receptor.

normal. The effects of thyroid hormones on growth are intimately entwined with GH, but T_3 and T_4 have little if any growth-promoting effect in the absence of GH. There are at least three levels at which T_3 interacts with GH: GH synthesis, GH secretion, and GH action (Fig. 12).

Dependence of GH Synthesis and Secretion on T_3

Concentrations of GH are severely reduced in the plasma of hypothyroid individuals, and in experimental animals, they fall to low levels within a few days after thyroidectomy. This decrease is due to decreased amplitude of secretory pulses and possibly to a decrease in their frequency as well. The pituitary glands of such animals are severely depleted of GH as a consequence of an almost complete cessation of GH synthesis. Treatment of hypothyroid animals with T_3 or T_4 restores the GH content of the pituitary within a few days. In rodents, this action of T_3 appears to be exerted directly at the level of gene transcription. Transcription of the human

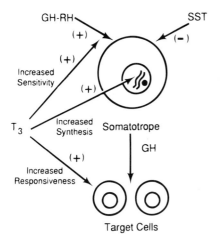

FIG. 12. Interactions of T_3 with growth hormone.

GH gene may not be directly activated by T_3, but T_3 may nevertheless affect GH synthesis indirectly by maintaining normal responsiveness of somatotropes to GHRH. Insulin-induced hypoglycemia and other stimuli for GH secretion produce abnormally small increases in the concentration of GH in the plasma of hypothyroid subjects. Such blunted responses to provocative signals probably reflect decreased sensitivity to GHRH as well as depletion of GH stores.

Importance of T_3 for Expression of GH Actions

Failure of growth in thyroid-deficient individuals is largely due to a deficiency of GH. Treatment of thyroidectomized animals with GH alone can reinitiate growth, but even large amounts cannot sustain a normal rate of growth unless some thyroid hormone is also given. In rats that were both hypophysectomized and thyroidecto-mized, T_4 decreased the amount of GH needed to stimulate growth (increased sensi-tivity) and exaggerated the magnitude of the response (increased efficacy). Both T_3 and T_4 potentiate the effects of GH on growth of long bones and increase its effects on protein synthesis in muscle and liver. Concentrations of IGF-I are reduced in the blood of hypothyroid individuals, partly because of decreased circulating GH and partly because of decreased hepatic responsiveness to GH. In addition, tissues iso-lated from thyroidectomized animals are less responsive to IGF-I.

INSULIN

Although neither GH nor T_4 appear to be important determinants of fetal growth, many investigators have suggested that insulin may serve as a growth-promoting hormone during the fetal period. Infants born of diabetic mothers are often larger than normal, especially when the diabetes is poorly controlled. Because glucose readily crosses the placenta, high concentrations of glucose in maternal blood increase fetal blood glucose and stimulate the fetal pancreas to secrete insulin. In the rare cases of congenital deficiency of insulin that have been reported, fetal size is below normal. Structurally, insulin is closely related to IGF-I and IGF-II, and when present in adequate concentrations, it can react with IGF receptors in some tissues. We do not know if the effects of insulin on fetal growth are mediated by the insulin receptor or IGF receptors, nor has the importance of the IGFs for growth during the fetal period been established.

Optimal concentrations of insulin in blood are required to maintain normal growth during postnatal life, but it has been difficult to obtain a precise definition of the role of insulin. Because life cannot be maintained for long without insulin, dramatic effects of sustained deficiency on final adult size are not seen. Insulin stimulates protein synthesis and inhibits protein degradation, and in its absence, protein breakdown is severe. Consequently, without insulin, normal responses to GH are not seen; the anabolic effects of GH on body protein either cannot be expressed or are masked by simultaneous, unchecked catabolic processes. Studies in pancreatectomized rats indicate a direct relationship between the effectiveness of GH and the dose of insulin administered. Treatment with GH sustained a rapid rate of growth so long as the daily dose of insulin was adequate, but growth progressively decreased as the dose of insulin was reduced (Fig. 13). Conversely, insulin cannot sustain growth in the absence of GH.

We still do not know how insulin participates in the growth process. Its action as a regulator of protein synthesis and degradation is clearly of great importance. In addition, it increases the number of receptors for GH and IGF on the surfaces of some cells and can even increase the production of IGF-I, but the relevance of these effects to the growth process is not understood. Although insulin is used diagnostically to provoke GH secretion, it is the resulting hypoglycemia, rather than insulin *per se*, that stimulates GH release. At least part of the influence of insulin on growth must relate to its central role in the regulation of energy metabolism. Clearly, growth requires not only nutrients to form the substance of body mass, but also fuels to provide the needed energy.

GONADAL HORMONES

The awakening of the gonads at the onset of sexual maturation is accompanied by a dramatic acceleration of growth. The adolescent growth spurt, like other changes at puberty, is attributable to steroid hormones of the gonads and perhaps the adrenals. Androgens, produced in the testes and adrenal glands, are called anabolic steroids because, in addition to their effects on the accessory sexual organs, they stimulate linear growth in the adolescent and can promote nitrogen retention and growth of muscle even after the epiphyses have closed. Because the development of pubic and axillary hair at the onset of puberty is a response to increased secretion of adrenal

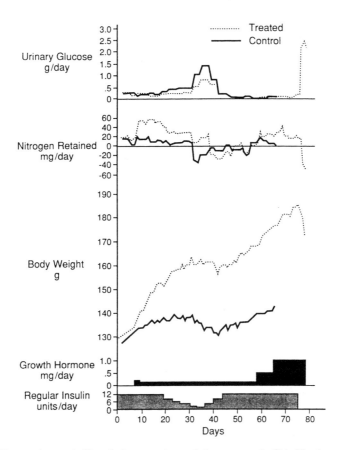

FIG. 13. The requirement of insulin for normal growth in response to GH. All rats were pancreatectomized 3 to 7 weeks before the experiment was begun. Each rat was fed 7 g of food per day. The treated group was injected with GH daily. Note the failure to respond to GH in the period between 20 and 44 days, coincident with the decrease in daily insulin dose, and the resumption of growth when the daily dose of insulin was restored. From Scow, R.O., Wagner, E.M., and Ronov, E. (1958): Effect of growth hormone and insulin on body weight and nitrogen retention in pancreatectomized rats. *Endocrinology.*, 62:593.

androgens, this initial stage of sexual maturation is called *adrenarche*. The physiological mechanisms that trigger increased secretion of adrenal androgens and the awakening of the gonadotropic secretory apparatus are poorly understood; they are considered further in Chapter 11.

Androgens

Androgens are potent promoters of linear growth in children whose epiphyses are not yet fused. Some stimulation of growth can usually be produced with androgens alone in GH-deficient children, and children suffering from isolated deficiency of GH often experience a small pubertal growth spurt even without GH replacement therapy. At least for a short while, combined treatment with GH and androgen produces more rapid growth than the sum of the responses to either androgen alone or GH alone, suggesting that the two hormones may interact in effector cells. Nevertheless, much of the growth-promoting effect of androgen appears to result from enhanced secretion of GH. During the pubertal growth spurt or when androgens are given to prepubertal children, there is an increase in both frequency and amplitude of secretory pulses (Fig. 14). Concentrations of GHRH are increased in the peripheral blood of boys and girls during puberty. The concentration of IGF-I in the blood also increases during the pubertal growth spurt or after androgens are given to prepubertal children (Fig. 15). This increase is probably a consequence of increased secretion of GH.

In addition to promoting linear growth, androgens stimulate the growth of muscle,

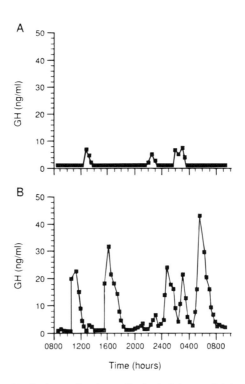

FIG. 14. The effects of testosterone in a boy with short stature and delayed puberty. **a:** Before testosterone. **b:** During therapy with long-acting testosterone. Note the increase in frequency and amplitude of GH secretory episodes in the treated subjects. From Link, K., Blizzard, R.M., Evans, W.S., et al. (1986): The effect of androgens on the pulsatile release and the twenty-four hour mean concentration of growth hormone in peripubertal males. *J. Clin. Endocrinol. Metab.*, 62:159.

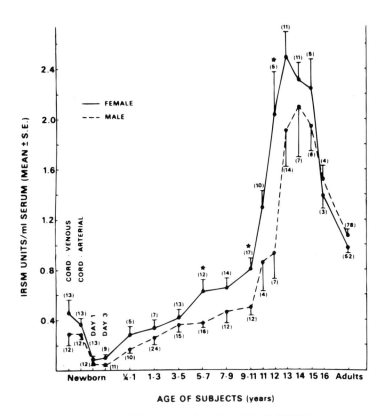

FIG. 15. The effects of age on IGF-I concentrations in the blood. *IRSM*, immunoreactive soma-tomedin. Note the abrupt increase during the adolescent growth spurt. *Numbers in parentheses* indicate numbers of subjects. *Asterisks* indicate statistically significant differences between male and female subjects. From Bala, R.M., Lopatka, J., Leung, A., et al. (1981): Serum immunoreactive somatomedin levels in normal adults, pregnant women at term, childhood at various ages, and children with constitutionally delayed growth. *J. Clin Endocrinol. Metab.*, 52:508.

particularly in the upper body. Androgen secretion during puberty in boys produces a doubling of muscle mass by increasing the size and number of muscle cells. This stimulation of muscle growth can occur in the absence of GH or thyroid hormones and appears to be mediated by specific androgen receptors that have all of the properties of receptors seen in other androgen-sensitive tissues (see Chapter 11). Stimulation of muscle growth is most pronounced in androgen-deficient or hypopituitary subjects, and only small effects, if any, are seen in men with normal testicular function.

Estrogens

Although the relationship of testicular androgens to pubertal growth in boys is straightforward, the corresponding actions of estrogens in girls is complex. Treatment with estrogen, even at the relatively low doses used therapeutically in adult women, inhibits growth in children and experimental animals. However, estrogen doses that were too low to stimulate growth of the mammary glands accelerated linear growth in girls suffering from ovarian dysgenesis (congenital absence of ovaries). These girls generally do not experience an adolescent growth spurt unless estrogen is given. In normal girls, the adolescent growth spurt usually occurs before estrogen secretion is sufficient to initiate the growth of breasts, and is probably attributable to the very low concentrations of estrogens produced by the awakening ovary.

We still do not understand the basis for either the stimulatory or inhibitory effects of estrogen on linear growth. At the same concentrations that inhibit growth, estrogens increase GH secretion. The GH secretory apparatus tends to be more sensitive to environmental influences in women than in men, and the circulating concentrations of GH tend to rise more readily in women in response to provocative stimuli. Although we do not understand its molecular basis, the inhibitory effects on growth appear to result from interference with the action of GH at the level of its target cells. Estrogens, which are not catabolic, also antagonize the effects of GH on nitrogen retention and minimize the increase in IGF-I in the blood of hypophysectomized or hypopituitary individuals treated with GH. Neither estrogens nor androgens affect the ability of IGF-I to act.

At the same time that gonadal steroids promote linear growth, they accelerate closure of the epiphyses and, therefore, limit the final height that can be attained. The mechanistic basis for this effect is not understood but it is probably exerted directly on the epiphyseal plates, which lose their capacity to replenish cartilage progenitor cells. Deficiency of gonadal hormones, if left untreated, delays epiphyseal closure, and despite the absence of a pubertal growth spurt, such hypogonadal individuals tend to be tall and have unusually long arms and legs. Children who undergo early puberty and, hence, experience their growth spurt while their contemporaries continue to grow at the slower prepubertal rate are likely to be the tallest and most physically developed in grade school or junior high but among the shortest in their high school graduating class. On occasion, pediatricians give estrogen to retard growth and hasten epiphyseal closure in young girls whose tall stature threatens to produce emotional and social difficulties.

GLUCOCORTICOIDS

Normal growth requires normal secretion of glucocorticoids, whose widespread effects promote optimal function of a variety of organ systems (see Chapter 4), a sense of health and well-being, and a normal appetite. Glucocorticoids are required for the synthesis of GH and have complex effects on GH secretion. When given acutely, they may enhance GH gene transcription and increase the responsiveness of somatotropes to GHRH. However, GH secretion is reduced by excessive glucocorticoids, probably as a result of increased somatostatin production. Children suffering

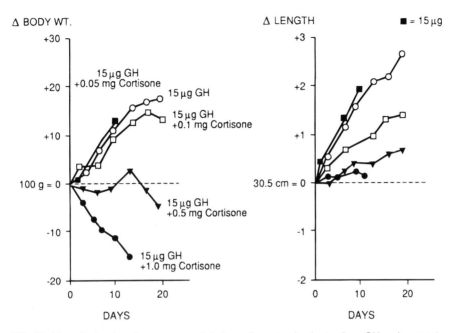

FIG. 16. The effects of cortisone on growth in hypophysectomized rats given GH replacement. The growth-promoting response to GH, measured as a change in either body weight or length, decreased progressively as the dose of cortisone was increased from 0.1 to 1.0 mg per day. The decrease in body weight seen when 1.0 mg per day of cortisone was given probably results from net breakdown of muscle mass (see Chapter 4). From Soyka, L.F. and Crawford, J.D. (1965): Antagonism by cortisone of the linear growth induced in hypopituitary patients and pypophysectomized rats by human. *J. Clin. Endocrinol. Metab.*, 25:469.

from overproduction of glucocorticoids (Cushing's disease) experience some stunting of their growth. Similar impairment of growth is seen in children treated chronically with high doses of glucocorticoids to control asthma or inflammatory disorders. Consistent with their catabolic effects in muscle and lymphoid tissues, glucocorticoids also antagonize the action of GH. Hypophysectomized rats grew less in response to GH when cortisone was given simultaneously (Fig. 16). Glucocorticoids similarly blunt the response to GH administered to hypopituitary children. The cellular mechanisms for this antagonism are not yet understood. Production of IGF-Imay be reduced by treatment with glucocorticoids, but we do not know if this is a cause or an effect of the decreased action of GH.

OTHER HORMONES AND GROWTH FACTORS

The IGFs belong to just one family of growth factors that appear to operate as autocrine, paracrine, and sometimes systemic, promoters of cell division and differentiation. A partial list of well-established growth factors and their principal actions is given in Table 1. Many of these factors were discovered and studied

TABLE 1. *Some local growth factors and their principal actions*

Factor	Principal effects
Epidermal growth factor (EGF)	Accelerates eyelid opening and tooth growth in neonatal mice, maintenance of epithelial tissues
Platelet-derived growth factor (PDGF)	Facilitates wound healing, attracts macrophages, stimulates fibroblast and endothelial cell division
Transforming growth factors (TGFα, TGFβ)	"Transforms" cells to grow in soft agar instead of monolayers, may inhibit or stimulate cell growth depending on the presence of other factors
Fibroblast growth factors (basic FBGF, acid FBGF)	Stimulate cell division, may serve as "angiogenesis factor" and promote formation of blood vessels and revascularization of tissues
Nerve growth factor (NGF)	Promotes differentiation of sympathetic and sensory neurons
Cytokines Interleukins-1 to -11 Colony-stimulating factors Tumor necrosis factor (TNF)	Regulate growth and function of lymphocytes and other cells; regulate growth and function of white blood cells; variable actions on growth, differentiation, and death, depending on cell type and the presence of other factors

because of their role in promoting division or differentiation of cells in tissue culture. Most appear to be local regulators of the immune response and such processes as wound healing, tissue repair, regeneration, or ordinary replacement of aged cells, but some are also found in the circulation and may function as true hormones. Some factors may be important primarily during the embryonic period. A discussion of all the growth factors is beyond the scope of this chapter, but the student must recognize that, in fulfilling our definition of growth as ''the organized addition of new tissue as occurs normally from infancy to adulthood,'' local growth factors undoubtedly play an important and probably decisive role.

SUGGESTED READING

Baumann, G. (1991): Growth hormone heterogeneity: genes, isohormones, variants and binding proteins. *Endocr. Rev.*, 12:424–449.

Davidson, M. (1987): Effect of growth hormone on carbohydrate and lipid metabolism. *Endocr. Rev.*, 8:115–131.

Froesch, E. R., Schmid, C., Schwander, J., and Zapf, J. (1985): Actions of insulin-like growth factors. *Annu. Rev. Physiol.*, 47:443–468.

Frohman, L. A., and Jansson, J.-O. (1986): Growth hormone-releasing hormone. *Endocr. Rev.*, 7:223–253.

Isaksson, O. G. P., Edén, S., and Jansson, J.-O. (1985): Mode of action of growth hormone on target cells. *Annu. Rev. Physiol.*, 47:483–500.

Sara, V. R., and Hall, K. (1990): Insulin-like growth factors and their binding proteins. *Physiol. Rev.*, 70:591–614.

11

Hormonal Control of Reproduction in the Male

OVERVIEW

The testes serve the dual function of producing sperm and hormones. The principal testicular hormone is the steroid testosterone which has an intratesticular role in sperm production and an extratesticular role in promoting delivery of sperm to the female genital tract. In this respect, testosterone promotes the development and maintenance of accessory sexual structures responsible for nurturing gametes and ejecting them from the body, development of secondary sexual characteristics that make men attractive to women, and those behavioral characteristics that promote successful procreation. Testicular function is driven by the pituitary through the secretion of two gonadotropic hormones: follicle-stimulating hormone (FSH) and luteinizing hormone (LH). Secretion of these pituitary hormones is controlled by (a) the central nervous system through secretion of the gonadotropin-releasing hormone (GnRH) by hypothalamic neurons and (b) the testes through the secretion of testosterone and inhibin. These hormones and an additional testicular secretion called anti-müllerian factor, also function as determinants of sexual differentiation during fetal life.

MALE REPRODUCTIVE TRACT

The testes are paired ovoid organs located in the scrotal sac outside the body cavity. The extraabdominal location, coupled with vascular countercurrent heat exchangers and muscular reflexes that retract the testes toward the abdomen, permits testicular temperature to be maintained constant at about 2°C below body temperature. For reasons that are not understood, this small reduction in temperature is crucial for normal *spermatogenesis* (sperm production). Failure of the testes to descend into the scrotum results in failure of spermatogenesis, although production of testosterone may be maintained. The two principal functions of the testis—sperm production and steroid hormone synthesis—are carried out in morphologically distinct compartments. Sperm are formed and develop within the *seminiferous tubules*, which comprise the bulk of testicular mass, and testosterone is produced by the *interstitial cells of Leydig*, which lie between the seminiferous tubules (Fig. 1). The entire testis is encased in an inelastic fibrous capsule consisting of three layers of dense connective tissue and some smooth muscle.

Blood reaches the testes primarily through the paired spermatic arteries, and is first cooled by heat exchange with returning venous blood in the *pampiniform plexus*. This complex tangle of blood vessels is formed by the highly tortuous and convoluted artery intermingling with equally tortuous venous branches that converge to form the spermatic vein. This arrangement provides a large surface area for warm arterial

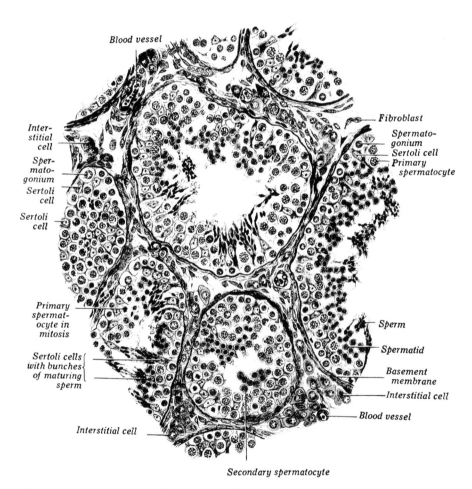

FIG. 1. A histological section of human testis. The transected tubules show various stages of spermatogenesis. From Fawcett, D.W. (1986): *A Textbook of Histology*, 11th ed., p. 804. WB Saunders, Philadelphia.

blood to transfer heat to cooler venous blood across thin vascular walls. Rewarmed venous blood returns to the systemic circulation primarily through the internal spermatic veins.

The Leydig cells are embedded in loose connective tissue that fills the spaces between seminiferous tubules. They are large polyhedral cells with an extensive smooth endoplasmic reticulum characteristic of steroid-secreting cells. Although extensive at birth, Leydig cells virtually disappear after the first 6 months of postnatal life, only to reappear more than a decade later with the onset of puberty.

The seminiferous tubules are highly convoluted loops that range from about 120 to 300 mm in diameter and from 30 to 70 cm in length. They are arranged in lobules bounded by fibrous connective tissue. Each testis has hundreds of such tubules that are connected at both ends to the *rete testis* (Fig. 2). It has been estimated that, if laid end to end, the seminiferous tubules of the human testes would extend more than 250 meters. The seminiferous epithelium that lines the tubules consists of three types of cell: *spermatogonia*, which are stem cells; *spermatocytes* in the process of becoming sperm; and *Sertoli cells*, which nurture developing sperm and secrete a variety of products into the blood and the lumens of the seminiferous tubules. The seminiferous tubules are surrounded by a thin coating of peritubular epithelial cells, which in some species, are contractile and help propel the nonmotile sperm through the tubules toward the rete testis.

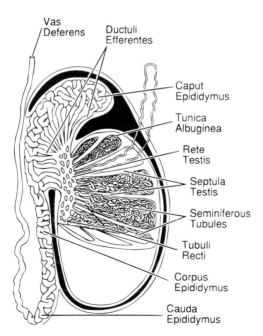

FIG. 2. Cutaway diagram of the architecture of the human testis. From Fawcett, D.W. (1986): *A Textbook of Histology*, 11th ed., p. 797. WB Saunders, Philadelphia; modified from Hamilton (1957): *Textbook of Human Anatomy*, Macmillan, London.

Spermatogenesis goes on continuously from puberty to senescence along the entire length of the seminiferous tubules. Though a continuous process, spermatogenesis can be divided into three discrete phases: (a) *mitotic divisions*, which replenish the spermatogonia and provide the cells destined to become mature sperm; (b) *meiotic divisions*, which reduce the chromosome number and produce a cluster of haploid spermatids; and (c) transformation of spermatids into mature sperm (*spermiogenesis*), a process involving the loss of most of the cytoplasm and the development of flagella. These events occur along the length of the seminiferous tubules in a definite temporal and spatial pattern. A *spermatogenic cycle* includes all of the transformations from spermatogonium to spermatozoan and requires about 64 days. As the cycle progresses, the germ cells move from the basal portion of the germinal epithelium toward the lumen. Successive cycles begin before the previous one has been completed, so that, at any given point along a tubule, different stages of the cycle are seen at different depths of the epithelium (Fig. 3). Spermatogenic cycles are synchronized in adjacent groups of cells, but the cycles are slightly advanced in similar groups of cells located immediately upstream, so that cells at any given stage of the spermatogenic cycle are spaced at regular intervals along the length of the tubules. This spatial organization is called the *spermatogenic wave*. This complex series of events ensures that mature spermatozoa are produced continuously. About two million spermatogonia, each giving rise to 64 sperm cells, begin this process in each testis every day. Hundreds of millions of spermatozoa are thus produced daily throughout six or more decades of reproductive life.

The Sertoli cells are remarkable polyfunctional cells whose activities are intimately related to many aspects of the formation and maturation of spermatozoa. They extend through the entire thickness of the germinal epithelium from the basement membrane to the lumen and, in the adult, take on exceedingly irregular shapes determined by the changing conformation of the developing sperm cells embedded in their cytoplasm (Fig. 4). Differentiating sperm cells are isolated from the blood stream and must rely on Sertoli cells for their sustenance. Adjacent Sertoli cells arch above the clusters of spermatogonia that nestle between them at the level of the basement membrane. Adjacent Sertoli cells form a series of tight junctions that limit passage of physiologically relevant molecules into or out of the seminiferous tubules. This so-called *blood–testis barrier* actually has selective permeability that allows rapid entry of testosterone, for example, but virtually completely excludes cholesterol. The physiological significance of the blood–testis barrier has not been established, but it is probably of some importance that spermatogonia are located on the blood side of the barrier, whereas developing spermatids are restricted to the luminal side. In addition to harboring developing sperm, Sertoli cells secrete a watery fluid that transports the spermatozoa through the seminiferous tubules and into the epididymis, where 99% of the fluid is reabsorbed.

The remaining portion of the male reproductive tract consists of modified excretory ducts that ultimately deliver sperm to the exterior along with secretions of accessory glands that promote sperm survival and fertility. Sperm leave the testis through multiple *ductuli efferentes* whose ciliated epithelium facilitates their passage

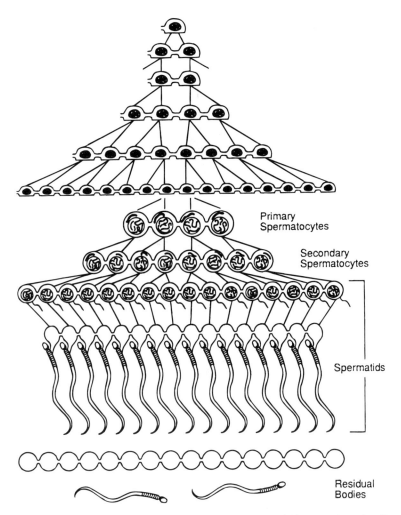

Primary
Spermatocytes

Secondary
Spermatocytes

Spermatids

Residual
Bodies

FIG. 3. The formation of mammalian germ cells. Each primary (A_1) spermatogonia ultimately gives rise to 64 sperm cells. Cytokinesis is incomplete in all but the earliest spermatogonial divisions, resulting in expanding clones of germ cells that remain joined by intercellular bridges. From Fawcett, D.W. (1986): *A Textbook of Histology*, 11th ed., p. 815. WB Saunders, Philadelphia.

from the rete testis into the highly convoluted and tortuous duct of the *epididymis*. The epididymis is the primary area for maturation and storage of sperm, which remain viable within its confines for months.

Sperm are advanced through the epididymis, particularly during sexual arousal, by rhythmic contractions of circular smooth muscle surrounding the duct. At ejaculation, sperm are expelled into the *vas deferens* and, ultimately, through the *urethra*. An accessory storage area for sperm lies in the ampulla of the vas deferens, posterior

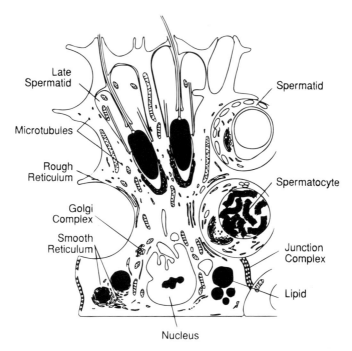

FIG. 4. Ultrastructure of the Sertoli cell and its relationship to the germ cells. The spermatocytes and early spermatids occupy niches in the sides of the columnar supporting cell, whereas the late spermatids reside in deep recesses in its apex. From Fawcett, D.W. (1986): *A Textbook of Histology*, 11th ed., p. 84. WB Saunders, Philadelphia.

to the *seminal vesicles*. These elongated, hollow evaginations of the deferential ducts secrete a fluid rich in citric acid and fructose that provides nourishment for the sperm after ejaculation. Metabolism of fructose provides the energy for sperm motility. Additional citrate and a variety of enzymes are added to the ejaculate by the prostate, which is the largest of the accessory secretory glands. Sperm and the combined secretions of the accessory glands make up the semen, of which less than 10% is sperm.

CONTROL OF TESTICULAR FUNCTION

The physiological activity of the testis is governed by two pituitary hormones, FSH and LH (see Chapter 2). The same gonadotropic hormones are produced in pituitary glands of men and women, but because these hormones have been studied more extensively in women, names that describe their activity in the ovary (see Chapters 12 and 13) have been adopted. The two gonadotropins FSH and LH are closely related and appear to be secreted by a single class of pituitary cells. Their sites of stimulation of testicular function, however, are discrete, i.e., FSH acts on the germinal epithelium and LH, on the Leydig cells.

Leydig Cells

The principal role of Leydig cells is the synthesis and secretion of the hormone testosterone in response to stimulation by LH. Interaction of LH with specific glyco-protein receptors on the surface of Leydig cells activates adenylyl cyclase through mediation of the stimulatory guanine nucleotide-binding protein (Gs). These events are typical of hormones whose actions are mediated by cyclic adenosine monophosphate (AMP, see Chapter 1). Cyclic AMP activates protein kinase A, which catalyzes the phosphorylation of proteins whose specific functions, though still unknown, promote the synthesis of testosterone. Some evidence indicates that the phospholipid–calcium–calmodulin system (see Chapter 1) may also mediate actions of LH.

As in the adrenal cortex (see Chapter 4), the rate-determining step in the synthesis of testicular steroids is conversion of cholesterol to pregnenolone. This process requires mobilization of cholesterol from storage droplets and its translocation from the cytosol to the intramitochondrial compartment, where side chain cleavage (des-molase reaction) occurs. Stored cholesterol may derive either from *de novo* synthesis within the Leydig cell or from circulating cholesterol, which apparently enters by receptor-mediated endocytosis of low density lipoproteins. The other crucial reaction in androgen biosynthesis involves cleavage of the side chain at carbon 17 to form the 19-carbon steroid nucleus. Cleavage at carbon 17 does not appear to be affected directly by LH or cyclic AMP. The biochemical pathway for testosterone biosynthesis is shown in Fig. 5. Although LH is the primary regulator of testosterone production, studies in rodents indicate that FSH may increase testicular responsiveness to it by increasing LH receptors on Leydig cells. Because Leydig cells apparently lack FSH receptors, these effects must follow indirectly from an action of FSH on some other testicular cell. Prolactin also enhances testosterone production in rodents by a direct interaction with specific receptors on the Leydig cells, but it is not yet known if prolactin has similar effects in humans.

Stimulation of testosterone secretion is not the only effect of LH on Leydig cells. Also, LH controls the availability of its own receptors (down regulation) and governs growth and differentiation. After hypophysectomy of experimental animals, the Leydig cells atrophy and lose their extensive smooth endoplasmic reticulum. Administration of LH restores them to normal and can produce frank hypertrophy if given in excess. Increased secretion of LH at the onset of puberty causes dormant juvenile Leydig cells to reawaken, hypertrophy, and reconstruct their testosterone synthetic apparatus. In the fetus, growth and development of Leydig cells depend on LH secreted by the fetal pituitary gland and on the placental hormone chorionic gonadotropin, which has LH-like activity.

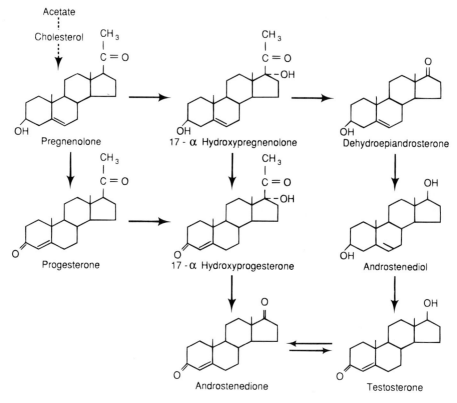

FIG. 5. Biosynthesis of androgens.

TESTOSTERONE

Testosterone is the principal androgen secreted by the mature testis. The normal young man produces about 7 mg each day, of which less than 5% is derived from adrenal secretions. This amount decreases somewhat with age, so that, by the seventh decade and beyond, testosterone production may have decreased to 4 mg per day, but in the absence of illness or injury, there is no sharp drop in testosterone production akin to the abrupt cessation of estrogen production in the postmenopausal woman. The testis also secretes androstenedione, which is considerably less potent than testosterone, and some estrogens. The Leydig cell is the chief source of testicular estrogens, but Sertoli cells have the capacity to convert testosterone to estradiol.

As with the other steroid hormones, testosterone in blood is largely bound to plasma proteins, with only about 2% to 3% present as free hormone. About 50% is bound to albumin, and about 45% to sex hormone-binding globulin (SHBG), which is also called testosterone–estradiol-binding globulin (TeBG). This glycoprotein binds both estrogen and testosterone, but its single binding site has a higher affinity for testosterone. Its concentration in plasma is increased by estrogens and decreased by androgens. Consequently, SHBG is more than twice as abundant in the circulation of women as of men.

Testosterone that is not bound to plasma protein diffuses out of capillaries and into nontarget as well as target cells. In some respects, testosterone can be considered to be a prohormone because it is converted in extratesticular tissues to other steroids and returned to the blood. In the skin and target cells of the male reproductive tract, testosterone may be reduced to the more potent androgen dihydrotestosterone in a reaction catalyzed by the enzyme 5α-reductase. Dihydrotestosterone is only about 5% as abundant in blood as testosterone and is largely derived from peripheral metabolism of testosterone. Some testosterone is also metabolized to estradiol (Fig. 6). A variety of cells, including some in brain, breast, and adipose tissue, can convert testosterone and androstenedione to estradiol and estrone. These estrogens may produce cellular effects that are different from, and sometimes opposite to, those of testosterone. The concentration of estrogens in blood of normal men is similar to that of women in the early follicular phase of the menstrual cycle (see Chapter 12). About two thirds of these estrogens are formed from androgen outside of the testis. We do not understand how or even if this process is regulated. In other tissues, including liver, reduction catalyzed by 5β-reductase destroys androgenic potency. The liver is the principal site of degradation of testosterone and releases water-soluble sulfate or glucuronide conjugates into the blood for excretion in the urine.

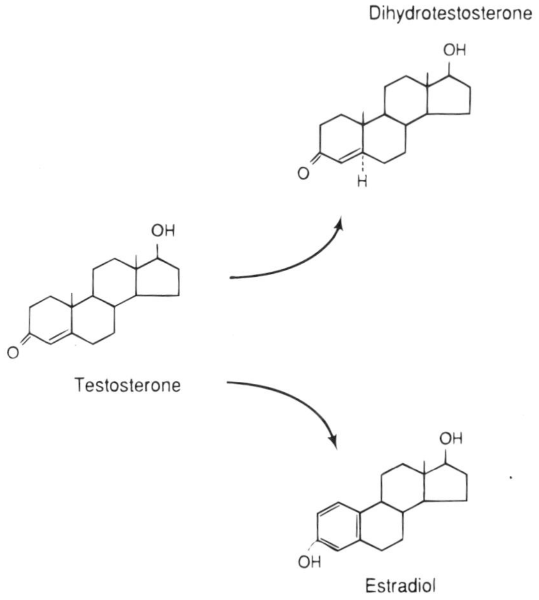

FIG. 6. Metabolism of testosterone.

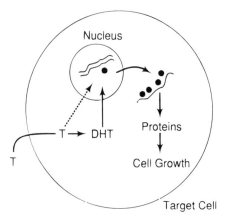

FIG. 7. Action of testosterone. Testosterone (*T*) enters its target cell and is converted to dihydrotestosterone (*DHT*), which binds to its intracellular receptor. The hormone–receptor complex binds to chromatin and induces formation of the RNA that encodes for the proteins that express the effects of the hormone.

Mechanism of Action

Like other steroid hormones, testosterone penetrates the target cells whose growth and function it stimulates (see Chapter 1). Androgen binds to an intracellular protein receptor and the complex then binds to specific response elements in target genes and activates transcription. Most target cells affected by testosterone contain 5α-reductase in their cytosol and convert testosterone to 5α-dihydrotestosterone before it binds to the androgen receptor. Actually, the human genome encodes two different enzymes with 5α-reductase activity. Both testosterone and dihydrotestosterone bind to the same cellular receptor, but the dihydro form dissociates from the receptor much more slowly than testosterone and, therefore, is the predominant androgen associated with DNA. It is possible that the higher affinity of dihydrotestosterone for the androgen receptor accounts for the differences in biological activity of testosterone and dihydrotestosterone. These events are summarized in Fig. 7.

Physiological Actions: Male Genital Tract

Testosterone promotes the growth, differentiation, and function of the accessory organs of reproduction. Its effects on the genital tract begin early in embryonic life and are not completed until adolescence, after an interruption of more than a decade. Maintenance of normal function in the adult also depends on continued testosterone secretion; the secretory epithelia of the seminal vesicles and prostate atrophy after castration but can be restored with injections of androgen.

Effects on Prenatal Development

Primordial components of both male and female reproductive tracts are present in early embryos of both sexes, and their development is either stimulated or suppressed by humoral factors. The primitive gonad becomes distinguishable as a testis by about the seventh week of embryonic life when cords of cells that give rise to seminiferous tubules appear. Leydig cells appear about 10 days later and undergo rapid proliferation for the next 6 to 8 weeks, presumably in response to chorionic gonadotropin produced in large amounts at this time by the placenta and perhaps also in response to LH secreted by the fetal pituitary gland. Fetal Leydig cells secrete sufficient testosterone to raise the blood concentrations to the same levels as those seen in adult men.

Regardless of its genetic sex, the embryo has the potential to develop phenotypically either as male or female. The pattern for female development is expressed unless overridden by the secretions of the fetal testis. The early embryo develops two sets of ducts that are the precursors of either male or female internal genitalia (Fig. 8). Seminal vesicles, epididymes, and vasa deferens arise from the primitive *mesonephric*, or *wolffian, ducts*. The internal genitalia of the female, including the uterus, fallopian tubes, and upper vagina, develop from the *müllerian ducts*. When stimulated by testosterone, the wolffian ducts differentiate into male reproductive structures, but in the absence of androgen, they regress and disappear. In contrast, the müllerian ducts develop into female reproductive structures unless actively sup-

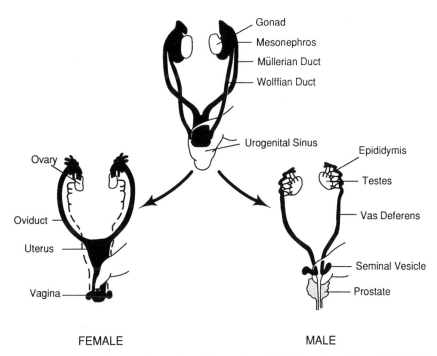

FEMALE   MALE

FIG. 8. Development of the male and female internal genitalia. From Yen, S.C. and Jaffe, R.B. (1986): Disorders of sexual development. In: *Reproductive Endocrinology*, edited by Boyd, S., p. 285, WB Saunders, Philadelphia.

pressed. Testosterone does not stimulate müllerian regression. Sertoli cells in newly differentiated seminiferous tubules secrete a glycoprotein called *müllerian regression factor* or *antimüllerian hormone*, which is responsible for reabsorption of the müllerian ducts. In experiments in which only one testis was removed from embryonic rabbits, the müllerian duct regressed only on the side with the remaining gonad, indicating that antimüllerian hormone must act locally as a paracrine factor. The wolffian duct regressed on the opposite side, suggesting that testosterone too must act locally to sustain the adjacent wolffian duct because the amounts that reached the contralateral duct through the circulation were inadequate to prevent its regression (Fig. 9).

The urogenital sinus and the genital tubercle are the primitive structures that give

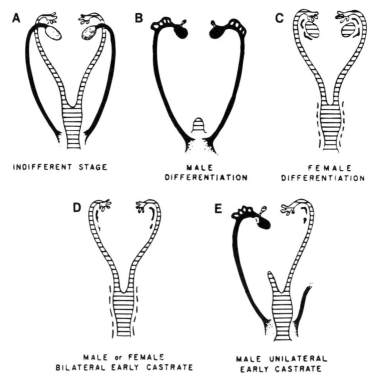

FIG. 9. Normal development of the male and female reproductive tracts. *Dark lines* indicate tissues destined to be the male tract; *cross-hatched area* represents tissues that develop into the female tract. Bilateral castration of either male or female embryos results in development of the female pattern (*second from right*). Early unilateral castration of male embryos results in the development of the normal male duct system on the side with the remaining gonad but female development on the contralateral side (*far right*). This pattern develops because both testosterone and antimüllerian factor act as paracrine factors. Modified from Jost (1971): Embryonic sexual differentiation. In: *Hermaphroditism, Genital Anomalies and Related Endocrine Disorders,* 2nd ed., edited by Jones, H.W. and Scott, W.W., p. 16, Williams & Wilkins, Baltimore.

rise to the external genitalia in both sexes. Masculinization of these structures to form the penis, scrotum, and prostate gland depends on secretion of testosterone by the fetal testis. Unless stimulated by androgen, these structures develop into female external genitalia. When there is insufficient androgen in male embryos, or too much androgen in female embryos, differentiation is incomplete, and the external genitalia are ambiguous. Differentiation of the masculine external genitalia depends on dihydrotestosterone rather than testosterone. The 5α-dehydrogenase enzyme responsible for conversion of testosterone to dihydrotestosterone is present in tissues destined to become external genitalia even before the testis starts to secrete testosterone. In contrast, this enzyme does not appear in tissues derived from the wolffian duct until after they differentiate, indicating that dihydrotestosterone was not the signal for differentiation of these tissues.

The importance of androgen action in sexual development is highlighted by a fascinating human syndrome called *testicular feminization*, which can be traced to an inherited defect in a single gene on the X chromosome. Afflicted individuals have a normal female phenotype but have sparse pubic and axillary hair and no menstrual cycles. Genetically, they are male and have intraabdominal testes and circulating concentrations of testosterone and estrogen that are characteristic of normal men, but their tissues are totally unresponsive to androgens. Absolute end-organ insensitivity has been traced to the absence of androgen receptors. Their external genitalia are female because, as already mentioned, the primordial tissues develop in the female pattern unless stimulated by androgen. Because antimüllerian hormone production and responsiveness were normal and their wolffian ducts were unable to respond to androgen, both of these duct systems regress and neither male nor female internal genitalia develop. Secondary sexual characteristics, including breast development, appear at puberty in response to unopposed action of estrogens formed extragonadally from testosterone.

Effects on Postnatal Development

Aside from a brief surge in androgen production during the immediate neonatal period, testicular function enters a period of quiescence, and further development of the male genital tract is arrested until the onset of puberty. Increased production of testosterone at puberty promotes growth of the penis and scrotum and increases pigmentation of the genitalia as well as the depth of rugal folds in scrotal skin. Further growth of the prostate, seminal vesicles, and epididymes also occurs at this time. Although differentiation of the epididymes and seminal vesicles was independent of dihydrotestosterone during the early fetal period, later acquisition of 5α-reductase makes this more active androgen the dominant form that stimulates growth and secretory activity during the pubertal period.

The importance of some of the foregoing information is highlighted by another interesting genetic disorder that has been described as *"penis at twelve."* Affected individuals have a deletion or mutation in one of the genes that code for 5α-reductase, and hence, their ability to convert testosterone to dihydrotestosterone is limited. Although the testes and wolffian derivatives develop normally, the prostate gland is absent, and the external genitalia at birth are ambiguous or overtly feminine. Affected children have been raised as girls. With the onset of puberty and the consequent increase in testosterone production, significant growth of the phallus occurs. Presumably, there is enough dihydrotestosterone formed at this time by the other 5α-reductase enzyme, which appears to be expressed in increased amounts at puberty.

Effects on Development of Secondary Sexual Characteristics

In addition to its effect on organs directly related to transport and delivery of sperm, testosterone affects a variety of other tissues and thus contributes to the morphological and psychological components of masculinity. These characteristics are clearly an integral part of reproduction, for they are related to the attractiveness of the male to the female. During early adolescence, androgens that may arise from the adrenals or testes stimulate growth of pubic hair. Growth of chest, axillary, and facial hair is also stimulated, but scalp hair is affected in the opposite manner. Recession of hair at the temples is a typical response to androgen, and adequate amounts allow expression of genes for baldness. Growth and secretion of sebaceous glands in the skin are also stimulated, a phenomenon undoubtedly related to the acne of adolescence. Dihydrotestosterone is the important androgen for recession of scalp hair and stimulation of the sebaceous glands.

Androgen secretion at puberty stimulates growth of the larynx and thickening of the vocal chords and thus lowers the pitch of the voice. At this time also, the characteristic adolescent growth spurt results from an interplay of testosterone and growth hormone (see Chapter 10) that promotes growth of the vertebrae and long bones. Development of the shoulder girdle is pronounced. This growth is self-limiting because androgens also accelerate epiphyseal closure. Androgens promote the formation of muscle, especially in the upper torso. Indeed, men have almost half again as much muscle mass as women. In some animals, the temporal and masseter muscles are particularly sensitive to androgenic stimulation. This anabolic action of androgens is exerted through nuclear androgen receptors and activation of the protein synthetic apparatus of muscle. Growth and nitrogen retention, of course, are also related to the stimulation of appetite and increased food intake. Accordingly, androgens bring about increased physical vigor and a feeling of well-being. In both men and women androgens increase sexual drive (*libido*).

Effects on Spermatogenesis

It has been known for many years that both FSH and LH are needed to stimulate spermatogenesis. The action of LH is limited to stimulating testosterone secretion by the Leydig cells, which are the only testicular cells known to have LH receptors. Testosterone diffuses from the Leydig cells to adjacent tubules and acts in a paracrine manner to mediate the effects of LH on spermatogenesis. Sertoli cells have androgen receptors, suggesting that they are targets for testosterone or one of its metabolites. Testosterone readily passes through the blood–testis barrier and is found in high concentrations in seminiferous fluid. We do not yet know what direct effects, if any, testosterone exerts on developing sperm cells. The concentration of testosterone in testicular venous blood, which reflects its concentration in testicular interstitial fluid, is 40 to 50 times that found in peripheral blood.

The administration of FSH alone to immature or hypophysectomized animals for several days produces testicular enlargement accompanied by increased cell division in the seminiferous epithelium. Sertoli cells, which are richly endowed with FSH receptors, are likely to be the target cells for FSH action. FSH is indispensable for initiating spermatogenesis at puberty and for restoring spermatogenesis after hypophysectomy. Meiosis does not begin until the germinal epithelium of the seminiferous tubules has been stimulated by both FSH and testosterone, but once initiated, sperm formation can be maintained indefinitely with very high doses of testosterone alone or with LH alone. If treatment with testosterone is not begun soon enough, however, spermatogenesis decreases, and FSH once again becomes essential. It is likely, but not certain, that FSH plays an ongoing role in spermatogenesis in the normal man.

The Sertoli cell is central to the regulation of spermatogenesis. In immature rats, binding of FSH to specific receptors on the surface of Sertoli cells is followed by increased adenylyl cyclase activity and synthesis of ribonucleic acid (RNA) and proteins (Fig. 10). Stimulated Sertoli cells produce a number of proteins. The most thoroughly studied of these is the androgen-binding protein (ABP), which is secreted into the lumens of seminiferous tubules and may preserve high androgen concentrations in the fluid surrounding maturing sperm in the rete testis and epididymis. Both testosterone and FSH stimulate the production of ABP, but how this joint action is related to initiation or maintenance of the spermatogenic process is still not understood. Local growth factors secreted by Sertoli cells, perhaps working in concert with testosterone, may regulate mitosis and meiosis in the germ cells.

REGULATION OF TESTICULAR FUNCTION

Testicular function, as we have seen, depends on stimulation by two pituitary hormones, FSH and LH. Without them, the testes lose their functional capacity, and either atrophy or fail to develop. Secretion of these hormones by the pituitary gland is driven by the central nervous system through its secretion of GnRH, which reaches the pituitary by way of the hypophyseal portal blood vessels. Separation of the pituitary gland from its vascular linkage to the hypothalamus results in total cessation of gonadotropin secretion and testicular atrophy. The central nervous system and the pituitary gland are kept apprised of testicular activity by signals related to each of the testicular functions: steroidogenesis and gametogenesis. The signals from the testis are inhibitory, characteristic of a negative feedback relationship. Castration

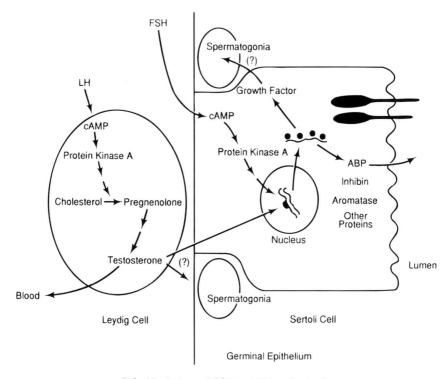

FIG. 10. Actions of FSH and LH on the testis.

results in a prompt increase in secretion of both FSH and LH. The central nervous system also receives and integrates other information from the internal and external environments and modifies GnRH secretion accordingly.

GnRH and the Hypothalamic Pulse Generator

Gonadotropin-releasing hormone is a decapeptide produced by neurons whose perikarya lie in the arcuate nuclei in the medial basal hypothalamus and whose axons terminate in the vicinity of the hypophyseal portal capillaries. GnRH-secreting neurons also project to other parts of the brain and may mediate some aspects of sexual behavior. GnRH is released into the hypophyseal portal circulation in discrete pulses at regular intervals ranging from about one every hour to one every 3 hours or longer. Each pulse lasts only a few minutes. Secretion of GnRH is difficult to monitor directly because obtaining samples of hypophyseal portal blood is problematic and because GnRH concentrations are usually too low to measure in peripheral blood after dilution by the general circulation. The pulsatile nature of GnRH secretion has been inferred from the results of frequent measurements of LH concentrations

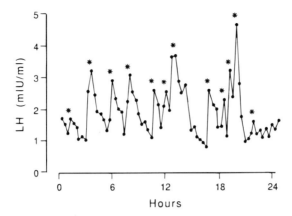

FIG. 11. The LH secretory pattern observed in a normal 36-year-old man. *, statistically significant discrete pulse. From Crowley, W.F., Jr. (1985): In: *Current Topics in Endocrinology and Metabolism*, edited by Krieger, D.T. and Bardin, C.W., p. 157, Marcel Dekker, New York.

in peripheral blood (Fig. 11). Concentrations of FSH tend to fluctuate much less, largely because FSH has a longer half-life than does LH.

Pulsatile secretion requires synchronous firing of many neurons, which therefore, must be in communication with each other or with a common pulse generator located nearby. Because pulsatile secretion of GnRH continues even after experimental disconnection of the medial basal hypothalamus from the rest of the central nervous system, the pulse generator must be located within this small portion of the hypothalamus and may be the network of GnRH neurons themselves. There is good correspondence between electrical activity in the arcuate nuclei and LH concentrations in blood as determined in rhesus monkeys fitted with permanently implanted electrodes. The frequency and amplitude of secretory pulses and corresponding electrical activity can be modified experimentally (Fig. 12). These parameters are regulated physiologically by gonadal steroids and probably by other information processed within the central nervous system.

The significance of the pulsatile nature of GnRH secretion became evident in studies of reproductive function in rhesus monkeys whose arcuate nuclei had been destroyed and whose secretion of LH and FSH therefore came to a halt. When GnRH was given as a constant infusion, it restored gonadotropin secretion only for a short while. Secretion of FSH and LH soon decreased and stopped even though the infusion of GnRH continued. Only when GnRH was administered intermittently for a few minutes of each hour was it possible to sustain normal gonadotropin secretion in these monkeys. Desensitization of the gonadotropes after prolonged uninterrupted exposure to GnRH appears to result from the combined effects of down regulation of GnRH receptors, a decrease in the calcium channels associated with secretion, and a decrease in releasable gonadotropin.

The necessity for pulsatile stimulation of the pituitary gland with GnRH for normal

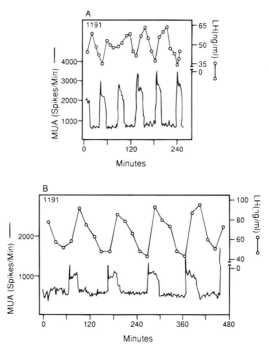

FIG. 12. Recording of multiple unit activity (*MUA*) in the arcuate nuclei of conscious (**A**) and anesthetized (**B**) monkeys fitted with permanently implanted electrodes. Simultaneous measurements of LH in peripheral blood are shown in the upper tracings. From Wilson, R.C., Kesner, J.S., Kaufman, J.M., et al. (1984): Central electrophysiologic correlates of pulsatile luteinizing hormone secretion in the rhesus monkey. *Neuroendocrinology.*, 39:256.

gonadotropin secretion has been confirmed in humans and applied therapeutically. Persons who are deficient in GnRH fail to experience pubertal development and remain sexually juvenile. Treating them with a long-acting analogue of GnRH that provides constant stimulation to the pituitary is ineffective in restoring normal function. Treating GnRH deficiency with the aid of a pump that delivers GnRH under the skin in intermittent pulses every 2 hours induces pubertal development and normal reproductive function. Treatment with a long-acting analogue of GnRH desensitizes the pituitary gland and blocks gonadotropin secretion. In fact, such a regimen has been used successfully to arrest premature sexual development in children suffering from precocious puberty.

Negative Feedback Regulators

Both gonadotropic hormones originate in the same pituitary cell whose secretory activity is stimulated by the same hypothalamic hormone. Nevertheless, FSH secretion is controlled independently of LH secretion by negative feedback signals that relate to the separate functions of the two gonadotropins. Although castration is followed by increased secretion of both FSH and LH, only LH is restored to normal when physiological amounts of testosterone are given. Failure of testicular descent into the scrotum (*cryptorchidism*) may result in destruction of the germinal epithelium without affecting the Leydig cells. With this condition, blood levels of testosterone and LH are normal, but FSH is elevated. Thus, testosterone, which is secreted in response to LH, acts as a feedback regulator of LH and, hence, of its own secretion. By this reasoning, we would expect that spermatogenesis, which is stimulated by FSH, might be associated with the secretion of a substance that reflects gamete production. Indeed, FSH stimulates the Sertoli cells to secrete a glycoprotein called *inhibin* that acts as a feedback inhibitor of FSH. Inhibin is a heterodimer comprised of an α subunit and either of two forms of a β subunit, β_A or β_B. At present, little is known about the significance of alternate β subunits or the factors that determine when each form is produced. All three subunits are encoded in separate genes, and presumably, each can be regulated independently. The β subunits belong to the gene family that includes the müllerian inhibiting factor. Of additional interest is the finding that dimers formed from two β subunits have effects that are opposite those of the α,β dimer and stimulate FSH release. This compound has been called *activin*. Its physiological importance is unknown.

The feedback relationships that fit best with our current understanding of the regulation of testicular function in the adult man are shown in Fig. 13. Pulses of GnRH originating in the arcuate nuclei evoke secretion of both FSH and LH by the anterior pituitary. Both FSH and LH are positive effectors of testicular function

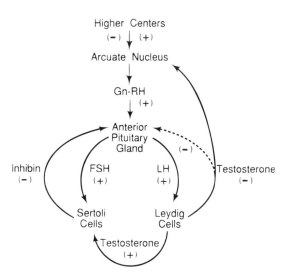

FIG. 13. Negative feedback regulation of testicular function. +, stimulation; −, inhibition. Direct effects of testosterone on the pituitary gland are still uncertain and, hence, indicated by a *dashed line*.

and stimulate release of inhibin and testosterone, respectively. Testosterone has an intratesticular action that reinforces the effects of FSH. It also travels through the circulation to the hypothalamus, where it exerts its negative feedback effect, primarily by slowing the frequency of GnRH pulses. Decreased frequency of GnRH pulses results in a decreased ratio of LH to FSH in the gonadotropic output. In the castrated monkey, the hypothalamic pulse generator discharges once per hour and slows to once every 2 hours after testosterone is replaced. This rate is about the same as that seen in normal men. The higher frequency in the castrated animal triggers more frequent bursts of gonadotropin secretion, resulting in higher blood levels. Testosterone may decrease the amplitude of the GnRH pulses somewhat and may also have a small restraining effect on LH release from gonadotropes. In high enough concentrations, testosterone may decrease GnRH sufficiently to shut off secretion of both gonadotropic hormones. The negative feedback effect of inhibin appears to be exerted exclusively on the gonadotropes, inhibiting FSH secretion in response to GnRH. Some evidence indicates that inhibin may also exert local effects on Leydig cells to enhance testosterone production.

Prepubertal Period

Testicular function is critical for development of the normal masculine phenotype early in the prenatal period. All of the elements of the control system are present in the early embryo. Both GnRH and gonadotropins are detectable at about the time that androgen begins stimulating wolffian duct development. The hypothalamic GnRH pulse generator and its negative feedback control are functional in the newborn. After about the sixth month of postnatal life and for the remainder of the juvenile period, gonadotropin secretion is low, although a pulsatile pattern of LH secretion is evident. The low amplitude of the pulses is probably due to both low amplitude of the GnRH pulses and the experimentally demonstrated low sensitivity of the pituitary to GnRH. It is evident that negative feedback regulation is operative because blood levels of gonadotropins increase after gonadectomy in prepubertal subjects and fall with gonadal hormone administration. The system is extremely sensitive to feedback inhibition during this time, but suppression of the pulse generator cannot be explained simply as a change in the set point for feedback inhibition. Concentrations of gonadotropins are high in juvenile subjects whose testes failed to develop and who consequently lack testosterone, but they rise even higher when these subjects reach the age when puberty would normally occur. Thus, with the onset of puberty, there is an increased positive input to the GnRH pulse generator as well as an increase in the threshold for feedback inhibition.

Early stages of puberty are characterized by the appearance of high-amplitude pulses of LH during sleep (Fig. 14). Testosterone concentrations in plasma follow the gonadotropins, and there is a distinct day–night pattern. As puberty progresses, high-amplitude pulses are distributed throughout the day at the adult frequency of about one every 2 hours. Sensitivity of the pituitary gland to GnRH increases during

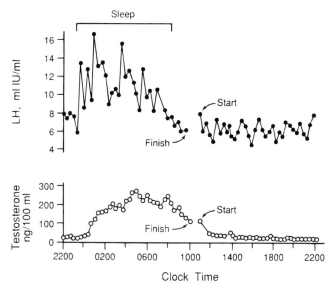

FIG. 14. Plasma LH and testosterone measured every 20 minutes reveal nocturnal pulsatile secretion of GnRH in a pubertal 14-year-old boy. From Boyar, R.M., Rosenfeld, R.S., Kapen, S., et al. (1974): Simultaneous augmented secretion of luteinizing hormone and testosterone during sleep. *J. Clin. Invest.*, 54:609.

puberty, possibly as a result of a priming effect of GnRH on the gonadotropes. GnRH may increase the number of its receptors expressed on the surface of gonadotropes (up regulation) and the amount of releasable gonadotropin. The low sensitivity of the pituitary gland to GnRH during the prepubertal period may therefore be secondary to hypothalamic suppression of GnRH. The underlying neural mechanisms for suppression of the GnRH pulse generator in the juvenile period are not understood. We also do not know what biological event signals readiness for reproductive development and function.

SUGGESTED READING

Crowley, W. F., Jr., Filicori, M., Spratt, D. I., and Santoro, N. F. (1985): The physiology of gonadotropin-releasing hormone (GnRH) in men and women. *Recent Prog. Horm. Res.*, 41:473–526.

George, F. W., and Wilson, J. D. (1986): Hormonal control of sexual development. *Vitam. Horm.*, 43: 145–196.

Josso, N. (1986): Anti-mullerian hormone: new perspectives for a sexist molecule. *Endocr. Rev.*, 7: 421–433.

Mooradian, A. D., Morley, J. E., and Korenman, S. G. (1987): Biological actions of androgens. *Endocr. Rev.*, 8:1–28.

Plant, T. M. (1986): Gonadal regulation of hypothalamic releasing hormone release in primates. *Endocr. Rev.*, 7:75–88.

Preslock, J. P. (1980): Steroidogenesis in the mammalian testis. *Endocr. Rev.*, 1:132–139.

Styne, D. M., and Grumbach, M. M. (1986): Puberty in the male and female—its physiology and disorders. In: *Reproductive Endocrinology*, 2nd ed., edited by Yen, S. C., and Jaffe, R. B. pp. 313–384, Saunders, Philadelphia.

Wilson, J. D. (1988): Androgen abuse by athletes. *Endocr. Rev.*, 9:181–199.

Ying, S.-Y. (1988): Inhibins, activins, and folliculostatins: gonadal proteins modulating the secretion of follicle-stimulating hormone. *Endocr. Rev.*, 9:267–293.

12

Hormonal Control of Reproduction in the Female

I. Menstrual Cycle

OVERVIEW

The ovaries serve the dual function of producing eggs and hormones. Unlike men, in whom large numbers of gametes are produced continuously from stem cells, women release only one gamete at a time from a limited pool of preformed gametes in a process that is repeated at regular monthly intervals. Each interval encompasses the time needed for the ovum to develop and the time allotted for that ovum to become fertilized and pregnancy established. If the ovary does not receive a signal that development of an embryo has begun, the process of gamete maturation begins anew.

The principal ovarian hormones are the steroids, estradiol and progesterone, which orchestrate the cyclic series of events that unfold in the ovary, pituitary, and reproductive tract. As the ovum develops within its follicle, estradiol stimulates growth of the structures of the reproductive tract that receive the sperm, facilitate fertilization, and ultimately, house the developing embryo. Estradiol also acts within the ovarian follicle to stimulate proliferation of granulosa cells and, thereby, enhances its own production. Progesterone is produced by the corpus luteum that develops from the follicle after the egg is shed. It prepares the uterus for successful implantation and growth of the embryo and is absolutely required for the maintenance of pregnancy.

Ovarian function is driven by the two pituitary gonadotropins follicle-stimulating hormone (FSH) and luteinizing hormone (LH), which stimulate ovarian steroid production, growth of the follicle, ovulation, and development of the corpus luteum. Secretion of these hormones depends on stimulatory input from the hypothalamus through the gonadotropin-releasing hormone (GnRH) and complex inhibitory and stimulatory input from the ovarian steroids.

FEMALE REPRODUCTIVE TRACT

Ovaries

The adult human ovaries are paired, flattened ellipsoid structures that measure about 5 cm in their longest dimension. They lie within the pelvic area of the abdominal cavity attached to the broad ligaments that extend from either side of the uterus by peritoneal folds called the *mesovaria*. The outer, or cortical, portion contains *primordial follicles*, *developing follicles, corpus luteum*, and *stromal or interstitial* cells. The inner portion, or medulla, consists chiefly of vascular elements that arise from anastomoses of the uterine and ovarian arteries. A rich supply of unmyelinated nerve fibers also enters the medulla along with blood vessels.

The ovarian follicles in which the ova develop, and the corpora lutea derived from them, are the sites of ovarian hormone production. The human female is born with an estimated two to four million primordial follicles, each consisting of a primary oocyte surrounded by a single layer of *granulosa cells*, enclosed in a basement membrane that separates it from cortical stroma. Primary oocytes are arrested in prophase of the first meiotic division from about the third month of embryonic life. Meiosis does not resume until the time of ovulation and is not completed until the second polar body is extruded at the time of fertilization, which may be more than four decades later for some oocytes. Unlike the male, in whom sperm production is continuous, development and release of mature gametes in the female occurs episodically. Only a small fraction of follicles is recruited in each episode, and normally, only one ovulates. The remaining follicles are quiescent and arrested in an immature state. Follicular development continues until the stockpile of primordial follicles is exhausted at menopause.

Early development of the follicle involves growth of the primary oocyte from a diameter of perhaps 15 mm to about 80 mm, and is accompanied by proliferation of granulosa cells (Fig. 1). The innermost granulosa cells are in intimate contact with the oocyte and form gap junctions with its plasma membrane. Granulosa cells also form gap junctions with each other. They may function as nurse cells for the oocyte and remain in physical contact with it by way of long cytoplasmic processes that penetrate the layer of mucopolysaccharide and protein called the *zona pellucida* that surrounds the oocyte. As a primordial follicle develops into a primary follicle, stromal cells immediately outside the basement membrane differentiate to form the *theca folliculi*. The inner layer, or *theca interna*, is composed of secretory cells with an extensive smooth endoplasmic reticulum characteristic of steroidogenic cells. Throughout development of the follicle, the oocyte and the granulosa cells are separated from direct contact with capillaries by the basal lamina, but the theca interna is richly vascularized.

As follicular development continues, there is further proliferation of granulosa cells and gradual elaboration of fluid within the follicle. Accumulation of this follicular fluid is associated with enlargement of the follicle and the formation of a central cavity called the *antrum*. At this stage, the follicle is called an antral or *graafian*

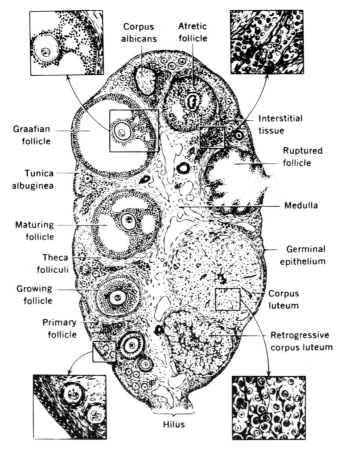

FIG. 1. A mammalian ovary showing the various stages of follicular and luteal development. Obviously, the events depicted occur sequentially and are not all present in any section of a human ovary. From Turner, C.D. and Bagnara, J.T. (1976): *General Endocrinology*, 6th ed., p. 453. Saunders, Philadelphia.

follicle. Follicular fluid is derived from blood plasma and contains plasma proteins, including hormones, as well as various proteins and steroids secreted by the granulosa cells. As the follicle matures, the fluid content in the antrum increases rapidly, possibly in response to increased colloid osmotic pressure created by partial hydrolysis of dissolved mucopolysaccharides. The ripe, preovulatory follicle reaches a diameter of 10 to 20 mm and bulges into the peritoneal cavity. At this time, it consists of multiple layers of granulosa cells around the periphery that connect by a narrow bridge of cells to the ovum and its surrounding layers of granulosa cells, the *corona radiata*, that are suspended in a sea of follicular fluid. At ovulation, the follicle ruptures, and the ovum with its corona of granulosa cells is extruded into the peritoneal cavity in a bolus of follicular fluid (Fig. 2).

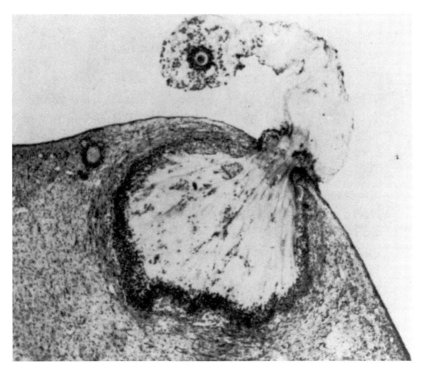

FIG. 2. Ovulation in a rabbit. Follicular fluid, granulosa cells, some blood, and cellular debris continue to ooze out of the follicle even after the egg mass has been extruded. From Hafez, E.S.E. and Blandau, R.J. (1969): Gamete transport–comparative aspects. In: *The Mammalian Oviduct*, edited by Hafez, E.S.E. and Blandau, R.J., University of Chicago Press, Chicago.

Many follicles are recruited during each cycle, but only one ovulates. Any follicle can be arrested at any stage of its development and undergo degenerative changes known as *atresia*. This fate is suffered by most follicles. During the reproductive lifetime of the normal woman, only about 500 follicles ovulate. More than 90% of the primordial follicles that were present at birth undergo partial development and atresia during the prepubertal period, and most of the remaining 200,000 to 400,000 remaining at puberty ultimately suffer a similar fate. The physiological mechanisms that control this seemingly wasteful process are poorly understood.

Following ovulation, there is ingrowth and differentiation of the remaining granulosa cells, thecal cells, and some stromal cells, which fill the cavity of the collapsed follicle to form a new endocrine structure, the *corpus luteum*. The process by which granulosa and thecal cells are converted to luteal cells is called *luteinization* (meaning yellowing) and is the morphological reflection of the accumulation of lipid. Luteinization also involves biochemical changes that enable the corpus luteum to become the most active of all steroid-producing tissues per unit weight. The corpus luteum consists of large polygonal cells containing smooth endoplasmic reticulum and a rich supply of fenestrated capillaries. Unless pregnancy ensues, the corpus luteum regresses after 2 weeks, leaving a scar on the surface of the ovary.

Oviducts and Uterus

The primitive müllerian ducts that develop during early embryonic life give rise to the duct system that, in primitive organisms, provides the route for ova to escape to the outside (Fig. 3). In mammals, these tubes are adapted to provide a site for fertilization of ova and nurturing of embryos. In female embryos, the müllerian ducts are not subjected to the destructive effects of the antimüllerian hormone (see Chapter 11) and, instead, develop into the oviducts, uterus, and upper portion of the vagina. Unlike the development of the sexual duct system in the male fetus (Chapter 11), this differentiation is independent of gonadal hormones.

The paired oviducts (*fallopian tubes*) are a conduit for transfer of the ovum to the uterus (see Chapter 13). The ovarian end comes in close contact with the ovary and has a funnel-shaped opening, *the infundibulum*, surrounded by finger-like projections called *fimbriae*. The oviduct, particularly the infundibulum, is lined with ciliated cells whose synchronous beating plays an important role in egg transport. The lining of the oviduct also contains secretory cells whose products provide nourishment for the zygote in its 3- to 4-day journey to the uterus. The walls of the oviducts contain layers of smooth muscle cells oriented both longitudinally and circularly.

Distal portions of the müllerian ducts fuse to give rise to the uterus. In the nonpreg-

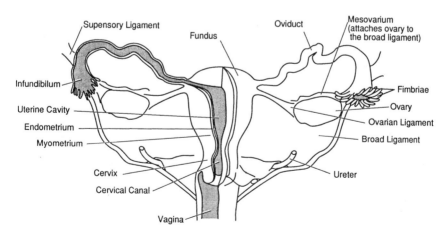

FIG. 3. The uterus and associated female reproductive structures. The *left* side of the figure has been sectioned to show the internal structures. Redrawn from Tortora, G.J. and Anagnostakos, N.P. (1981): *Principles of Anatomy and Physiology*, 3rd ed., p. 721. Harper & Row, New York.

nant woman, the uterus is a small, pear-shaped structure extending about 6 to 7 cm in its longest dimension. It is capable of enormous expansion, partly by passive stretching and partly by growth, so that at the end of pregnancy it may reach 35 cm or more in its longest dimension. Its thick walls consist mainly of smooth muscle and are called the *myometrium*. The secretory epithelial lining is called the *endometrium* and varies in thickness with changes in the hormonal environment, as discussed subsequently. The oviducts join the uterus at the upper, rounded end. The caudal end constricts to a narrow cylinder called the *uterine cervix*, whose thick wall is composed largely of dense connective tissue rich in collagen fibers and some smooth muscle. The cervical canal is lined with mucus-producing cells and is usually filled with mucus. The cervix bulges into the upper reaches of the vagina, which forms the final link to the outside. The lower portion of the vagina, which communicates with the exterior, is formed from the embryonic urogenital sinus.

OVARIAN HORMONES

The principal hormones secreted by the ovary are estrogens (*estradiol-17β* and *estrone*) and *progesterone*. These hormones are steroids and are derived from cholesterol by the series of reactions depicted in Fig. 4. Their biosynthesis is intricately interwoven with the events of the ovarian cycle, and is discussed in the next sections.

Estrogens

Unlike humans, of whom it has been said, "eat when they are not hungry, drink when they are not thirsty, and make love at all seasons of the year," most vertebrate animals mate only at times of maximum fertility of the female. This period of sexual receptivity is called *estrus*, derived from the Greek word for vehement desire. Estrogens are compounds that promote estrus and were originally isolated from follicular fluid of sow ovaries. Characteristic of steroid-secreting tissues, little hormone is stored within the secretory cells themselves. Estrogens circulate in blood loosely bound to albumin and tightly bound to the testosterone–estrogen-binding globulin, which is also called the sex hormone-binding globulin (see Chapter 11). Plasma concentrations of estrogen are considerably lower than those of other gonadal steroids and vary over an almost 20-fold range during the cycle.

The liver is the principal site of metabolic destruction of the estrogens. Estradiol and estrone are completely cleared from the blood by a single passage through the liver and are inactivated by hydroxylation and conjugation with sulfate and glucuronide. About half the protein-bound estrogen in blood is conjugated with sulfate and glucuronide. Although the liver may excrete some conjugated estrogens in the bile, they are reabsorbed in the lower gut and returned to the liver in portal blood in a typical enterohepatic circulatory pattern. The kidney is the chief route of excretion of estrogenic metabolites.

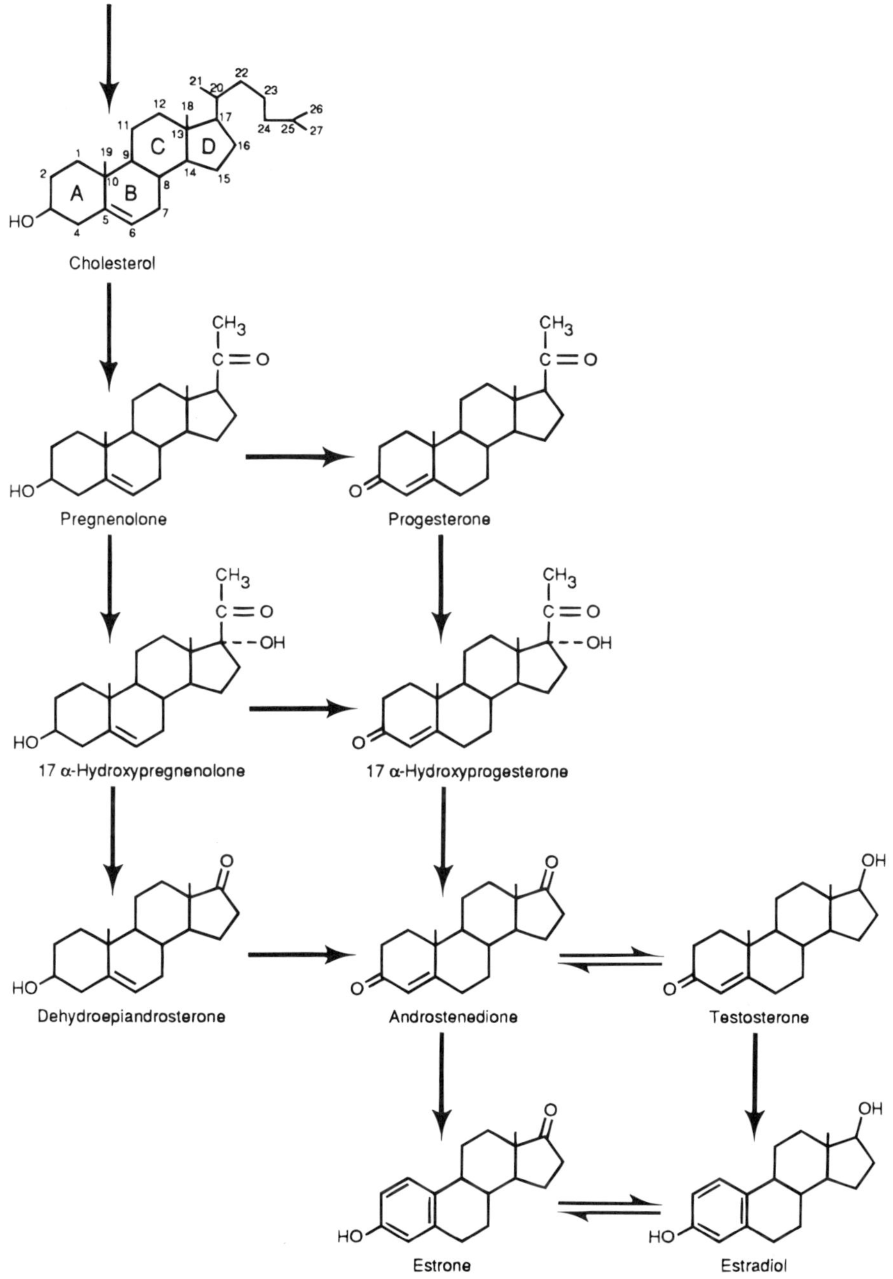

FIG. 4. The biosynthesis of the ovarian hormones. Cleavage of the cholesterol side chain between carbons 21 and 22 gives rise to 21-carbon progestins. Removal of carbons 20 and 21 produces the 19-carbon androgen series. Aromatization of ring A on the *far left* eliminates carbon 19 and yields 18-carbon estrogens.

Progesterone

Pregnancy, or gestation, requires the presence of another ovarian steroid hormone, progesterone. In the nonpregnant woman, progesterone secretion is largely confined to cells of the corpus luteum, but because it is an intermediate in the biosynthesis of all steroid hormones, small amounts may also be released from the adrenal cortex. Some progesterone is also produced by granulosa cells just before ovulation. The rate of progesterone production varies widely. Its concentration in blood ranges from virtually nil during the early preovulatory part of the cycle to as much as 2 mg/dl after the corpus luteum has formed. Progesterone circulates in blood in association with plasma proteins and has a high affinity for the corticosteroid-binding globulin. The liver is the principal site of progesterone inactivation, which is achieved by reduction of the A ring and the keto groups at carbons 3 and 20 to give pregnanediol, which is the chief metabolite found in urine. Considerable degradation also occurs in the uterus.

Ovarian Peptide Hormones

The ovary secretes peptide hormones as well as steroids. *Inhibin* (see Chapter 11) is produced by granulosa cells in the preovulatory period and released into follicular fluid where it is thought to play a paracrine role. It is also secreted into the systemic circulation throughout the ovarian cycle and is synthesized in the corpus luteum in the postovulatory period.

The corpus luteum also produces a peptide called *relaxin*, whose structure is closely related to those of insulin and the insulin-like growth factors. Relaxin was named for its ability to relax the pubic ligament of the pregnant guinea pig, but in other species, including humans, it also relaxes the myometrium. Because the function of this hormone in humans and other primates is not firmly established, it is not discussed further.

CONTROL OF OVARIAN FUNCTION

Follicular development beyond the antral stage depends on two gonadotropic hormones secreted by the anterior pituitary gland: FSH and LH. In addition to follicular growth, gonadotropins are required for ovulation, luteinization, and steroid hormone formation by both the follicle and the corpus luteum. The characteristics of these glycoprotein hormones are described in Chapter 2. Follicular growth and function also depend on the actions of estrogens and androgens, and possibly progesterone as well.

Follicles can develop up to the preantral stage in the absence of the pituitary gland, but little is understood about the regulation of early follicular growth or how primordial follicles are recruited for development at any given time. All follicles in both ovaries are exposed to the same circulating hormones; yet under normal circumstances, only a certain group, or cohort, develops during each cycle. Of these, only one becomes dominant and ovulates. The ovulatory follicle appears randomly in either the right or left ovary and is selected early in each cycle. Somehow, the other follicles of the cohort, located in both ovaries, are inhibited, presumably by the dominant follicle, and become atretic. Growth of the next cohort of follicles does not begin so long as the dominant follicle or its resultant corpus luteum is present and functional. Experimental destruction of either the dominant follicle or the corpus luteum is promptly followed by development of a new cohort of follicles.

The sequence of follicular development, ovulation, and the subsequent formation and degeneration of the corpus luteum is repeated about every 28 days and constitutes the ovarian cycle. The part of the cycle involving follicular development takes about 14 days and is called the *follicular phase*. The remainder of the cycle is dominated by the corpus luteum and is called the *luteal phase*. It too lasts about 14 days. Ovulation occurs at midcycle and requires only about 1 day.

Effects of FSH and LH on the Developing Follicle

The granulosa cell is the principal and perhaps only target for FSH in the ovary. No other ovarian cells are known to have FSH receptors. Granulosa cells secrete estrogens in response to FSH and proliferate in response to combined stimulation by FSH and estrogens. The administration of excessive FSH results in the development of a large number of follicles that are capable of ovulating. This finding indicates that many, and perhaps all, follicles in a cohort are able to respond to FSH but are less sensitive to it than the one follicle destined to ovulate.

Before the antrum forms, LH receptors are found only in cells of the theca interna and the stroma. LH stimulates these cells to synthesize and secrete steroid hormones and, in excess, can promote hypertrophy of the stromal cells. Early in each ovarian cycle, thecal cells surrounding the follicle that is destined to ovulate somehow become more sensitive to LH than those of other follicles of the cohort. Increased sensitivity probably results from increased density of LH receptors. When given to rhesus monkeys, LH labeled with a fluorescent dye selectively accumulated on thecal cells of the dominant follicle even before it was any larger than other follicles of the developing cohort.

Follicular development depends on production of estradiol, which acts within the follicle in an autocrine or paracrine manner. Estradiol promotes proliferation of granulosa cells and increases their responsiveness to FSH (Fig. 5). Because estradiol increases both the number of granulosa cells and their responsiveness to FSH, it is a powerful amplifier of FSH actions. Estradiol may also stimulate proliferation of theca interna cells. These events constitute a local positive feedback system that gives the follicle progressively greater capacity to produce estradiol and makes it increasingly sensitive to FSH as it matures. By these actions, estradiol increases its own production. Simultaneously, estradiol and FSH induce granulosa cells to synthesize receptors for LH. In preantral follicles, granulosa cells have few if any

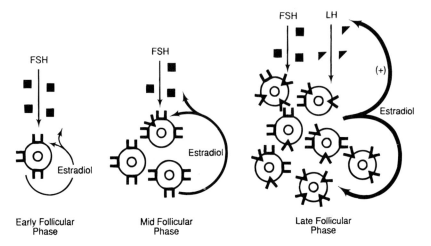

FIG. 5. The proliferation of granulosa cells during follicular development. *Solid squares* represent FSH, and *solid triangles* LH. Initially, the granulosa cells are few and have receptors only for FSH on their surfaces. In response to continued stimulation with both FSH and estradiol, the granulosa cells proliferate, and by midfollicular phase, LH receptors begin to appear. By late in the follicular phase, a large number of granulosa cells are present, and they are responsive to both LH and FSH. They are now competent to secrete sufficient estradiol to trigger the ovulatory surge of gonadotropins.

receptors for LH and are unresponsive to it. In contrast, granulosa cells of preovulatory follicles have abundant LH receptors and consequently have acquired sensitivity to LH.

Effects on Estradiol Production

Estrogen synthesis depends on complex interactions between the two gonadotropins and between theca and granulosa cells. Although theca and granulosa cells by themselves can synthesize some estrogens, cooperation of both cell types is required for optimal hormone production. Cells of the theca interna respond to LH by producing large amounts of androstenedione and testosterone, which are the precursors of estrogens (Fig. 4), but because these cells have little aromatase activity, they produce little estrogen. Granulosa cells, which synthesize aromatase in response to FSH, are deficient in the enzymes needed to convert 21-carbon precursors to 19-carbon androgens. Thus, granulosa cells can produce progesterone and pregnenolone, but these steroids cannot be used for estrogen synthesis until the side chain at carbon 17 is removed (Fig. 4). When stimulated with FSH, granulosa cells readily transform androgens produced by cells of the theca interna to estrogen. At the same time, 21-carbon steroids produced in granulosa cells can be converted to androgens by thecal cells. This two-cell interaction is illustrated in Fig. 6. The participation of two different cells, each stimulated by its own gonadotropin, accounts for the requirement of

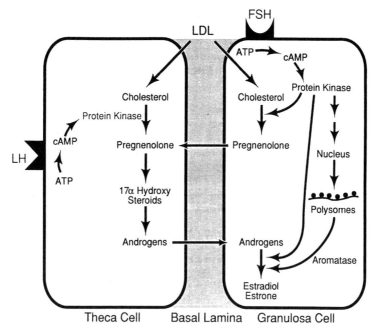

FIG. 6. Theca and granulosa cell cooperation in estrogen synthesis. The theca cells produce mainly androgens in response to *LH*. The granulosa cells respond to *FSH* by producing pregnenolone from cholesterol and by aromatizing androgens to estrogens. *LDL,* low density lipoproteins.

both pituitary hormones for adequate estrogen production and, hence, for follicular development.

Cellular Actions of FSH and LH

Follicle stimulating hormone and LH each bind to specific receptors on the surface of granulosa or theca cells and activate adenylyl cyclase in the manner described for other cyclic adenosine monophosphate (AMP)-dependent hormones (Chapter 1). Increased concentrations of cyclic AMP in the cytoplasm activate protein kinase, which catalyzes the phosphorylation of critical proteins, leading to steroidogenesis. As described for adrenal cortical cells (see Chapter 4) and Leydig cells (see Chapter 11), the rate-limiting step in steroid hormone synthesis is the conversion of cholesterol to pregnenolone in both theca and granulosa cells (Fig. 6). In theca cells, increased formation of androstenedione and testosterone results from increased availability of pregnenolone. In granulosa cells, the principal effect of cyclic AMP-mediated phosphorylation of protein is on the formation of aromatase, but cyclic AMP may also regulate the activity of aromatase after it is formed.

The actions of FSH and LH on the developing follicle appear to be enhanced by the autocrine and paracrine actions of the insulin-like growth factors (IGFs). Gonadotropins increase the availability of the IGFs to receptors on the granulosa cells by stimulating the synthesis of IGF-I and IGF-II by theca and granulosa cells and by inhibiting the synthesis of their binding proteins. In human ovarian cells studied in tissue culture, IGFs potentiate the actions of gonadotropins on granulosa cell proliferation, estradiol production, and synthesis of LH receptors.

Effects on Ovulation

Luteinizing hormone is the physiological signal for ovulation. Its concentration in blood rises sharply and reaches a peak about 16 hours before ovulation (see subsequent discussion). Blood levels of FSH also increase at this time, and although large amounts of FSH can also cause ovulation, the needed concentrations are not achieved during the normal reproductive cycle. The events that lead to follicular rupture are not fully understood, but the process is known to be initiated by increased production of cyclic AMP in theca and granulosa cells in response to LH.

As the follicle approaches ovulation, it accumulates follicular fluid. Despite the preovulatory swelling, intrafollicular pressure does not increase. The follicular wall becomes increasingly distensible, probably because of the activity of hydrolytic enzymes, which digest the collagen framework and other proteins of the intercellular matrix. Plasminogen activator is secreted by granulosa cells in response to hormonal stimulation and releases the active proteolytic enzyme from plasminogen that is present in follicular fluid. Because of their newly acquired receptors, granulosa cells of the preovulatory follicle respond to LH by secreting progesterone and prostaglandins. The finding that pharmacological blockade of their synthesis prevents ovulation indicates that prostaglandins and progesterone also play essential roles. Prostaglandins may activate contractile elements in the follicle wall and, thus, facilitate extrusion of the ovum and formation of the corpus luteum.

Although little or no progesterone is produced throughout most of the follicular phase, acquisition of the capacity for progesterone production by granulosa cells of the preovulatory follicle is the result of events already described. Newly acquired receptors enable granulosa cells to respond to LH with increased formation of cyclic AMP and, consequently, increased conversion of cholesterol to pregnenolone. Because of limited capacity to remove the side chain at carbon 17, 21-carbon steroids are formed faster than they can be processed and, hence, are secreted as progesterone. As granulosa cells acquire the ability to respond to LH, they also acquire increased capacity to convert pregnenolone to progesterone and begin to lose aromatase activity (Fig. 7). This is reflected in the abrupt decline in estrogen production that just precedes ovulation.

Effects on Corpus Luteum Formation

Luteinizing hormone was named for its ability to induce the formation of the corpus luteum after ovulation. However, as already mentioned, luteinization may

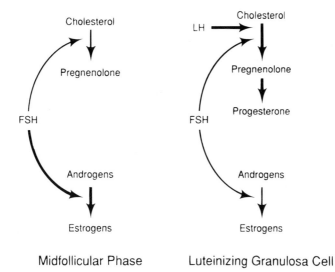

FIG. 7. The biochemical changes with luteinization of the granulosa cells. The thickness of the *arrows* represents the magnitude of effect.

actually begin before the follicle ruptures. Granulosa cells removed from mature follicles complete their luteinization in tissue culture without further stimulation by gonadotropin. Nevertheless, luteinization is absolutely dependent on LH, and the increased concentration of LH that precedes ovulation may accelerate the process. Sometimes, luteinization occurs in the absence of ovulation and results in the syndrome of luteinized unruptured follicles, which may be a cause of infertility in some women whose reproductive cycles seem otherwise normal.

Effects on Oocyte Maturation

The oocyte remains quiescent until the follicle begins to mature. It then increases about tenfold in diameter by the time the follicle reaches the antrum stage, after which little further growth occurs. The oocyte achieves this nearly 1,000-fold increase in mass even though it has no direct blood supply, and hence, it must rely on the granulosa cells to help provide the required nutrients. The granulosa cells may prevent the oocyte from completing its meiotic division until the time of ovulation. Granulosa cells are thought to secrete a substance called oocyte maturation inhibitor into the follicular fluid. LH may trigger the resumption of meiosis at the time of ovulation by blocking the production of this factor.

Effects on Corpus Luteal Function

The maintenance of steroid production by the corpus luteum depends on continued stimulation with LH. Decreased production of progesterone and premature demise of the corpus luteum is seen in women whose secretion of LH is blocked pharmaco-logically. In this respect, LH is said to be *luteotropic*. The corpus luteum has a finite life span, however, and about 1 week after ovulation, it becomes progressively less sensitive to LH and, finally, regresses, despite continued stimulation with LH. Estradiol and prostaglandin $F_{2\alpha}$, which are produced by the corpus luteum, can hasten luteolysis and may be responsible for its demise. We do not understand the mechanisms that limit the functional life span of the human corpus luteum.

Effects on Ovarian Blood Flow

Luteinizing hormone increases blood flow to the ovary and produces ovarian hyperemia. This effect may be secondary to the release of histamine or, perhaps, prostaglandins. Increased ovarian blood flow increases the opportunity for delivery of steroid hormones to the general circulation and for delivery to the ovary of low density lipoproteins containing cholesterol precursors of steroidogenesis. Increased blood flow may also be important for preovulatory swelling of the follicle, which depends on increased elaboration of follicular liquor from plasma.

PHYSIOLOGICAL ACTIONS OF OVARIAN STEROID HORMONES

Production of ovarian steroid hormones is intimately connected to production of the ovum and formation of the corpus luteum. In general, the extraovarian actions of these hormones ensure that the ovum reaches its potential to develop into a new individual. The ovarian steroids act on the reproductive tract to prepare it for fulfilling its role in fertilization, implantation, and development of the embryo, and they induce changes elsewhere that equip a woman physically and behaviorally to conceive, give birth, and rear the child. Although estrogens, perhaps in concert with progesterone, drive females of subprimate species to mate, androgens, rather than estrogens, are responsible for libido in humans of either sex.

Estrogens and progesterone tend to act in concert and sometimes enhance or antagonize each other's actions. Estrogen secretion usually precedes progesterone secretion and primes the target tissues to respond to progesterone. Estrogens induce the synthesis of progesterone receptors, and without them, progesterone has little biological effect. Conversely, progesterone accelerates the turnover of estrogen receptors in some tissues and, thereby, decreases responses to estrogens.

Effects on the Reproductive Tract

At puberty, estrogens promote growth and development of the oviducts, uterus, vagina, and external genitalia. Estrogens stimulate cellular proliferation in the mucosal linings as well as in the muscular coats of these structures. Even after they have matured, maintenance of the size and function of internal reproductive organs

TABLE 1. *Effects of estrogen and progesterone on the reproductive tract*

Organ	Estrogen	Progesterone
Oviducts		
Lining	↑Cilia formation and activity	↑Secretion
Muscular wall	↑Contractility	↓Contractility
Uterus		
Endometrium	↑Proliferation	↑Differentiation and secretion
Myometrium	↑Growth and contractility	↓Contractility
Cervical glands	Watery secretion	Dense, viscous secretion
Vagina	↑Epithelial proliferation	↑Differentiation
	↑Glycogen deposition	↓Proliferation

requires continued stimulation by estrogen and progesterone. Prolonged deprivation after ovariectomy results in severe involution of both the muscular and mucosal portions. Dramatic changes are also evident, especially in the mucosal linings of these structures, as steroid hormones wax and wane during the reproductive cycle. These effects of estrogen and progesterone are summarized in Table 1.

Menstruation

Nowhere are the effects of estrogen and progesterone more obvious than in the endometrium. Estrogens secreted by developing follicles increase the thickness of the endometrium by stimulating growth of epithelial cells in terms of both number and height. Endometrial glands form and elongate. Endometrial growth is accompanied by increased blood flow, especially through the spiral arteries, which grow rapidly under the influence of estrogens. This stage of the uterine cycle is known as the *proliferative phase* and coincides with the follicular phase of the ovarian cycle. Progesterone secreted by the corpus luteum causes the newly proliferated endometrial lining to differentiate and become secretory. This action is consistent with its role of preparing the uterus for nurture and implantation of the newly fertilized ovum if successful mating has occurred. The so-called uterine milk secreted by the endometrium is thought to nourish the blastocyst until it can implant. This portion of the uterine cycle is called the *secretory phase* and coincides with the luteal phase of the ovarian cycle (Fig. 8).

Maintaining the thickened endometrium depends on the continued presence of the ovarian steroid hormones. After the regressing corpus luteum loses its ability to produce adequate amounts of estradiol and progesterone, the outer portion of the endometrium degenerates and is sloughed into the uterine cavity. The mechanism for shedding the uterine lining is incompletely understood, although prostaglandins may play an important role, perhaps in producing vascular spasm and ischemia. Loss of the proliferated endometrium is accompanied by bleeding. This monthly vaginal discharge of blood is known as *menstruation*. The typical menstrual period lasts 3 to 5 days, and the total flow of blood seldom exceeds 50 ml. The first

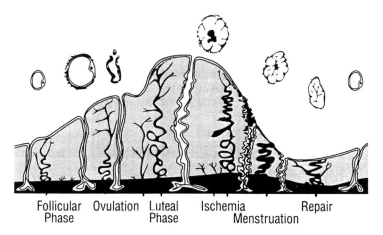

Follicular   Ovulation   Luteal   Ischemia   Repair
  Phase   Phase   Menstruation

FIG. 8. Endometrial changes during a typical menstrual cycle. Simultaneous events in the ovary are also indicated. The endometrium thickens during the follicular phase. Uterine glands elongate, and the spiral arteries grow to supply the thickened endometrium. During the early luteal phase, there is further thickening of the endometrium, marked growth of the coiled arteries, and increased complexity of the uterine glands. As the corpus luteum wanes, the endometrial thickness is reduced by loss of ground substance. Increased coiling of the spiral arteries causes ischemia and finally sloughing of the endometrium. From Bartelmez, G.W. (1957): The phases of the menstrual cycle and their interpretation in terms of the pregnancy cycle. *Am. J. Obstet. Gynecol.*, 74:931.

menstrual bleeding, called *menarche*, usually occurs at about 13 years of age. Menstruation continues at monthly intervals until late in the fifth decade, normally interrupted only by periods of pregnancy.

In the myometrium, estrogen increases contractile proteins and spontaneous muscular activity. In its absence, uterine muscle is insensitive to stretch or other stimuli for contraction. Further estrogen increases the irritability of uterine smooth muscle and, in particular, increases its sensitivity to oxytocin, in part as a consequence of inducing uterine receptors for oxytocin (see Chapter 13). The latter phenomenon may be of significance during parturition. Progesterone counteracts these effects and decreases both the amplitude and frequency of spontaneous contractions. Withdrawal of progesterone prior to menstruation is accompanied by increased myometrial prostaglandin formation. Myometrial contractions in response to prostaglandins are thought to account for the discomfort that precedes menstruation.

Effects on the Mammary Glands

Development of the breasts begins early in puberty and is due primarily to estrogen, which promotes the development of the duct system and the growth and pigmentation of the nipples and areolar portions of the breast. In cooperation with progesterone, estrogen may also increase the lobuloalveolar portions of the glands, but alveolar development also requires the pituitary hormone prolactin (see Chapter 13). Secretory components, however, account for only about 20% of the mass of the adult breast. The remainder is stromal tissue and fat. Estrogen also stimulates stromal proliferation and fat deposition. Responsiveness of all these tissue elements to the growth-promoting effects of estrogen is of significance in neoplastic breast disease. Some forms of breast cancer remain partially or completely dependent on estrogen for growth. Removal of the ovaries or treatment with estrogen antagonists may therefore have life-prolonging benefits in patients afflicted with such tumors.

Other Effects of Ovarian Hormones

Estrogen also acts on the rest of the body in ways that are less directly related to reproduction. As already indicated (see Chapter 10), it contributes to the pubertal growth spurt and stimulates epiphyseal closure. It can cause selective changes in bone structure, especially widening of the pelvis, which facilitates passage of the infant through the birth canal. It promotes deposition of subcutaneous fat and increases hepatic synthesis of steroid- and thyroid hormone-binding proteins. It also acts on the central nervous system and is responsible for some behavioral patterns, especially in lower animals.

Progesterone has a mild thermogenic effect and may increase basal body temperature by as much as 1°F. Because the appearance of progesterone indicates the presence of a corpus luteum, a woman can readily determine when ovulation has occurred and, hence, the time of maximum fertility, by monitoring her temperature daily. This simple, noninvasive procedure has been helpful for couples seeking to conceive a child or who are practicing the ''rhythm method'' of contraception. Progesterone also acts on the central nervous system and may produce changes in behavior or mood. It is curious that more dramatic effects may result from the withdrawal of progesterone than from administering it. Thus, withdrawal of progesterone may trigger menstruation, lactation, parturition, and the postpartum psychic depression experienced by many women.

Mechanism of Action

Estrogens and progesterone, like other steroid hormones, readily penetrate cell membranes and bind firmly to intranuclear receptors, which upon activation, bind to hormone response elements in the vicinity of promoter regions in target genes (see Chapter 1). The resulting synthesis of new ribosomal and messenger ribonucleic acid (RNA) is followed, in turn, by the formation of a variety of proteins that modify cellular activity. Because estrogens promote growth of most target tissues, it is likely that estrogens turn on genes that regulate cellular proliferation, including IGF-I

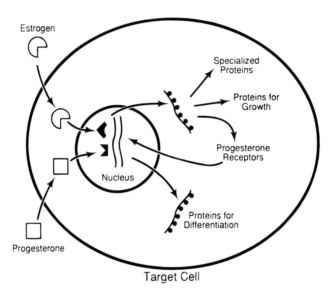

Estrogen

Specialized
Proteins

Proteins for
Growth

Progesterone
Receptors

Nucleus

Proteins for
Differentiation

Progesterone

Target Cell

FIG. 9. The actions of estradiol and progesterone. Estradiol and progesterone diffuse into target cells and bind to intracellular receptors. Interaction with the hormone transforms the receptor so that the hormone–receptor complex binds to DNA and induces the formation of RNA. The induced proteins express the hormone's effects.

(Chapter 10). In some tissues, induced proteins are receptors for other hormones, including progesterone, oxytocin, and LH (Fig. 9).

REGULATION OF THE REPRODUCTIVE CYCLE

The central event of each ovarian cycle is ovulation, which is triggered by a massive increase in LH concentration. This surge of LH secretion must be timed to occur when the ovum and its follicle are ready. The corpus luteum must secrete its hormones to optimize the opportunity for fertilization and establishment of pregnancy. The period after ovulation during which the ovum can be fertilized is brief and lasts only about 24 hours. If fertilization does not occur, a new follicle must be prepared. Coordination of these events requires two-way communication between the pituitary and the ovaries and between the ovaries and the reproductive tract. Let us examine the changing pattern of hormones in blood throughout the ovarian cycle to gain some insight into these communications.

Pattern of Hormones in Blood During Ovarian Cycle

Figure 10 illustrates daily changes in the concentrations of major hormones in a typical cycle extending from one menstrual period to the next. The only remarkable

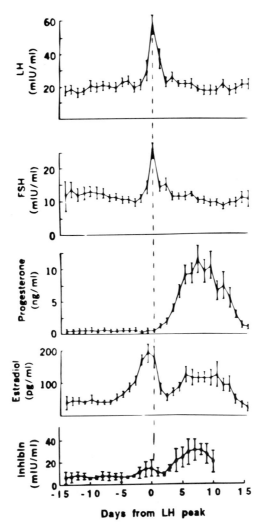

FIG. 10. The mean values of LH, FSH, progesterone, estradiol, and inhibin in daily serum samples of women during ovulatory menstrual cycles. Data from various cycles are combined, using the midcycle peak of LH as the reference point (day 0). *Vertical bars* indicate the standard error of mean. Redrawn from Thorneycroft, I.H., Mishell, D.R., Stone, S.C., et al. (1971): The revelation of serum 17-hydroxyprogesterone and estradiol-17 β levels during the human menstrual cycle. *Am. J. Obstet. Gynecol.*, 111:947; and McLachlan, R. I., Robertson, D.M., Healy, D.L., et al. (1987): Circulating immunoreactive inhibin levels during the normal human menstrual cycle. *J. Clin. Endocrinol. Metab.*, 65:954.

feature of the profile of gonadotropin concentrations is the dramatic peak in LH and FSH that precedes ovulation. Except for the 2 to 3 days of the midcycle peak, LH concentrations remain at nearly constant low levels throughout the follicular and luteal phases. The concentration of FSH is also low during both phases of the cycle, but some fluctuation is evident. The level of FSH tends to be higher early in the follicular phase and diminishes as ovulation approaches. Blood levels of FSH remain low throughout most of the luteal phase but begin to rise 1 or 2 days before the onset of menstruation, suggesting that the next ovarian cycle may begin before the previous uterine cycle has come to an end.

The ovarian hormones follow a different pattern. Early in the follicular phase, the concentration of estradiol is low. It then gradually increases at an increasing rate until it reaches its zenith about 12 hours before the peak in LH. Thereafter, estradiol levels fall abruptly and reach a nadir just after the LH peak. During the luteal phase, there is a secondary rise in estradiol concentration, which then falls to the early follicular level a few days before the onset of menstruation. Progesterone is barely or not at all detectable throughout most of the follicular phase and then begins to rise along with LH at the onset of the ovulatory peak. Progesterone continues to rise and reaches its maximum concentration several days after the LH peak has ended. Progesterone levels remain high for about 7 days and, then, gradually fall and reach almost undetectable levels 1 to 2 days before the onset of menstruation. Inhibin concentrations are low early in the follicular phase and then rise and fall in parallel with those of estradiol. They reach their highest levels in the luteal phase before declining along with progesterone.

Regulation of FSH and LH Secretion

At first glance, this pattern of hormone concentrations is unlike anything seen for other anterior pituitary hormones and the secretions of their target glands. Indeed, there are unique aspects, but during most of the cycle, gonadotropin secretion is under negative feedback control similar to that seen for thyroid-stimulating hormone (Chapter 3), corticotropin (Chapter 4), and the gonadotropins in men. The ovulatory burst of FSH and LH secretion is brought about by a positive feedback mechanism unlike any we have considered. In addition (see Chapter 11), the secretion of FSH and LH is also controlled by GnRH, which is secreted in synchronized pulsatile bursts by neurons whose cell bodies reside in the arcuate nuclei and the medial preoptic area of the hypothalamus.

Negative Feedback Aspects

As we have seen, FSH and LH stimulate the production of ovarian hormones (Fig. 11, follicular phase). Conversely, in the absence of ovarian hormones after ovariectomy or menopause, concentrations of FSH and LH in blood may increase as much as five- to tenfold. Treatment with low doses of estrogen lowers circulating

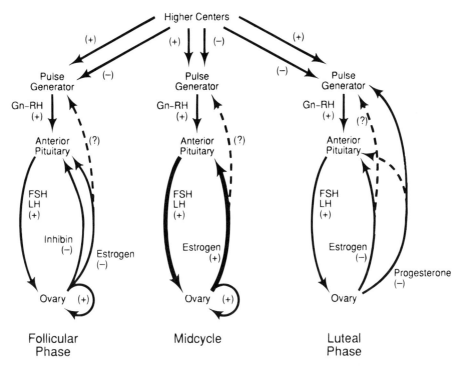

FIG. 11. Ovarian–pituitary interactions at various phases of the menstrual cycle. +, stimulation; −, inhibition. *Dashed arrows* indicate possible direct effects that have not been experimentally established. The thickness of the *arrows* indicates the intensity of stimulation.

concentrations of gonadotropins to levels seen during the follicular phase. When low doses of estradiol are given to subjects whose ovaries are intact, inhibition of gonadotropin secretion can produce failure of follicular development. Progesterone alone, unlike estrogen, is ineffective in lowering high levels of FSH and LH in the blood of postmenopausal women, but it can synergize with estrogen to suppress gonadotropin secretion. This exemplifies classic negative feedback. Inhibin may also provide some feedback inhibition of FSH secretion during the follicular phase, and may contribute the low level of FSH during the luteal phase. However, its effects are probably small. In ovariectomized rhesus monkeys, the pattern of gonadotropin concentrations can be reproduced by treating with only estradiol and progesterone. The rise in FSH concentration, which presumably initiates the next ovarian cycle, follows the fall in estrogen, progesterone, and inhibin at the end of the luteal phase. Throughout the follicular and luteal phases of the cycle, steroid concentrations appear to be sufficient to suppress LH.

Although the ovarian steroids and inhibin suppress FSH and LH secretion, their concentrations change during the cycle in ways that seem independent of gonadotropin concentrations. For example, estrogen rises dramatically as the follicular phase progresses, even though LH remains constant and FSH is diminishing. The mechanism is implicit in what has already been presented and is consistent with negative feedback. Estrogen production by the maturing follicle increases without a preceding increase in the gonadotropin concentration because the mass of responsive theca and granulosa cells increases. In fact, the decrease in FSH during the transition from early to late follicular phase probably results from feedback inhibition by the increasing concentration of estrogen, perhaps in conjunction with inhibin. Although luteinizing cells no longer divide, progesterone and estrogen concentrations continue to increase during the early luteal phase, well after FSH and LH have returned to basal levels. Increasing steroid hormone production at this time reflects completion of the luteinization process. Conversely, the gradual loss of sensitivity of luteal cells to LH accounts for the decrease in progesterone and estrogen secretion during the latter part of the luteal phase. Thus, one of the unique features of the female reproductive cycle is that changes in steroid hormone production result more from changes in the number or sensitivity of competent target cells than from changes in gonadotropin concentrations.

Positive Feedback Aspects

Rising estrogen levels in the late follicular phase trigger the massive burst of LH secretion that just precedes ovulation. This LH surge can be duplicated experimentally in monkeys and women given sufficient estrogen to raise their blood levels above a critical threshold level for 2 to 3 days. This compelling evidence implicates increased estrogen secretion by the ripening follicle as the causal event that triggers the massive release of LH and FSH from the pituitary (Fig. 11, midcycle)). It can be considered positive feedback because LH stimulates estrogen secretion, which in turn, stimulates more LH secretion in a self-generating explosive pattern.

Progesterone concentrations begin to rise somewhat before ovulation. This change is probably a response to the increase in LH rather than its cause. It is significant that large doses of progesterone given experimentally block the estrogen-induced surge of LH in women, which may account for the absence of repeated LH surges during the luteal phase, when the concentrations of estrogen might be high enough to trigger the positive feedback effect (Fig. 11, luteal phase). This action of progesterone contributes to its effectiveness as an oral contraceptive agent. In this regard, progesterone also inhibits follicular growth.

Neural Control of Gonadotropin Secretion

It is clear that secretion of gonadotropins is influenced to a large measure by ovarian steroid hormones. It is equally clear that secretion of these pituitary hormones is controlled by the central nervous system. Gonadotropin secretion ceases after the vascular connection between the anterior pituitary gland and the hypothalamus is interrupted or after the arcuate nuclei of the medial basal hypothalamus are destroyed.

Less drastic environmental inputs, including rapid travel across time zones, stress, anxiety, and other emotional changes, can also affect reproductive function in women, presumably through neural input to the medial basal hypothalamus. As we discussed in Chapter 11, the secretion of gonadotropins requires the operation of a hypothalamic pulse generator that produces intermittent stimulation of the pituitary gland by GnRH.

Sites of Feedback Control

The ovarian steroids might produce their positive or negative feedback effects by acting at the level of the hypothalamus or the anterior pituitary gland or both. The GnRH pulse generator in the medial basal hypothalamus drives gonadotropin secretion, regardless of whether negative or positive feedback prevails. Gonadotropin secretion falls to zero after bilateral destruction of the arcuate nuclei in rhesus monkeys and cannot be increased by either ovariectomy or treatment with the same amount of estradiol that evokes a surge of FSH and LH in normal animals. When such animals are fitted with a pump that delivers a constant amount of GnRH in brief pulses every hour, the normal cyclic pattern of gonadotropin is restored, and the animals ovulate each month. Identical results have been obtained in women suffering from Kallman's syndrome, in which there is a deficiency in GnRH production by the hypothalamus (Fig. 12). In both cases, administration of GnRH in pulses of constant amplitude and frequency was sufficient to produce ovulatory cycles. Because both positive and negative feedback aspects of gonadotropin secretion can be produced even when hypothalamic input is "clamped" at constant frequency and amplitude, these effects of estradiol must be exerted at the level of the pituitary.

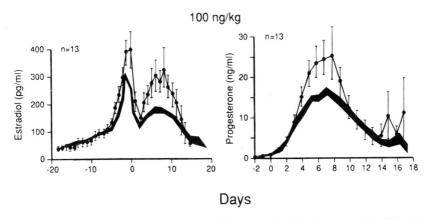

FIG. 12. The results of ovulation induction employing a physiological frequency of GnRH administration to hypogonadotropic hypogonadal women upon ovarian steroid secretion. The normal values are represented by the *shaded areas.* From Crowley, W.F., Jr., Filicori, M., Spratt, D.I., et al. (1985): The physiology of gonadotropin-releasing hormone (GnRH) secretion in men and women. *Recent Prog. Horm. Res.*, 41:473.

Although changes in amplitude and frequency of GnRH pulses are not necessary for the normal pattern of gonadotropin secretion during an experimental or therapeutic regimen, variations nevertheless occur physiologically. During the normal reproductive cycle, GnRH pulses are less frequent in the luteal phase than in the follicular phase. Estradiol may decrease the amplitude of GnRH pulses, and progesterone slows their frequency, perhaps by stimulating hypothalamic production of endogenous opioids. It is possible that an increase in GnRH precedes the LH surge, and there is good evidence that progesterone acts at the level of the hypothalamus to block the estradiol-induced LH surge. Thus, feedback effects of estradiol appear to be exerted primarily, but not exclusively, on the pituitary, and those of progesterone primarily, but probably not exclusively, on the hypothalamus.

We do not yet understand the intrapituitary mechanisms responsible for the negative and positive feedback effects of estradiol. As seen with the ovary, changes in hormone secretion may be brought about by changes in the sensitivity of target cells, as well as by changes in concentration of a stimulatory hormone. In the case of the pituitary, increases or decreases in sensitivity to GnRH are not accompanied by changes in either the number of gonadotropes or the number of receptors for GnRH. Nevertheless, women and experimental animals are more responsive to a test dose of GnRH at midcycle than at any other time.

Timing of Reproductive Cycles

Although the pacemaker for rhythmic release of GnRH resides in the hypothalamus, the timekeeper for the slower monthly rhythm of the ovarian cycle resides in the ovary. As already indicated, the corpus luteum has a built-in life span of about 12 days and involutes despite continued stimulation with LH. A new generation of follicles cannot arise so long as the corpus luteum remains functional. Its demise appears to relieve inhibition of follicular growth and FSH secretion, which increases sufficiently in blood to stimulate growth of the next cohort of follicles. Thus, the interval between the LH surge and the emergence of the new cohort of follicles is determined by the ovary. The principal event around which the menstrual cycle revolves is ovulation, which depends on an ovulatory surge of LH. The length of the follicular phase may be somewhat variable and may be influenced by extraovarian events, but the timing of the LH surge resides in the ovary. It is only when the developing follicle signals its readiness to ovulate with increasing blood levels of estradiol that the pituitary secretes the ovulatory spike of gonadotropin. Hence, throughout the cycle, it is the ovary that notifies the pituitary and hypothalamus of its readiness to proceed to the next stage.

The beginning and end of cyclic ovarian activity, called menarche and menopause, occur on a longer time scale. We considered the events associated with the onset of puberty in Chapter 11. Although we still do not know what biological phenomena signal readiness for reproductive development and the end of the juvenile period, it appears that the timekeeper for this process resides in the central nervous system, which initiates sexual development and function by activating the GnRH pulse generator. The termination of cyclic ovarian activity coincides with the disappearance or exhaustion of primordial follicles.

SUGGESTED READING

Ackland, J. F., Schwartz, N. B., Mayo, K. E., and Dodson, R. E. (1992): Nonsteroidal signals originating in the gonads. *Physiol. Rev.*, 72:731–788.

di Zerega, G. S., and Hodgen, G. D. (1981): Folliculogenesis in the primate ovarian cycle. *Endocr. Rev.*, 2:27–49.

Dorrington, J. H., and Armstrong, D. T. (1979): Effects of FSH on gonadal function. *Recent Prog. Horm. Res.*, 35:301–332.

Giudice, L. C. (1992): Insulin-like growth factors and ovarian follicular development. *Endocr. Rev.*, 13: 641–669.

Hsueh, A. J. W., Adashi, E. Y., Jones, P. B. C., and Welsh, T. H., Jr. (1984): Hormonal regulation of the differentiation of cultured ovarian granulosa cells. *Endocr. Rev.*, 5:76–127.

Knobil, E., and Hotchkiss, J. (1988): The menstrual cycle and its neuroendocrine control. In: *The Physiology of Reproduction*, edited by Knobil, E., and Neill, J. D. pp. 1971–1994, Raven Press, New York.

Marshall, J. C., Dalkin, A. C., Haisleder, D. J., Paul, S. J., Ortolano, G. A., and Kelch, R. P. (1991): Gonadotropin-releasing hormone pulses: regulators of gonadotropin synthesis and ovarian cycles. *Recent Prog. Horm. Res.*, 47:155–187.

Richards, J. S., Jahnsen, T., Hedin, L., Lifka, J., Ratoosh, S., Durica, J. M., and Goldring, N. B. (1987): Ovarian follicular development: from physiology to molecular biology. *Recent Prog. Horm. Res.*, 43: 231–270.

13

Hormonal Control of Reproduction in the Female

II. Pregnancy and Lactation

OVERVIEW

Successful reproduction depends, not only on the union of eggs and sperm, but also on survival of adequate numbers of the new generation to reach reproductive age and begin the cycle again. In some species, parental involvement in the reproductive process ends with fertilization of the ova; thousands or even millions of embryos may result from a single mating, with just a few surviving long enough to procreate. Higher mammals, particularly humans, have adopted the alternative strategy of producing only few or a single fertilized ovum at a time. Prolonged parental care during the embryonic and neonatal periods substitutes for huge numbers of unattended offspring as the means for increasing the likelihood of survival. Estrogen and, especially, progesterone prepare the maternal body for successful internal fertilization and hospitable acceptance of the embryo. The conceptus then takes charge. After lodging firmly within the uterine lining and gaining access to the maternal circulation, it secretes protein and steroid hormones that ensure continued maternal acceptance, and it directs maternal functions to provide for its development. Simultaneously, the conceptus withdraws whatever nutrients it needs from the maternal circulation. At the appropriate time, the fetus signals its readiness to depart the uterus and initiates the birth process. While *in utero*, placental hormones prepare the mammary glands to produce the milk needed for nurture after birth. Finally, suckling stimulates continued milk production.

FERTILIZATION AND IMPLANTATION

Gamete Transport

Fertilization takes place in a distal portion of the oviduct called the ampulla, far from the site of sperm deposition in the vagina. To reach the ovum, sperm must

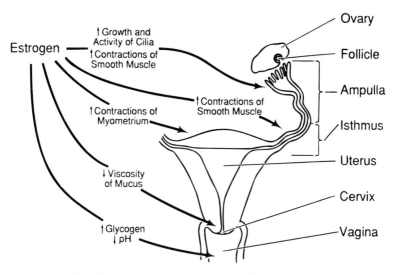

FIG. 1. The actions of estrogen to promote sperm transport.

swim through the cervical canal, cross the entire length of the uterine cavity, and then travel up through the muscular isthmus of the oviduct. Even with the aid of contractions of the female reproductive tract, the journey is formidable, and only about one of every million sperm deposited in the vagina reach the ampulla. Here, if they arrive first, they await the arrival of the ovum. Sperm usually remain fertile within the female reproductive tract for 1 to 2 days, but as long as 4 days is possible. Access to the upper reaches of the reproductive tract is heavily influenced by ovarian steroid hormones.

Estrogen is secreted in abundance late in the follicular phase of the ovarian cycle and prepares the reproductive tract for efficient sperm transport (Fig. 1). Glycogen deposited in the vaginal mucosa under its influence provides substrate for the production of lactate, which lowers the pH of vaginal fluid. An acidic environment increases the motility of sperm, which is essential for their passage through the cervical canal. In addition, the copious watery secretion produced by cells lining the cervical canal under the influence of estrogen increases access to the uterine cavity. When estrogen is absent or when its effects are opposed by progesterone, the cervical canal is filled with a viscous fluid that resists sperm penetration. Vigorous contractions of the uterus propel the sperm toward the oviducts, where they may appear anywhere from 5 to 60 minutes after ejaculation. Prostaglandins present in seminal plasma and oxytocin released from the pituitary in response to intercourse may stimulate contraction of the highly responsive estrogen-dominated myometrium.

Role of the Oviducts

The oviducts are uniquely adapted for facilitating the transport of sperm toward the ovary and transporting the ovum in the opposite direction toward its rendezvous with the sperm. It is also within the oviducts that sperm undergo a process called *capacitation*, which enables them to penetrate the ovum. Capacitation involves both enhancement of flagellar activity and dissolution of acrosomal membranes which permits the release of enzymes needed for the sperm to penetrate the zona pellucida and the adherent rim of cumulus cells. After fertilization, the oviduct retains the embryo for about 3 days and nourishes it with secreted nutrients before facilitating its entry into the uterine cavity. These complex events, orchestrated by the interplay of estrogen, progesterone, and autonomic innervation, require participation of the smooth muscle of the walls as well as secretory and ciliary activity of the epithelial lining. As crucial as these mechanical actions may be, however, the oviduct does not contribute in an indispensable way to fertility of the ovum or sperm or to their union; modern techniques of *in vitro* fertilization bypass it with no ill effects.

Propulsion of sperm through the isthmus toward the ampulla is accomplished largely by muscular contractions of the tubal wall. The circular smooth muscle of the isthmus is innervated with sympathetic fibers and has both α-adrenergic receptors, which mediate contraction, and β-adrenergic receptors, which mediate relaxation. Under the influence of estrogen, the α receptors predominate. Subsequently, as estrogenic effects are opposed by progesterone, the β receptors prevail, and isthmic smooth muscles relax. This reversal in the response to adrenergic stimulation may account for the ability of the oviduct to facilitate sperm transport through the isthmus toward the ovary and, subsequently, to promote passage of the embryo in the opposite direction toward the uterus.

In response to estrogens or perhaps other local signals associated with impending ovulation, muscular activity in the distal portion of the oviduct brings the infundibulum into close contact with the surface of the ovary. At ovulation, the ovum, together with its surrounding granulosa cells, the *cumulus oophorus*, is released into the peritoneal cavity and is swept into the ostium of the oviduct by the vigorous, synchronous beating of cilia on the infundibular surface. Development of cilia in the epithelial lining and their synchronized rhythmic activity are consequences of earlier exposure to estrogens. Movement of the egg mass through the ampulla toward the site of fertilization near the ampullar–isthmic junction depends principally on currents set up in tubal fluid by the beating of cilia and, to a lesser extent, by activity of the ampullar wall to produce a churning motion.

The period of fertility is short; from the time the ovum is shed until it can no longer be fertilized is only about 6 to 24 hours. As soon as a sperm penetrates the ovum, the second polar body is extruded, and the fertilized ovum begins to divide. By the time the fertilized egg reaches the uterine cavity, it has reached the blastocyst stage and consists of about 100 cells. Timing of the arrival of the blastocyst in the uterine cavity is determined by the balance between antagonistic effects of estrogen and progesterone on the contractility of the oviductal wall. Under the influence of estrogen, circularly oriented smooth muscle of the isthmus is contracted and bars passage of the embryo to the uterus. As the corpus luteum organizes and increases its capacity to secrete progesterone, β-adrenergic receptors gain ascendancy, muscles of the isthmus relax, and the embryonic mass is allowed to pass into the uterine cavity. Ovarian steroids can thus "lock" the ovum or embryo in the oviduct or cause its delivery prematurely into the uterine cavity.

Implantation and the Formation of the Placenta

The blastocyst floats freely in the uterine cavity for about 1 day before it implants, normally on about the fifth day after ovulation. Experience with *in vitro* fertilization indicates that there is about a 3-day period of uterine receptivity in which implantation leads to full-term pregnancy. Little can be said of the factors that determine uterine receptivity, except that high concentrations of progesterone, or a high progesterone–estrogen ratio, are essential. It should be recalled that this period of endometrial sensitivity coincides with the period of maximal progesterone output by the corpus luteum (Fig. 2).

At the time of implantation, the blastocyst consists of an inner mass of cells destined to become the fetus and an outer rim of cells called the *trophoblast*. It is

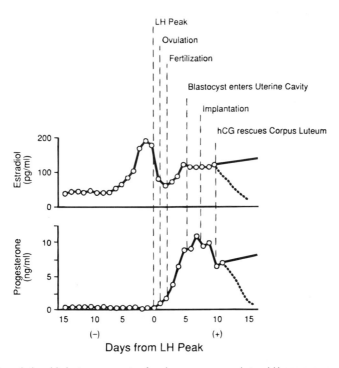

FIG. 2. The relationship between events of early pregnancy and steroid hormone concentrations in maternal blood. The estradiol and progesterone concentrations are redrawn from data given in Fig. 10 of Chapter 12. By the 10th day after the LH peak, there is sufficient hCG to maintain and increase estrogen and progesterone production, which would otherwise decrease (*dotted lines*) at this time.

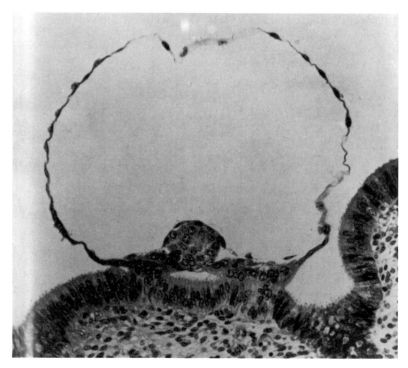

FIG. 3. Early implantation of a 9-day-old embryo of a rhesus monkey. In the two areas where the embryo and the uterus have joined, the trophoblast has begun to invade the endometrium. ×400.

the trophoblast that forms the attachment to maternal tissue and gives rise to the fetal membranes (Fig. 3). After prolonged stimulation with progesterone, endometrial cells accumulate glycogen and differentiate further to become *decidual cells*. The cells of the trophoblast proliferate and form the multinucleated *syncytial trophoblast* whose specialized functions enable it to destroy adjacent decidual cells and allow the blastocyst to penetrate deep into the uterine endothelium. Killed decidual cells are phagocytosed by the trophoblast as the embryo penetrates the subepithelial connective tissue and, eventually, becomes completely enclosed within the endometrium. Products released from degenerating decidual cells produce hyperemia and increased capillary permeability. Local extravasation of blood from damaged capillaries forms small pools of blood that are in direct contact with the trophoblast and provide nourishment to the embryo until the definitive placenta forms. From the time the ovum is shed until the blastocyst implants, metabolic needs are met by secretions of the oviduct and the endometrium.

The syncytial trophoblast and an inner cytotrophoblast layer of cells soon completely surround the inner cell mass and send out solid columns of cells that further erode the endometrium and anchor the embryo. These columns of cells differentiate into the placental villi. As they digest the endometrium, pools of extravasated maternal blood become more extensive and fuse into a complex labyrinth that drains into venous sinuses in the endometrium. These pools expand and, eventually, receive an abundant supply of arterial blood. By the third week, the villi are invaded by fetal blood vessels as the primitive circulatory system begins to function. As the placenta matures, the trophoblastic tissue thins, reducing the barrier to diffusion between maternal and fetal blood. The syncytial trophoblast takes on specialized functions of hormone production and active bidirectional transport of nutrients and metabolites (Fig. 4).

Although much uncertainty remains regarding the details of implantation in humans, it is perfectly clear that progesterone secreted by the ovary at the height of luteal function is indispensable for all of these events to occur. Removal of the corpus luteum at this time or blockade of progesterone secretion or activity prevents implantation. Progesterone is indispensable for maintenance of decidual cells, quiescence of the myometrium, and the formation of the dense, viscous cervical mucus that essentially seals off the uterine cavity from the outside. An interesting but still unresolved question is why the maternal immune system does not reject the implanted embryo as a foreign body. Some information suggests that progesterone may be essential for immunological acceptance of the embryo. The importance of progesterone for implantation is underscored by the development of a progesterone antagonist RU486 (mifepristone) that prevents implantation or causes an already

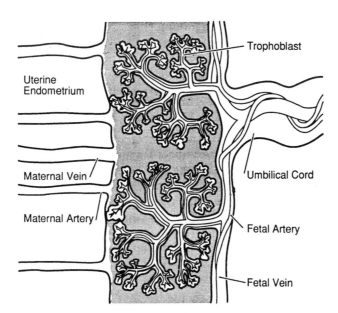

FIG. 4. Placental villae bathed in a lake of maternal blood. From Beer, A.E. and Billingham, R.E. (1974): The embryo as transport. *Sci. Am.*, 230(4):36.

implanted conceptus to be shed along with the uterine lining. Progesterone antagonists may become the next generation of oral contraceptives.

THE PLACENTA

The placenta is a complex, primarily vascular organ adapted to optimize exchange of gases, nutrients, and electrolytes between maternal and fetal circulations. In humans, the placenta is also a major endocrine gland capable of producing large amounts of both protein and steroid hormones. The placenta is the most recently evolved of all mammalian organs, and its endocrine function is highly developed in primates. It is unique among endocrine glands in that, as far as we know, its secretory activity is autonomous and not subject to regulation by maternal or fetal signals. In experimental animals, such as the rat, pregnancy is terminated if the pituitary gland is removed during the first half of gestation or if the ovaries, and consequently the corpora lutea, are removed at any time. In primates, the pituitary gland and ovaries are essential only for a brief period after fertilization. After about 7 weeks, the placenta can produce enough progesterone to maintain pregnancy. In addition, it also produces large amounts of estrogen, human chorionic gonadotropin (hCG), and human chorionic somatomammotropin (hCS), which is also called human placental lactogen (hPL). It can also secrete growth hormone (GH), thyroid-stimulating hormone (TSH), adrenocorticotropic hormone (ACTH), and probably other biologically active peptides. During pregnancy, there is the unique situation of hormones secreted by one individual, the fetus, regulating the physiology of another, the mother. By extracting needed nutrients and adding hormones to the maternal circulation, the placenta redirects some aspects of maternal function to accommodate the growing fetus.

Placental Hormones

hCG

As already discussed (see Chapter 12), the functional life of the corpus luteum during infertile cycles ends by the 12th day after ovulation. About 2 days later, the endometrium is shed, and menstruation begins. For pregnancy to develop, the endometrium must be maintained, and therefore, the ovary must be notified that fertilization has occurred. The signal to the ovary in humans is a luteotropic substance secreted by the conceptus called hCG, which rescues the corpus luteum (i.e., extends its life span) and stimulates it to continue secreting progesterone and estrogen. Continued secretion of these ovarian steroids maintains the endometrium in a state favorable for implantation and placentation (Fig. 5). The ovarian steroids also notify the pituitary gland of the pregnancy and inhibit secretion of the gonadotropin that would otherwise stimulate development of the next cohort of follicles. Pituitary gonadotropins are virtually undetectable in maternal blood during pregnancy.

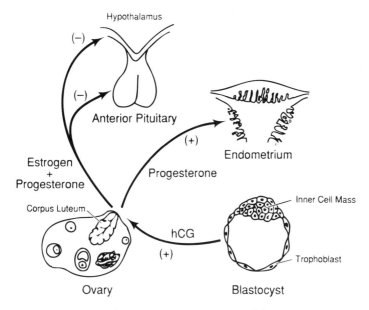

FIG. 5. Maternal responses to hCG.

Trophoblast cells of the developing placenta begin to secrete hCG early, with detectable amounts already present in blood by about the eighth day after ovulation, when luteal function is still at its height. The production of hCG increases dramatically during the early weeks of pregnancy (Fig. 6). Blood levels continue to rise and, during the third month of pregnancy, reach peak values that are perhaps 200 to 1,000 times that of luteinizing hormone (LH) at the height of the ovulatory surge. It is the appearance of hCG in large amounts in urine that is used as a test for pregnancy. Because its biological activity is like that of LH, urine containing hCG induces ovulation in the estrous rabbit in the classic rabbit test. Now, hCG can be measured with a simple sensitive immunological test, and pregnancy can be detected even before the next expected menstrual period.

Secretion of progesterone by the corpus luteum of pregnancy is short lived despite continued stimulation with high concentrations of hCG. Measurements of progesterone levels in human ovarian venous blood indicate that the corpus luteum remains functional throughout most of the first trimester of pregnancy and then involutes. Well before this time, placental production of progesterone is adequate to maintain pregnancy. Production of hCG, however, continues throughout pregnancy, but its role after luteal involution is unknown.

Human chorionic gonadotropin is a glycoprotein that is closely related to the pituitary glycoprotein hormones (see Chapter 2). Like them, it consists of α and β subunits. Although there are wide variations in carbohydrate components, the amino acid sequence of the α subunit is identical to that of α subunits of FSH, LH, and

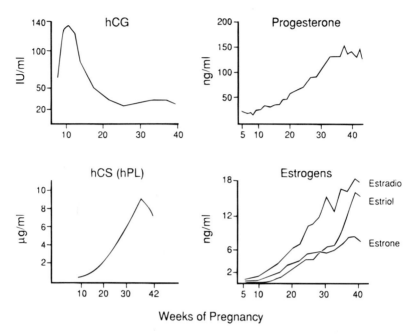

FIG. 6. Changes in plasma levels of "hormones of pregnancy" during normal gestation. From Freinkel, N. and Metzger, B.E. (1992): Metabolic changes in pregnancy. In: *Williams Textbook of Endocrinology*, 8th ed., edited by Wilson, J.D. and Foster, D.W., Saunders, Philadelphia.

TSH, and all are encoded by a single gene. In humans, seven genes or pseudogenes on chromosome 19 code for hCG β, but only two or three of them are expressed. The β subunit of hCG is almost identical to the β subunit of LH, except for a 32-amino acid extension at the carboxy terminus. It is not surprising, therefore, that hCG has LH-like bioactivity. However, hCG contains considerably more carbohydrate than its pituitary counterparts, which accounts for its extraordinary stability in blood. The half-life of hCG is of the order of 30 hours, as compared to just a few minutes for the pituitary glycoprotein hormones. The long half-life facilitates a rapid buildup of adequate concentrations of this vital signal produced by a few vulnerable cells.

hCS

The other placental protein hormone that is secreted in large amounts is hCS. Like hCG, hCS is produced by the syncytial trophoblast and becomes detectable in maternal plasma early in pregnancy. Its concentration in maternal plasma increases steadily from about the third week after fertilization, reaching a plateau by the last month of pregnancy (Fig. 6). The concentration achieved at this time is about 100 times higher than that normally seen for other protein hormones. The placenta produces about 1 g of hCS each day during late pregnancy, a rate far exceeding that for any other hormone in men or women. hCS has a short half-life and, despite its high concentration, is undetectable in plasma after the first postpartum day.

Despite its abundance and its ability to produce a number of biological actions experimentally, the physiological role of hCS has not been established definitively. It has strong prolactin-like activity and can induce lactation in test animals, but lactation normally does not begin until long enough after parturition for hCS to be cleared from maternal blood. It is likely that hCS promotes mammary growth in preparation for lactation. It is also likely that hCS contributes to the availability of nutrients for the developing fetus by operating like GH to mobilize maternal fat and decrease maternal glucose consumption. In this context, hCS may be responsible for the decreased glucose tolerance, the so-called *gestational diabetes*, experienced by many women during pregnancy. Although secretion of hCS is directed predominantly into maternal blood, appreciable concentrations are also found in fetal blood in midpregnancy. Receptors for hCS are present in human fetal fibroblasts and myoblasts, and these cells release insulin-like growth factor II when stimulated by hCS. As already discussed (see Chapter 10), fetal growth is independent of GH, but the role of hCS in this regard is uncertain.

Despite these observations, evidence from genetic studies makes it unlikely that hCS is indispensable for the successful outcome of pregnancy. hCS is a member of the GH–prolactin family (see Chapter 2) and shares large regions of structural homology with both of these pituitary hormones. Five genes of this family are clustered on chromosome 17, including three that encode hCS and two that encode GH. Two of the hCS genes are expressed and code for identical secretory products. The third hCS gene appears to be a pseudogene whose transcription does not produce fully processed messenger ribonucleic acid (RNA). No adverse consequences for pregnancy, parturition, or early postnatal development were seen in three cases in which a stretch of DNA that contains both hCS genes and one hGH gene was missing from both chromosomes. No immunoassayable hCS was present in maternal plasma, but it is possible that the remaining hCS pseudogene was expressed under these circumstances or that recombination of remaining fragments of these genes produced a chimeric protein with hCS-like activity. Regardless of whether or not hCS is indispensable for normal gestation, important functions are often governed by redundant mechanisms, and it is likely that hCS contributes in some way to a successful outcome of pregnancy.

Progesterone and Estrogen

Even while the corpus luteum is still operational, the trophoblast becomes the major producer of progesterone. By the time ovarian production shuts down, placental production of progesterone is substantial. It continues to increase as pregnancy progresses, so that during the final months, upward of 250 mg may be produced per day. This huge amount is more than ten times the daily ovarian production at the height of luteal function, and it may be even greater in women bearing more than one fetus.

The placenta has little capacity to synthesize cholesterol and, therefore, relies almost exclusively on maternal low density lipoproteins for substrate. In late pregnancy, progesterone production consumes an amount of cholesterol equivalent to about 25% of the daily turnover in a normal nonpregnant woman. The rate of progesterone production in the placenta is limited only by the availability of substrate. In contrast, steroidogenesis in the adrenals and gonads is limited by the hormonally dependent conversion of cholesterol to pregnenolone within the mitochondria (Fig. 7). In other words, the reaction step(s) that require(s) activation by tropic hormones through cyclic adenosine monophosphate (AMP)-mediated processes is constitutively active in placental tissue. Virtually all of the cholesterol that is converted to 21-carbon steroids by the placental desmolase reaction is secreted as progesterone.

The human placenta is also a major producer of estrogen, even though it totally lacks 17α-hydroxylase, the enzyme required to convert progesterone or pregnenolone to 19-carbon intermediates. Reminiscent of the interplay between granulosa and thecal cells of the ovary (see Chapter 12), estrogen synthesis by trophoblastic cells depends on receipt of androgen substrate from the maternal or fetal adrenals (Fig. 8), although most of the androgenic substrate originates in the fetal adrenal cortex. The trophoblast has an abundance of aromatase, whose activity is limited only by the availability of substrate. This conversion effectively protects a female fetus from the masculinizing effects of any androgens in the maternal circulation.

Estradiol and estrone are the major estrogens produced by the ovary, but together they account only for about 10% of the estrogens produced by the placenta. One of

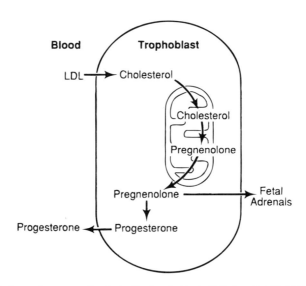

FIG. 7. Progesterone synthesis by the trophoblast. *LDL*, low density lipoproteins.

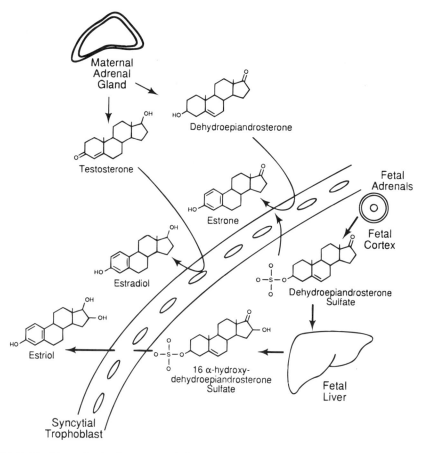

FIG. 8. The biosynthesis of estrogens during pregnancy. Note that androgens formed in either the fetal or maternal adrenals are the precursors for all three estrogens and that the placenta cannot convert progesterone to androgens. The hydroxylation of DHEA at carbon 16 by the fetal liver gives rise to estriol, which therefore originates in the placenta, whereas estrone and estradiol are primarily maternal in origin. The thickness of the *arrows* implies quantitative importance.

the placental estrogens is *estriol*, which is seen in significant amounts only during pregnancy. Estriol is a product of the combined activities of the fetal adrenal, fetal liver, and placenta (Fig. 8), and its rate of production is often used as an indicator of fetal well-being. The cortex of the fetal adrenal gland consists of an outer region (which will become the glomerulosa, fasciculata, and reticularis of the adult, see Chapter 4) and a huge, inner "fetal zone." The fetal adrenals during midpregnancy are large—larger, in fact, than the kidneys—and the fetal zone constitutes 80% of the adrenal mass. The chief product of the fetal zone is the weak androgen dehydro-epiandrosterone (DHEA), which is secreted as the inactive sulfate ester. DHEA sulfate is converted in the fetal liver to 16α-DHEA sulfate, which upon aromatization in the placenta becomes estriol. The placenta is rich in sulfatase activity and readily removes the sulfate group prior to aromatization. Any DHEA sulfate that escapes 16α-hydroxylation in the liver is converted to estradiol in the placenta.

Production of placental estrogens and progesterone is driven by the fetal pituitary gland through the action of ACTH on the fetal zone of the adrenal cortex. Estrogens may increase low density lipoprotein receptors in the placenta and, therefore, increase the availability of the cholesterol precursor needed for biosynthesis of steroid hormones. The physiological importance of large-scale production of 16α-DHEA sulfate to the fetus is not apparent nor is the physiological importance of large-scale production of estriol. Although estriol can bind to estrogen receptors, its estrogenic activity is exceedingly weak. All of the estrogens, including estriol, promote uterine blood flow. It is possible that the fetus uses this elaborate mechanism of estriol production to ensure that uterine blood flow remains adequate for its survival.

PARTURITION

Pregnancy in the human lasts about 40 weeks. The process of birth, or *parturition*, involves expulsion of the fetus at the end of pregnancy and is the culmination of all the processes discussed in this and the previous two chapters. It is therefore most unsatisfying that we do not yet understand the events that bring about this climactic event in reproductive physiology. In theory, the signal to terminate pregnancy could originate with either the mother or the fetus, but despite the paucity of supporting evidence, many investigators favor the idea that the fetus, which has essentially controlled events during the rest of pregnancy, somehow signals its readiness to be born. This idea appears to be valid for sheep, the only species for which reasonably solid information is available. The triggering event for parturition in sheep is an ACTH-dependent increase in cortisol production by the fetal adrenals. In this species, cortisol increases the activity of 17α-hydroxylase in the placenta and, therefore, shifts the production of steroids away from progesterone and toward estrogen. As already indicated, progesterone causes relaxation of the uterine musculature and suppresses spontaneous contractions of the myometrium. An increased estrogen–progesterone ratio favors the production of prostaglandins $F_{2\alpha}$ and E_2, which in turn, promote the formation of gap junctions between myometrial cells and softening of the uterine cervix just prior to parturition. These agents may also be the immediate instigators of uterine contractions.

Although it seems reasonable that an event as fundamental as the initiation of parturition would be regulated in the same stereotyped way in all species, it is clearly not the case. The human fetus does not signal its readiness to be born by increasing its production of cortisol, which in any event would be of little use because the human placenta lacks 17α-hydroxylase. There is no evidence for increased production of DHEA as an alternate way of increasing placental production of estrogen. It is possible that some other signal for parturition in humans originates within the uterus, but progress in understanding is slow because fundamental differences, even among closely related species, make it difficult to draw inferences from animal experiments.

Few, if any, answers have been forthcoming from studies of maternal blood constituents. Progesterone concentrations are high and do not change at the onset of labor, and hence, withdrawal of its inhibitory effects on myometrial contraction cannot be the precipitating event. This finding is consistent with clinical observations that parturition cannot be delayed by administration of progesterone. Similarly, in humans, unlike ruminants, blood estrogens are not increased at this time. However, a localized change in the concentration of estrogens or progesterone in some part of the interface between the placenta and the myometrium may not be reflected in changes in blood levels of these hormones. Along these same lines, it has been suggested that local production of cytokines, prostaglandins, and even oxytocin might initiate parturition.

Role of Oxytocin

Oxytocin is a neurohormone secreted by nerve endings in the posterior lobe of the pituitary gland in response to neural stimuli received by cell bodies in the paraventricular and supraoptic nuclei of the hypothalamus. It produces powerful synchronized contractions of the myometrium at the end of pregnancy, when uterine muscle is highly sensitive to it. Oxytocin is sometimes used clinically to induce labor. As parturition approaches, responsiveness to oxytocin increases in parallel with increases in oxytocin receptors in both the endometrium and myometrium. It is unlikely that oxytocin is the physiological trigger for parturition, however, because its concentration in maternal blood normally does not increase until after labor has begun. Oxytocin is secreted in response to stretching of the uterine cervix and hastens expulsion of the fetus and the placenta (see Chapter 1), but probably, it plays little role in the earlier stages of labor. As a consequence of its action on myometrial contraction, oxytocin protects against hemorrhage after expulsion of the placenta. Just prior to delivery, the uterus receives 10% of the cardiac output, most of which flows through the low resistance pathways of the maternal portion of the placenta. Intense contraction of the newly emptied uterus acts as a natural tourniquet to control the loss of blood from the massive wound left when the placenta is torn away from the uterine lining.

LACTATION

The mammary glands are specialized secretory structures derived from the skin. As the name implies, they are unique to mammals. The secretory portion of the mammary glands is arranged in lobules consisting of branched tubules, the *lobuloal-*

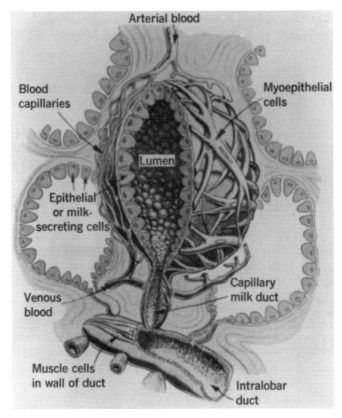

FIG. 9. Mammary alveolus consisting of milk-producing cells surrounded by a meshwork of contractile myoepithelial cells. The milk-producing cells are the targets for prolactin, while the myoepithelial cells are the targets for oxytocin. From Turner, C.W. (1969): *Harvesting your Milk Crop*, p. 17. Babson Bros., Oak Brook, IL.

veolar ducts, from which multiple evaginations or *alveoli* emerge (Fig. 9). The alveoli consist of a single layer of secretory epithelial cells surrounded by a meshwork of contractile *myoepithelial cells*. Many lobuloalveolar ducts converge to form a *lactiferous duct*, which carries the milk to the nipple. A mammary gland consists of perhaps 20 lobules, each with its own lactiferous duct opening separately to the outside. In the inactive, nonlactating gland, alveoli are present only in rudimentary form, with the entire glandular portion consisting almost exclusively of lobuloalveolar ducts. The mammary glands have an abundant vascular supply and are innervated with sympathetic nerve fibers and a rich supply of sensory fibers to the nipple and areola.

Milk secreted by the mammary glands provides nourishment and immunoglobulins to the offspring during the immediate postnatal period and for varying times thereafter, depending on culture and custom. Milk provides all of the basic nourishment, vitamins, minerals, fats, carbohydrates, and proteins needed by the infant until the teeth erupt. The extraordinarily versatile cells of the mammary alveoli simultaneously synthesize large amounts of protein, fat, and lactose and secrete these constituents by different mechanisms, along with a large volume of aqueous medium whose ionic composition differs substantially from blood plasma. Human milk consists of about 1% protein, principally in the form casein and lactalbumin, about 4% fat, and about 7% lactose. Each liter of milk also contains about 500 mg of calcium. After lactation is established, the well-nourished woman suckling a single infant may produce about 1 liter of milk per day and as much as 3 liters per day if suckling twins. It should be apparent therefore that, in addition to hormonal regulation at the level of the mammary glands, milk production requires extramammary regulation by all those hormones responsible for compensatory adjustments in intermediary metabolism (see Chapters 6 and 9), calcium balance (see Chapter 8), and salt and water balance (see Chapter 7).

Growth and Development of the Mammary Glands

Prenatal growth and development of the mammary glands appear to be independent of sex hormones and genetic sex. Until the onset of puberty, there are no differences in the male and female breast. With the onset of puberty, the duct system grows and branches under the influence of estrogen. Surrounding stromal and fat tissue also proliferate. Progesterone, in combination with estrogen, promotes growth and branching of the lobuloalveolar tissue, but for these steroids to be effective, prolactin, GH, and cortisol must also be present. Lobuloalveolar growth and regression occur to some degree during each ovarian cycle. There is pronounced growth, differentiation, and proliferation of mammary alveoli during pregnancy, when estrogen and progesterone levels are high and pituitary prolactin and hCS levels are also elevated.

Milk Production

Once the secretory apparatus has developed, production of milk depends primarily on continued episodic stimulation with high concentrations of prolactin, but adrenal glucocorticoids and insulin are also important in a permissive sense that needs to be defined more precisely. All of these hormones and hCS are present in abundance during late stages of pregnancy, yet lactation does not begin until after parturition. High concentrations of estrogen and progesterone in maternal blood inhibit lactation by interfering with the action of prolactin on the mammary epithelium. With parturition, the precipitous fall in estrogen and progesterone levels relieves this inhibition, and prolactin receptors in alveolar epithelium may increase as much as 20-fold. Development of secretory capacity, however, takes some time. Initially, the mammary glands put out only a watery fluid called *colostrum*, which is rich in protein but poor in lactose and fat. It takes more than 1 week for the mammary gland to secrete mature milk with a full complement of nutrients. It is not clear whether this delay reflects a slow acquisition of secretory capacity or a regulated sequence of events timed to coincide with the infant's capacity to utilize nutrients.

Mechanism of Prolactin Action

Prolactin acts directly on the alveolar epithelium and stimulates it to synthesize and secrete milk, but little is known of how it acts at the molecular level. Prolactin binds to receptors on the surface of mammary epithelial cells and induces transcription of genes for milk constituents such as casein. We do not know how prolactin binding to receptors at the surface of the alveolar cell activates gene transcription in the nucleus. The prolactin receptor, which is closely related to the GH receptor, has no structural component that resembles any known signaling mechanism. Like insulin and GH, prolactin does not utilize cyclic AMP as a second messenger.

Neuroendocrine Mechanisms

Continued lactation requires more than just the right complement of hormones. Milk must also be removed regularly by suckling. Failure to empty the mammary alveoli causes lactation to stop within about 1 week and the lobuloalveolar structures to involute. Suckling triggers two neuroendocrine reflexes critical for the maintenance of lactation: the so-called *milk let-down reflex* and surges of prolactin secretion.

Milk Let-Down Reflex

Because each lactiferous duct has only a single opening to the outside and the alveoli are not readily collapsible, application of negative pressure at the nipple does not cause milk to flow. The milk let-down reflex, also called the milk ejection reflex, permits the suckling infant to obtain milk. This neuroendocrine reflex involves the hormone oxytocin, which is secreted in response to suckling. Oxytocin stimulates the myoepithelial cells that surround each alveolus to contract, which creates a positive pressure of about 10 to 20 mmHg in the alveoli and the communicating duct system. Suckling merely distorts the valve-like folds of tissue in the nipple and allows the pressurized milk to be ejected into the infant's mouth. Sensory input from nerve endings in the nipple are transmitted to the hypothalamus by way of the spinal cord and stimulate hypothalamic neurons to release oxytocin from terminals in the posterior lobe (Fig. 10). These neurons can also be activated by higher brain centers, so that the mere sight of the baby or hearing it cry is often sufficient to produce milk let down (Fig. 11). Conversely, stressful conditions may inhibit oxytocin secretion, preventing the suckling infant from obtaining milk even though the breast is full.

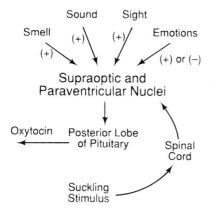

FIG. 10. The control of oxytocin secretion during lactation.

Control of Prolactin Secretion

Suckling is also an important stimulus for secretion of prolactin. During suckling, the prolactin concentration in blood may increase by tenfold or more within just a few minutes (Fig. 12). Although suckling evokes secretion of oxytocin and prolactin, the two secretory reflexes are processed separately in the central nervous system, and the hormones are secreted independently. Emotional signals that release oxytocin and produce milk let down are not followed by prolactin secretion. It is unlikely

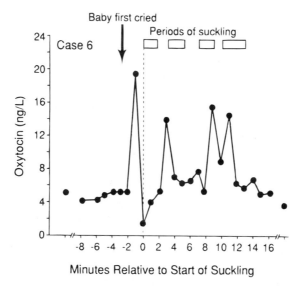

FIG. 11. The relationship of blood oxytocin concentrations to suckling. Note that the initial rise in oxytocin preceded the initial period of suckling. From McNeilly, A.S., Robinson, I.C.A., Houston, M.J., et al. (1983): Release of oxytocin and prolactin in response to suckling. *BMJ.*, 286:257.

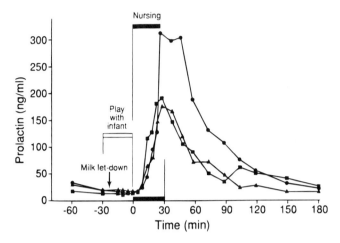

FIG. 12. Plasma prolactin concentrations during nursing and anticipation of nursing. Note that, although anticipation of nursing apparently resulted in oxytocin secretion, increased prolactin secretion did not occur until well after suckling began. From Noel, G.L., Suh, H.K., and Frantz, A.G. (1974): Prolactin release during nursing and breast stimulation in postpartum and nonpostpartum subjects. *J. Clin. Endocrinol. Metab.*, 38:413.

that the prolactin secreted during suckling can act quickly enough to increase milk production to meet current demands. Rather, such episodes of secretion are important for producing the milk needed for subsequent feedings. Milk production is thus related to frequency of suckling, which gives the newborn some control over its nutritional supply, and is an extension into the postnatal period of the self-serving control over maternal function that the fetus exercised *in utero.*

Increased secretion of prolactin and even milk production do not require a preceding pregnancy. Repeated stimulation of the nipples can induce lactation in some women who have never borne a child. In some cultures, postmenopausal women act as wet nurses for infants whose mothers produce inadequate milk. This fact underscores the lack of involvement of the ovarian steroids in lactation once the glandular apparatus has been formed.

Prolactin is unique among the anterior pituitary hormones in the respect that its secretion is increased rather than decreased when the vascular connection between the pituitary gland and the hypothalamus is interrupted. Prolactin secretion is controlled primarily by an inhibitory hypophysiotropic hormone, most likely dopamine. Surgical transsection of the human pituitary stalk increases plasma prolactin concentrations and may lead to the onset of lactation. Stimulation of prolactin secretion by suckling probably follows from the inhibition of dopamine secretion into the hypophyseal portal circulation by dopaminergic neurons whose cell bodies are located in the arcuate nuclei. It is likely that prolactin secretion is also under positive control by way of a prolactin-releasing factor. Experimentally, prolactin secretion is increased by neuropeptides such as thyrotropin-releasing hormone (TRH), vasoactive inhibitory peptide (VIP), and an undefined factor that may arise in the posterior or intermediate lobe of the pituitary gland. In spite of its potency as a prolactin releasing agent, it is unlikely that TRH is a physiological regulator of prolactin secretion. Normally, TSH and prolactin are secreted independently; TSH secretion does not increase during lactation. The physiological importance of VIP as a prolactin-releasing hormone has not been established.

Even though it blocks the effects of prolactin on milk production, estradiol increases prolactin secretion. Lactotropes have estrogen receptors and, in response to estradiol, increase their synthesis of both prolactin messenger RNA and prolactin. Estradiol, which stimulates hypertrophy and proliferation of lactotropes, is probably responsible for the increased number of lactotropes in the pituitary and their prolactin content during pregnancy. Estradiol may therefore increase prolactin secretion by increasing its availability. In addition, although it does not act directly as a prolactin-releasing factor, estradiol decreases the sensitivity of lactotropes to dopamine. Paradoxically, however, estradiol also increases dopamine synthesis and its concentration in the hypothalamus and may therefore increase dopamine secretion (Fig. 13).

To date, there is no known product of prolactin action that produces feedback regulation of prolactin secretion. The effects of suckling and estrogen on prolactin secretion are open loops. Experiments in animals suggest that prolactin itself may act as its own ''short-loop'' feedback inhibitor by acting at the level of the hypothalamus. It is not certain that such an effect is applicable to humans. If prolactin is a negative effector of its own secretion, it is not clear what mechanisms override feedback inhibition to allow prolactin to rise to high levels during pregnancy.

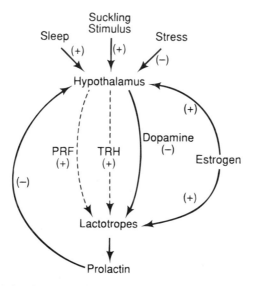

FIG. 13. The control of prolactin secretion. *Dashed lines* indicate uncertainty of the physiological importance of *TRH* and prolactin-releasing factor (*PRF*). +, stimulates; −, inhibits.

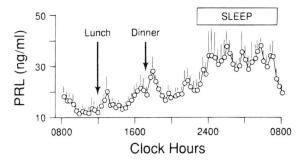

FIG. 14. Around-the-clock prolactin concentrations in eight normal women. An acute elevation of prolactin level occurs shortly after the onset of sleep and begins to decrease shortly before awakening. From Yen, S.C. (1986): Prolactin in human reproduction. In: *Reproductive Physiology*, 2nd ed., edited by Boyd, S., p. 246. Saunders, Philadelphia.

Prolactin in Blood

Prolactin is secreted continuously at low basal rates throughout life regardless of sex. Its concentration in blood increases during nocturnal sleep in a diurnal rhythmic pattern. Basal values are somewhat higher in women than in men and prepubertal children, presumably reflecting the effects of estrogens. Episodic increases in response to eating and stress are superimposed on this basal pattern (Fig. 14). Prolactin concentrations rise steadily in maternal blood throughout pregnancy to about 20 times the nonpregnant value (Fig. 15). After delivery, prolactin concentrations remain elevated, even in the absence of suckling, and slowly return to the prepregnancy range usually within less than 2 weeks. Prolactin also increases in fetal blood as

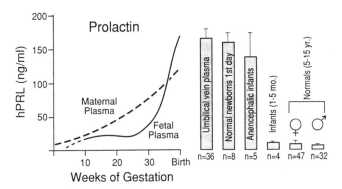

FIG. 15. Left: Comparison of the pattern of change of prolactin concentrations in fetal and maternal plasma during gestation. **Right**: Plasma levels in normal and anencephalic newborns are compared with those of normal infants and adults. The high concentrations seen in anencephalic babies presumably reflects prolactin secretion by an anterior pituitary gland uninhibited by influences of the brain. From Aubert, M.L., Grumbach, M.M., and Kaplan, S.L. (1975): The ontogenesis of human fetal hormones. *J. Clin. Invest.*, 56:155.

pregnancy progresses and, during the final weeks, reaches levels that are higher than those seen in maternal plasma. The fetal kidney apparently excretes prolactin into the amniotic fluid where, at midpregnancy, the prolactin concentration is five to ten times higher than that of either maternal or fetal blood. Although some of the prolactin in maternal blood is produced by decidual cells of the maternal placenta, prolactin in fetal blood originates in the fetal pituitary and does not cross the placental barrier. The high prolactin concentration seen in the newborn decreases to the low levels of childhood within the first week after birth. We do not understand the physiological importance of any of these changes in prolactin concentration in either prenatal or postnatal life. Although prolactin receptors are present in the gonads and reproductive tract of both sexes, the physiological consequences of prolactin binding to these tissues in humans remains unknown.

Lactation and Resumption of Ovarian Cycles

Menstrual cycles resume as early as 6 to 8 weeks after delivery in women who do not nurse their babies. With breast-feeding, however, the reappearance of normal ovarian cycles may be delayed for many months. This delay serves as a natural but unreliable form of birth control. The delay in resumption of cyclicity is related to high plasma concentrations of prolactin. Delayed resumption of fertile cycles therefore is most pronounced when breast milk is not supplemented with other foods, and consequently, the frequency of suckling is high. Ovarian activity is largely limited to varying degrees of incomplete follicular development, and even in those women who ovulate, luteal function is deficient. High concentrations of prolactin are associated with suppression of gonadotropin secretion, but the mechanisms are not yet understood. Some studies suggest that prolactin acts at the level of the hypothalamus to slow the gonadotropin-releasing hormone (GnRH) pulse generator. Other studies suggest that the positive feedback effects of estradiol on the pituitary are diminished, and still others suggest that prolactin interferes with the actions of gonadotropins at the level of the gonads. Hyperprolactinemia, often resulting from a small prolactin-secreting pituitary tumor (*microadenoma*), is now recognized as a common cause of infertility and abnormal or absent menstrual cycles. Treatment with bromocriptine, a drug that activates dopamine receptors, suppresses prolactin secretion and restores normal reproductive function.

SUGGESTED READING

Ben-Jonathan, N. (1985): Dopamine: a prolactin inhibiting hormone. *Endocr. Rev.*, 6:564–589.
Hodgen, G. D. (1986): Hormonal regulation in *in vitro* fertilization. *Vitam. Horm.*, 43:251–282.
Jaffe, R. B. (1986): Endocrine physiology of the fetus and fetoplacental unit. In: *Reproductive Physiology*, 2nd ed., edited by Yen, S. S. C., and Jaffe, R. B. pp. 737–757, Saunders, Philadelphia.
Jansen, R. P. S. (1984): Endocrine response in the fallopian tube. *Endocr. Rev.*, 5:525–552.
Shull, J. D., and Gorski, J. (1986): The hormonal regulation of prolactin gene expression: an examination

of mechanisms controlling prolactin synthesis and the possible relationship of estrogen to these mechanisms. *Vitam. Horm.*, 43:197–242.

Tucker, H. A. (1988): Lactation and its hormonal control. In: *The Physiology of Reproduction*, edited by Knobil, E., and Neill, J. D. pp. 2235–2264, Raven Press, New York.

Yen, S. S. C. (1986): Prolactin in human reproduction. In: *Reproductive Physiology*, 2nd ed., edited by Yen, S. S. C., and Jaffe, R. B. pp. 237–263, Saunders, Philadelphia.

Subject Index

NOTE: Page numbers in *italics* refer to illustrations; page numbers followed by t refer to tables.